AF837616

"By bringing together accounts of how group analysis has developed, and how research is viewed, in various European contexts, the editors address an aspect of practice that is rarely acknowledged. Our theory holds that human interaction is shaped – mostly unconsciously – by the groups and communities of which we are part, while at the same time those interactions shape the group. This must also be true of our own practice, and here is a book that takes this issue seriously and, importantly, asks, 'What can we learn from each other?'"

Dr Linde Wotton, IGA London Faculty, EGATIN Committee, International Consulting Board of the Croatian *Journal of Psychotherapy*, previously GASi Scientific Chair, Editorial Board of Group Analysis

"This timely and scholarly volume offers a rigorous examination of Group analytic psychotherapy as it is practiced, researched, and reformulated across diverse European contexts. It addresses critical questions concerning cultural embeddedness, clinical adaptation, and the integration of evidence-based principles within contemporary mental health systems. By situating current developments in dialogue with the foundational contributions of S. H. Foulkes, the editors successfully bridge historical depth and conceptual innovation. An important and substantive contribution to the literature for mental health professionals and anyone interested in the healing potential of 'we'."

Konstantinos Liolios, MD, Psychiatrist, Group Analyst, IAGP (International Association for Group Psychotherapy and Group Processes) Secretary

"Generous contributions from colleagues across different countries offer a rich and varied picture of how group analytic psychotherapy is developing in Europe. They reveal how training and practice shape Foulkesian group analysis within diverse historical, cultural and institutional contexts. As group analysis continues to expand, this book provides valuable guidance for training programs, trainers, trainees, and clinicians. It brings together unique experiences, challenges and modern applications, while highlighting research as a 'challenge that touches professional identity, training, and values'."

Egle Pauziene, Clinical Psychologist, Psychotherapist, Group Analyst, Chair of EGATIN

Exploring Perspectives in Group Analytic Psychotherapy in Europe

Exploring Perspectives in Group Analytic Psychotherapy in Europe examines the theory, practice, research, and prospective developments of group analytic psychotherapy across European contexts. The volume brings together contributions from authors working in a range of European countries, offering an overview of current approaches within the field.

Individual chapters address the ways in which group analytic psychotherapy is practised in culturally specific settings, with attention to the adaptation of the approach to local conditions and changing mental health demands. The book also considers the status of research within national clinical communities and outlines possible directions for further development.

The volume is intended for practitioners of group analytic psychotherapy but also group psychotherapists and for those in training.

Anna Zajenkowska is an Associate Professor at VIZJA University in Warsaw, Poland. She is a trained group analyst, head of the Center for Personality Disorders at an outpatient clinic, and a supervisor applicant. She has served as a Board Member and as Head of the Group Section of the European Federation for Psychoanalytic Psychotherapy (EFPP), and is currently Head of the Polish Psychological Association.

Hanne-Sofie Johnsen Dahl is a psychologist, psychoanalyst, and training group analyst at IGA-Norway. She combines clinical practice within the public health sector with psychotherapy research and teaching at the University of Oslo. She is also co-chairing a psychoanalytic training program for therapists in China and has served as a board member of the Group Section of EFPP.

The EFPP Monograph Series

Series Editor: Anne-Marie Schlösser

A series of Monographs produced in conjunction with the European Federation for Psychoanalytic Psychotherapy (EFPP). Each volume brings together writings on a particular topic by authors from several European countries. The EFPP promotes communication and discussion between psychotherapists across national boundaries in the child and adolescent, adult, family and group sections of the organisation, through its conferences and seminars on topics of interest in contemporary psychoanalytic psychotherapy. The organisation represents some 13,000 psychoanalytic psychotherapists in twenty-two countries in Western, Central and Eastern Europe and is concerned with many matters which are relevant to the profession, such as training and registration.

Recent titles in the series include:

Families in Transformation
A Psychoanalytic Approach
Edited by Anna Maria Nicolo, Pierre Benghozi and Daniela Lucarelli

A Psychoanalytic Exploration of Social Trauma
The Inner Worlds of Outer Realities
Edited by Cristina Călărăşanu, Ulrich Schultz-Venrath and Hansjorg Messner

Psychoanalytic Psychotherapy Between Identity and Change
Edited by Luigia Cresti and Isabella Lapi

Exploring Perspectives in Group Analytic Psychotherapy in Europe
Assessing Current Status and Shaping Future Directions
Edited by Anna Zajenkowska and Hanne-Sofie Johnsen Dahl

For further information about this series please visit: https://www.routledge.com/The-EFPP-Monograph-Series/book-series/KARNACEFPPPM

Exploring Perspectives in Group Analytic Psychotherapy in Europe

Assessing Current Status and Shaping Future Directions

Edited by
Anna Zajenkowska and
Hanne-Sofie Johnsen Dahl

Routledge
Taylor & Francis Group
LONDON AND NEW YORK

Designed cover image: Getty Images

First published 2027
by Routledge
4 Park Square, Milton Park, Abingdon, Oxon OX14 4RN

and by Routledge
605 Third Avenue, New York, NY 10158

Routledge is an imprint of the Taylor & Francis Group, an informa business

© 2027 selection and editorial matter, Anna Zajenkowska and Hanne-Sofie Johnsen Dahl; individual chapters, the contributors

The right of Anna Zajenkowska and Hanne-Sofie Johnsen Dahl to be identified as the authors of the editorial material, and of the authors for their individual chapters, has been asserted in accordance with sections 77 and 78 of the Copyright, Designs and Patents Act 1988.

All rights reserved. No part of this book may be reprinted or reproduced or utilised in any form or by any electronic, mechanical, or other means, now known or hereafter invented, including photocopying and recording, or in any information storage or retrieval system, without permission in writing from the publishers.

For Product Safety Concerns and Information please contact our EU representative GPSR@taylorandfrancis.com. Taylor & Francis Verlag GmbH, Kaufingerstraße 24, 80331 München, Germany.

Trademark notice: Product or corporate names may be trademarks or registered trademarks, and are used only for identification and explanation without intent to infringe.

British Library Cataloguing-in-Publication Data
A catalogue record for this book is available from the British Library

ISBN: 978-1-032-98221-2 (hbk)
ISBN: 978-1-032-98220-5 (pbk)
ISBN: 978-1-003-59767-4 (ebk)

DOI: 10.4324/9781003597674

Typeset in Times New Roman
by Taylor & Francis Books

Contents

Illustrations

Figures

Tables

Contributors

Agnieszka Chrzczonowicz-Stępień is a psychologist, a psychotherapist certified by the Polish Psychological Association, and a trained group analyst. She has completed training in psychotherapy supervision at the Laboratory of Psychoeducation. She is a specialist clinical psychologist, trained at the Institute of Psychiatry and Neurology, where she worked for many years in inpatient units. She holds a PhD in Psychiatry. For several years, she worked as an assistant professor at SWPS University. She currently teaches at university level and in psychotherapy training programmes. Her research interests focused on psychotic disorders and currently concentrate on personality disorders. She has a strong interest in the psychoanalytic understanding of social and cultural phenomena. She is actively involved in the Poland on the Couch project, a series of workshops exploring societal reflection.

Almudena Sanahuja is a professor of clinical psychology and psychopathology at Marie and Louis Pasteur University in Besançon, France, and a clinical psychologist and family and couples therapist. She is vice president of the SFPPG board, the AIPCF (International Association for Couples and Family Psychoanalysis) and the SFTFP (French Society for Psychoanalytic Family Therapy).

Andrey Sklizkov is Chairman of the Training Committee of the Moscow Institute of Group Analysis (MIGA, iga.msk.ru), training group analyst, supervisor, psychiatrist, and clinical psychologist.

Anna Tsapenko is Director of the Moscow Institute of Group Analysis (MIGA, iga.msk.ru), training group analyst, supervisor, clinical psychologist, and author of articles and books on group analytic psychotherapy.

Anna Zajenkowska is an Associate Professor at VIZJA University in Warsaw. She is a trained group analyst, head of the Center for Personality Disorders at an outpatient clinic, and a supervisor applicant. She has served as a Board Member and as Head of the Group Section of the European Federation for Psychoanalytic Psychotherapy (EFPP) and is currently Head of the Polish Psychological Association. Her research interests focus on social information processing, particularly hostile attributions, and she applies group analytic knowledge to better understand social dynamics. She is also actively involved in the "Poland on the Couch – Reflective Citizens Workshops" project, which explores societal reflection and civic engagement.

Apostolis Angelopoulos, MSc, is a psychologist, a group analyst, and a couple and family analyst in private practice in Athens. He has also worked in the fields of migration, social exclusion, addiction prevention, adult education, and social research, where he developed various models for group analytic psychosocial interventions. His clinical and research interests include family dynamics, community-based psychotherapy, transcultural processes, large-group dynamics, and social unconscious functions in social problems. For the past decade, he has been actively involved in the teaching of group analysis and is a training group analyst. He is a founding member of the Hellenic Organization for Psychotherapy and Education in Group Analysis (HOPE in GA), a member of its Training Committee, and the Director of its Group-Analytic Training Programme.

Aurélie Maurin Souvignet is Professor of Clinical Psychology and Psychopathology at Lyon2 University, CRPPC (Centre for Research in Psychopathology and Clinical Psychology), a psychotherapist, St Cyr Hospital, and a member of the SFPPG board.

Christer Sandahl is a licensed psychologist and psychotherapist, a member of the Group Analytic Institute in Stockholm, and Professor Emeritus of Social and Behavioral Sciences at the Karolinska Institutet, a medical university in Stockholm, Sweden. He is a former President of the International Association for Group Psychotherapy and Group Processes (IAGP). Christer has extensive practical experience in both clinical and organizational psychology. Over the past 25 years, he has worked as a full-time researcher, focusing on group psychotherapy and organizational psychology. Additionally, he is a member of the Royal Swedish Academy of Engineering Sciences.

Clarisse Vollon is Associate Professor of Clinical Psychology and Psychopathology, Aix-Marseille University, LPCPP, a psychotherapist, and expert psychotherapist at tribunal. She is also a Member of the SFPPG board.

Daniela Březnová is an IPA psychoanalyst, group analyst, and clinical psychologist. She is a co-founder and coordinator of the Slovak Society for Psychoanalytic Psychotherapy (SSPAP), where she teaches and supervises candidates in individual psychoanalytic psychotherapy and group analytic training. She is based in Prague, where she works in private practice and at a psychosomatic clinic.

Darina Ilyanina is a psychoanalytic psychotherapist, group analyst, member of the SGA Coordinating Council, head of the "Secretary" psychological space, and in private practice.

Dolores Britvić, MD, PhD, is a psychiatrist, a group analyst, with subspecialization in psychotherapy and forensic psychiatry at the University Hospital Split, and Professor of Psychiatry and Psychological medicine in the School of Medicine, Split, Croatia. She is the President of the Institute of Group Analysis Zagreb, Croatia.

Édith Lecourt is Professor Emeritus at Paris Cité University, President of the SFPPG (French Society for Psychoanalytic Group Psychotherapy), Secretary General of the EFPPFrance, clinical psychologist, and psychoanalyst for groups and institutions.

Eirini Ioannovich is a psychiatric social worker, a training group analyst, and a psychoanalytic psychotherapist specializing in couple and family therapy. She has served in clinical posts at the Psychiatric Clinic of the University of Athens in Aiginiteio Hospital, where she coordinated the Clinic's inaugural Department of Group Analytic Psychotherapy for five years and has continued her affiliation as an external associate since 2011. Her professional experience includes extensive involvement in intensive treatment programs for individuals with borderline personality disorders at the Personality Study Clinic in Aiginiteio Hospital, as well as contributions to the Vocational Training Workshops of the Community Mental Health Center of Vyronas (Athens). She has delivered numerous presentations at national and international psychoanalytic conferences and has contributed chapters to collective academic volumes. She is Delegate of Greece in the Group Psychotherapy Section of the European Federation for Psychoanalytic Psychotherapy (EFPP). She is also a founding member and the current President of the Hellenic Society for Psychoanalytic Group Psychotherapy.

Elvir Bećirović, MD, PhD, is a specialist in neuropsychiatry with subspecialization in clinical psychiatry and subspecialization in psychotherapy. He is a group analyst, certified group psychotherapist, and EMDR practitioner. He works at the Clinic for Psychiatry as Chief of Department for Acute Psychiatry and Semi-intensive Care as well as in private practice.

Esmina Avdibegović is a Professor Emeritus, neuropsychiatrist, subspecialist in social psychiatry, and training group analyst in Bosnia and Herzegovina. She is a member of the Institute for Group Analysis Zagreb, President of the Association of Group Analysts in BiH, and Chair of the Executive Committee of the Union of Psychotherapy Associations in BiH.

Eugenijus Laurinaitis, MD, PhD, is a renowned Lithuanian psychiatrist and psychotherapist, recognized for his significant contributions to the fields of mental health, psychotherapy, and academic teaching. He is a partnership professor at the Faculty of Medicine, Vilnius University, a member of the Lithuanian Psychiatric Association, and an honorary member of the Lithuanian Group Analytic Society. Eugenijus Laurinaitis was a coordinator, a trainer, and a leader of a group analysis training programme in Lithuania. He is also past President of the European Association for Psychotherapy (2011–13), and author of numerous articles and publications in psychiatry and psychotherapy.

Galina Stepanova is a psychoanalytic psychotherapist, training group analyst, supervisor and member of the MIGA Training Committee, MIGA Large Group leader, and guest lecturer at SGA. She has led 'Codependency in Relationships' groups for a long time and has written articles on this topic.

Hanne-Sofie Johnsen Dahl, PhD, is a psychologist, psychoanalyst, and group analyst. She works within the public health system as a clinical psychologist, running analytic groups and doing individual psychotherapy. For the last ten years she has been a training group analyst, supervisor, theory lecturer, and one of the large group conductors at the group analytic training program in Norway. She supervises psychotherapy at the University of Oslo as well as doing psychotherapy research. She is a previous director of IGA-Norway and a former member of the EFPP board.

Ilona Laurinaitytė is a psychodynamic group psychotherapist and a professor of psychology at the Institute of Psychology, as well as the head of the Forensic Psychology Research Centre at the Faculty of Philosophy, Vilnius University, Lithuania. Her research interests focus on understanding the nature, causes, and management of violence and mental health problems across different settings. She is a member of the Lithuanian Group Analytic Society. From 2013 to 2025, she served as Lithuania's national representative on the Board of Ethics of the European Federation of Psychologists' Associations.

Ingalill Pagliettini Johnsen is a group analyst, an art therapist, and the current director of Institute of Group Analysis and Group Psychotherapy, Norway. She is a teacher at the group analytic training program in Norway over the last nine years, including small group leader, supervisor, theory lecturer, and large group conductor. She is a practising group analyst, art therapist, and clinical supervisor in private practice. She has worked within the public health system for 20 years, and she has co-edited a book on psychodynamic psychotherapy for eating disorders.

Iryna Frankova, MD, PhD, is a clinical psychologist, group analyst, and training analyst in the educational programme for group analysis at the Association of Psychoanalysts and Psychotherapists of Ukraine, and Ukrainian delegate to the European Federation for Psychoanalytic Psychotherapy. She is a psychologist and senior researcher at the Outpatient Child and Family Unit, Centrum 45, the ARQ National Psychotrauma Centre in Oegstgeest, Netherlands. Additionally, she is an Affiliated Assistant Professor at the Educational and Research Institute of Mental Health, Bogomolets National Medical University, Kyiv, Ukraine.

Isaura Manso Neto is an MD, psychiatrist, training and supervisory member, past-President, of the Portuguese Society of Groupanalysis (SPGPAG), GASi full-member, member of the Portuguese Society of Psychoanalysis (SPP) and of the Portuguese Association of Relational Psychoanalysis (PsiRelacional). She has worked in a psychiatric hospital applying group analytic and psychoanalytic conceptualizations in the treatment framework of severe cases as well as teaching residents. She currently works in private practice as a group analyst, psychoanalytic psychotherapist, and supervisor, and represents the SPGPAG as a Delegate for the Group Section at EFPP. She has organized international and national conferences on Group Analysis (GA) and Psychoanalytic Psychotherapy (PP) and also written papers and contributed chapters to published books on GA and PP, and is the co-editor of the book *The Portuguese School of Group Analysis: Towards a Unified and Integrated Approach to Theory, Research and Clinical Work* (Routledge, 2021).

Ivanka Dunjić, MD, is a psychiatrist, training group analyst, training analyst, President of IGAB, and member of TC PBD (IPA).

Karina Nahr is a psychological psychotherapist specializing in psychodynamic and psychoanalytic therapy for adults (individual and group treatment). She established her own practice in Munich (Germany) in 2008, financed by health insurance funds. She is a lecturer, supervisor, training therapist, and group training analyst (D3G), and a delegate to the EFPP in the Group Section.

Katarzyna Czajkowska-Łukasiewicz is an individual and group psychotherapist and sexologist. She is a PhD candidate and currently works as a teaching and research assistant at VIZJA University in Warsaw. Her psychotherapeutic training was completed at the Rasztów Institute of Group Analysis. She holds a Master's degree in Psychology and a Bachelor's degree in Ethnology. For the past five years, she has taught psychotherapy at university level as well as in psychotherapy training programs. Her scientific interests focus on narcissistic personality pathology and the dynamics of change in group psychotherapy.

Lila Mitsopoulou-Sonta, Associate Professor (HDR) in Psychopathology and Clinical Psychology, Group Analyst, member of the SFPPG and the SHPPG, and SFPPG delegate to the EFPP.

Ljiljana Moro, PhD, is a neuropsychiatrist, a training group analyst, and psychoanalytic therapist. She is also a co-founder of the Institute of Group Analysis Zagreb, Croatia. She is a former president of the Institute of Group Analysis Croatia. Ljiljana Moro has served as the editor of the journal *Psychotherapy* since 2016.

Maja Brkić, PhD, is a group analyst, supervisor and educator from Tuzla, Bosnia and Herzegovina. She is a member of the Association of Group Analysts of Bosnia and Herzegovina, as well as member of the Institute for Group Analysis in Zagreb, Croatia. Maja Brkić is a delegate in EGATIN on behalf of the Association of Group Analysts of Bosnia and Herzegovina. As a psychotherapist Maja Brkić is employed full time in Day Hospital of the Clinic for Psychiatry of the University Clinical Center Tuzla.

Margarida França is a clinical psychologist and specialist in Clinical Psychology, Community Psychology, and Psychotherapy; Master of Clinical Psychology (ISPA – Instituto Superior de Psicologia Aplicada); member of the Portuguese Society of Groupanalysis and Analytic Group Psychotherapy (SPGPAG) and associate member of GASi. She represents the SPGPAG as a Delegate for the Group Section at EFPP. She has worked in a social care institution with the homeless and other victims of social exclusion for several years and as a teacher in the context of vocational training courses for economically disadvantaged young people. and is currently working as a psychotherapist in private practice, in Lisbon, with adults, young children and adolescents. She recently became responsible for coordinating monthly seminars in SPGPAG and is the co-editor of the book *The Portuguese School of Group Analysis: Towards a Unified and integrated approach to theory, research and clinical work* (Routledge, 2021).

Margarita Kritikou, MD, is a psychiatrist and group analyst with extensive experience in clinical practice, teaching, and institutional leadership. Her work is grounded in advancing group analytic training and fostering intercultural dialogue within the field. She is a founding member and President of the Hellenic Organization for Psychotherapy and Education in Group Analysis (HOPE in GA). She has been a member of the Board of the International Association for Group Psychotherapy and Group Processes (IAGP) (2001–9), chair of its Membership Committee, and founder of its Transcultural Section. She has been a long-standing representative in the European Group Analytic Training Institutions Network (EGATIN) and is currently Delegate of Greece in the European Federation for Psychoanalytic Psychotherapy (EFPP), Group Psychotherapy Section.

Maria Tvorogova is a clinical psychologist, a private practice psychotherapist specializing in psychoanalysis, a group analyst, and head of the theoretical and supervision training unit, training analyst, and supervisor at the Moscow Institute of Group Analysis.

Marina Mojović, MA, MD, psychiatrist, training group analyst, psychoanalytic psychotherapist, supervisor, and organizational consultant in Serbia. She is the founder of: the Reflective Citizens Koinonia Method (RC) and of the International Reflective Citizens (IRC); the School of Integrative Group Analysis "Koinonia-Art; the Belgrade Trainings for 'Psychoanalytic and

Group Analytic Approach to Understanding Institutions, Organizations and Society', for Social Dreaming Hosts, and for Large Group Conductors. In the Serbian Medical Society, she is the President of the Psychotherapy Section. Internationally, she is a full member of: the Group Analytic Society International, where she was a member of the management committee, the International Association for Group Psychotherapy and Group Processes and currently a member of its Group Analytic Section team, the International Society for Psychoanalytic Studies of Organizations, the Organization for Promoting Understanding of Society, the International Association for Relational Psychoanalysis and Psychotherapy and a section delegate in the European Society of Psychoanalytic Psychotherapy. She presents, and publishes in areas of social trauma, the social unconscious, field theory, and large groups, as well as conceptualized 'social-psychic retreats' and 'conception trauma' of organizations and societies.

Milijana Niskanović is a psychologist, training group analyst, and member of Group Analytic Society Belgrade.

Nadezhda Mitryashkina is a clinical psychologist, psychoanalytic psychotherapist (EFPP), training group analyst and a supervisor in group analysis. She is head of the Group Analysis Section of the Association for the Development of Psychotherapy and Psychoanalysis (Stavropol), an EFPP and EGATIN delegate, visiting lecturer at MIGA, NIGRA, IGA, and DPP, and maintains a private practice.

Paul Benér is a licensed psychologist and psychotherapist, a psychotherapy supervisor, and a member of the Group Analytic Institute in Stockholm and the Institute of Group Analysis in Copenhagen. He has maintained a private practice for 20 years, following 20 years of public service in psychiatry in Malmö and Lund, Sweden. His areas of expertise include neuropsychology, psychodynamic psychotherapy, psychotherapy training, and supervision. He completed his group analytic training in 2010 and currently works with group psychotherapy, individual psychotherapy with a specialization in ISTDP, and supervises psychology students at Lund University, Sweden and at the group psychotherapy training at Teheran University, Iran.

Pia Litzell Berg is a sociologist and holds a Bachelor of Science in Social Work. She is a licensed psychotherapist, group analyst, teacher and supervisor in psychotherapy. She is a member of the Group Analytic Institute in Stockholm. She has worked with children, adolescents, and adults within psychiatric services in Stockholm for 35 years and has maintained a private practice for 30 years. She has also served as a course coordinator and lecturer in psychotherapy for more than 20 years. Pia has previously been the director of the The Psychotherapy Society Inc. where the Swedish group analytic training program was offered. She is currently a delegate in the Group Section of the European Federation for Psychoanalytic Psychotherapy (EFPP).

Rafał Styła is a psychologist, psychotherapist, group analyst, and psychotherapy supervisor. He is an academic teacher and researcher at the Faculty of Psychology, University of Warsaw, Head of the Chair of Clinical Psychology and Psychotherapy, and a member of the e-MPAT Lab (e-Mindfulness, Psychotherapy, and Technology Lab). He is also a member of the "Rasztów" Institute of Group Analysis, the Psychotherapy Section of the Polish Psychological Association, and the Society for Psychotherapy Research, as well as co-founder of the Psychotherapy and Psychiatry Center PSYCHE PLUS. Rafał is author of numerous publications on psychotherapy, psychometrics, and psychopathology.

Rūta Klimašauskienė is a doctor of social sciences, a graduate of studies in organizational group psychodynamics, and an expert in human resource management. In her role as an organizational consultant, she applies a psychodynamic approach and way of thinking. In the study programme for Working with Adult Groups in Organisations, she has been a supervisor for several years. Ruta Klimašauskienė is also a member of the board of the Lithuanian Group Analytic Society (LGAS) and a delegate of the European Federation for Psychoanalytic Psychotherapy (EFPP) Group Section.

Sigmund Karterud, MD, PhD, is a professor of psychiatry, formerly at the University of Oslo, and formerly head of The Norwegian Institute for Mentalization. He is trained in psychoanalytic psychotherapy, in particular self psychology, group analysis and mentalization-based treatment (MBT). He has published around 200 scientific papers and 20 books on self psychology, day hospital treatment, MBT, personality, personality psychiatry, personality-focused psychotherapy, and group analysis. Available in English is *Mentalization-based Group Therapy (MBT-G)* (Oxford University Press, 2015), *Group Analysis: A Modern Synthesis* (Routledge, 2024), and *Mentalizing and Group Analysis* (Routledge, 2026). Karterud maintains a private practice in Oslo for personality assessment, individual psychotherapy, group analysis, supervision, and MBT training. He supervises and lectures internationally.

Steinar Lorentzen is Professor Emeritus in Psychiatry at the University of Oslo, Norway. He is a psychoanalyst and group analyst and a founding member of the Institute of Group Analysis, Norway. He has done research and published papers and books in the field of psychotherapy, psychodynamic group psychotherapy, and group analysis. He is honorary member of EGATIN and the Group Analytic Society of Lithuania. He is co-founder and honorary member of the Norwegian Group Psychotherapy Association and honorary member of the European Group Analytic Training Institutions Network (EGATIN). He has been a member of the management committee of Group Analytic Society international (GASi), and previous member of the Board of Directors of International Association for Group Psychotherapy and Group

Processes (IAGP), and is currently co-editor of the IAGP Globeletter. He has published papers on large groups and on group analytic training.

Susanne Vosmer is a clinical psychology and group analytic psychotherapist, who practises in Britain. She has worked clinically for 30 years in the field of mental health and was involved in many research projects. In addition to being a research supervisor and examiner, she teaches and sits on editorial boards.

Tanja Frančišković, MD, PhD, psychiatrist, a training group analyst, Professor in Psychiatry and Psychological Medicine, University of Rijeka.

Taras Levin, MD, is a psychiatrist, psychoanalytic psychotherapist, and group analyst. He serves as First Vice-President for Organisational Affairs of the Association of Psychotherapists and Psychoanalysts of Ukraine (APPU) and is Head of its Section for Group Psychoanalytic Psychotherapy. He is a training analyst and supervisor in the APPU educational programme in group analysis, co-founder and head of the Kyiv School of Group Analysis, and the Ukrainian delegate to both the European Federation for Psychoanalytic Psychotherapy and the European Group Analytic Training Institutions Network (EGATIN), where he is also a committee member. He is currently completing his doctoral studies at the Shupyk National University of Health of Ukraine and maintains a private clinical practice in Kyiv.

Thor Kristian Island, MD, is a psychiatrist, psychotherapist, and group analyst from Oslo, Norway. He is co-founder and previous director of the Institute of Group Analysis (Norway). He has been a training group analyst, supervisor, and theory lecturer, as well as one of the large group conductors at the group analytic training program in Norway for more than 25 years.

Tija Despotović is a psychiatrist and training group analyst in Group Analytic Society Belgrade, training analyst and President of the Belgrade Psychoanalytic Society IPA, training committee member of the Serbian Association of Psychoanalytic Psychotherapists, staff member of Group Analysis India, and lives and works in Belgrade Serbia.

Tomasz Wyrzykowski is a group analyst and a psychotherapist at the Polish Psychiatric Association, a supervisor and training analyst at the Rasztów Institute of Group Analysis. He holds a Master's degree in Psychology and a Masters degree in Archaeology, and is a former chairman of the board of the Rasztów Institute. He has been running a private psychotherapy practice for over 20 years. From the beginning, he has also been associated with the Public Health Service. He is interested in the functioning of teams providing support, treatment, and counselling, as well as the social application of psychoanalytic theories. He utilizes analytic psychodrama and nonverbal techniques in his work with teams and groups. He is interested in Wilfred Bion's psychoanalytic theory and for seven years, he has co-led a seminar on this idea.

Taru Kaivola is a Helsinki-based group analyst, senior training therapist, and clinical supervisor who works in private practice. She is one of the founding members of the Finnish Group Analytic Society, where she has played a central role in developing group analytic thinking, training structures, and professional community in Finland. Over the course of her career, Kaivola has written extensively on psychotherapy, group analysis, and clinical supervision, contributing to both Finnish and international professional literature. In addition to her clinical and teaching work, Kaivola has been an active participant in professional organizations. She served for many years on the Finnish board of the European Federation for Psychoanalytic Psychotherapy (EFPP), where she worked to strengthen the position of psychoanalytic psychotherapy and to promote dialogue between European member states. Her long-standing engagement in training, supervision, and organizational development has made her a significant figure in advancing psychoanalytic and group analytic practice in Finland.

Ulrich Schultz-Venrath is Prof. Dr med., Emeritus for Psychosomatics and Psychotherapy at the University of Witten/Herdecke. Psychoanalyst (DPV / DGPT / IPA), Group Analyst and Group Training Analyst (D3G/ EFPP to GASi), MBT-Practitioner and -Supervisor (MBT-D-A-CH). He was head of the Clinic of Psychiatry, Psychotherapy and Psychosomatics, Evangelisches Krankenhaus Bergisch Gladbach from 1999 to 2019. He has been working in private practice in Cologne since 2019. He was the former Vice-Chair and Chair of the Group Section of EFPP, and a delegate to the EFPP in the Group Section. He has been editor and co-editor of the Journal *Gruppenpsychotherapie und Gruppendynamik. Zeitschrift für Theorie und Praxis der Gruppenanalyse* since 2010, Chair of the Institute of Group Analysis and Mentalizing in Groups, and a board member of MBT-D-A-CH.

Vladislava Stamos is a licensed psychiatrist in Slovenia, group analyst, a member of the Group Analytic Society of Slovenia and its former President, management member of the Institute of Group Analysis Ljubljana, and full member of the Group Analytic Society International.

Zoya Shargalina is a clinical psychologist of the highest category, training group analyst and supervisor in the field of group analysis. She is President of SGA, an ex-delegate of EGATIN, member of GASI, visiting lecturer at MIGA, VEIP, IGA, and DPP, and is in private practice.

Chapter 1

Introduction

Examining the Contemporary Context of Group Analytic Psychotherapy: Factors Impacting Practice and Patient Care

Anna Zajenkowska and Hanne-Sofie Johnsen Dahl

In recent years, Europe has experienced a significant deterioration in population mental health, a trend markedly intensified by the COVID-19 pandemic. During the first year of the pandemic alone, rates of anxiety and depression increased by approximately 25%, accompanied by a 22% rise in reported loneliness across the European Union. Even prior to this period, mental health challenges were widespread: in 2019, over 14 million young people aged 15–29 were living with mental health difficulties. However, the reported increases may also reflect growing awareness of mental health issues and the need for psychotherapeutic treatment. Therefore, particularly concerning is the substantial gap between mental health needs and access to care. Nearly half of young people in the EU (49%) reported unmet mental health care needs, a problem that also affected almost one quarter of the adult population (23%) (Council of the European Union, 2024).

The Rationale for Group Psychotherapy and the Foundations of Group Analysis: *"We" Rather Than Solely "I" or "You"*

Health professionals increasingly recommend group psychotherapy as a response to the growing demand for mental health care and the limited availability of individual treatment (Whittingham et al., 2023). One of the central therapeutic factors in group therapy is *universality*, which fosters a sense of belonging and helps participants recognize that they are not alone in their struggles (Yalom, 1975). Group psychotherapy has also been described as a "triple-E treatment" – efficient, effective, and equivalent to individual therapy in clinical outcomes (Rosendahl et al., 2021).

A wide range of group-based interventions is currently available and evaluated in research, including, among others, cognitive-behavioural therapy (CBT) groups, dialectical behaviour therapy (DBT) groups, psychoeducational groups, and a great variety of self-help formats. In addition to these approaches, one form of group psychotherapy that is particularly widespread in Europe is group analysis. Foulkes (1975, p. 3) described group analysis as "not only the therapy of an individual *in* the group, but also a form of psychotherapy *by* the group, *of* the group, including its conductor".

DOI: 10.4324/9781003597674-1

S.H. Foulkes (1898–1976), a German-British psychiatrist and psychoanalyst, is regarded as the founder of group analysis. Having fled Nazi Germany, Foulkes developed the group analytic approach in England during the 1940s while working with soldiers suffering from combat fatigue. Shortly after the Second World War, he presented his ideas on group analysis for the first time to the British Psychoanalytic Society (Foulkes, 1946/1990). To clarify what he meant by a *group* in this context, Foulkes (1946) invited his audience to imagine five to ten people – preferably seven or eight – gathered informally around a table, a fireplace, or in a circle, guided by a conductor (the therapist). The group meets to address difficulties and mental distress, using language as the primary medium of treatment. Sessions typically last one to two hours and take place once or twice a week. Over time, dynamic relationships emerge between individual members and the conductor, among the members themselves, and between the group-as-a-whole and any single participant. Subgroups or factions may form, relationships may shift or stabilize, and members become increasingly engaged in one another's concerns – expressing opinions, judgements, tolerance or intolerance, moods, and characteristic emotional reactions. Gradually, the group begins to think, feel, and act more in terms of "we" rather than solely "I" or "you". Importantly, this emerging group identity does not erase individuality. On the contrary, Foulkes emphasized that personal characteristics often become more clearly defined within the group's evolving and sometimes intense interactions.

Foulkes' use of the term *analysis* was shaped by three major influences. The first was *psychological analysis*, including Gestalt and related holistic tradition. Before Foulkes started training as a psychoanalyst he spent two years as an assistant to the neurologist Kurt Goldstein. They worked on rehabilitation of brain-damaged soldiers from the First World War, who were studied neurologically with methods derived from Gestalt psychology. Goldstein's holistic approach to the function of the central nervous system later influenced Foulkes' concept of the group as a whole where each person represents a nodal point in the group's network, analogous to the function of the neurone in the cortical network of the central nervous system, where all observable phenomena are to be treated as meaningful, and the observer is seen as an integral part of the situation (Gelb & Goldstein, 1920). The second influence was *psychoanalysis*, particularly its focus on unconscious processes, meaning, and dynamics. Like psychoanalysis, group analysis does not primarily aim at the direct removal of symptoms; rather, it seeks to approach underlying emotional conflicts through insight into behaviour, symptoms, transference, defences, and resistance, with the hope of achieving enduring change. The third influence was *sociological analysis*, or socio-analysis, which examines how social forces and cultural currents permeate the group. This perspective allows the group to question prevailing norms and, through collective reflection, potentially revise what is considered "normal" within the community.

Across the chapters in this volume, written by authors from all over Europe, a shared image emerges: people are meeting without a predetermined topic, engaging in free-floating discussion, where thoughts and feelings – about oneself and about others – are welcomed and explored. In such settings, relationships inevitably form. Participants gradually learn about unconscious forces, about being both individual subjects and members of a larger social and cultural matrix. Contemporary group analysis is, however, a dynamic and evolving field. It has been influenced by other group theories, adapted to diverse clinical and organizational contexts, and subjected to empirical, conceptual, and methodological critique. Developments include brief and manualized forms of treatment (see for example Lorentzen, 2025), and the emergence of digital group formats (Weinberg et al., 2023). Group analysis has become institutionalized through training programmes across Europe and is increasingly gaining ground in other regions, including India and China.

Despite shared theoretical roots – most notably in the work of Foulkes (1975) and Bion (1961) – significant differences exist in how group analytic psychotherapy is understood, adapted, and practised across countries. Most contributions in this volume remain anchored in group analytic traditions while responding to local cultural, historical, and institutional conditions. For example, in Portugal the term *groupanalysis* is commonly used to describe slow-open, small groups meeting with high frequency – often two to three sessions per week, and in some cases up to four sessions weekly over several years – aimed at treating the individual *in and through* the group. While in Norway *groupanalytic* training encompasses both the traditional once-a-week, slow open groups, in addition to modified time limited group analytic psychotherapy adapted to specific populations within the public health system. Each chapter, therefore, presents a locally grounded understanding of group analytic psychotherapy, illustrating both shared foundations and meaningful diversity in practice – essentially offering a *glocalized approach* (Radjuni, 2021).

Aims of the Book

This book focuses primarily on group analytic psychotherapy, encompassing group analysis, which has undergone significant evolution in recent years. Karterud's (2024) recent work on modern group analysis addresses contemporary challenges and compares this approach with other group-based therapies, such as CBT groups and mentalization-based therapy groups (MBT-G). Both Lorentzen (2025) and Karterud (2024), contributors to the book, emphasize the importance of research in group analytic psychotherapy, in line with World Health Organization (WHO) guidelines, which stress the need for evidence-based, manual-guided psychotherapeutic treatments (WHO, 2024). Lorentzen (2013) has developed manuals for short- and long-term group analysis and introduced a new model based on group analysis that is more directly focused (Lorentzen, 2022). At the same time, some voices within the field caution against over-reliance on manuals.

The current book aims to achieve two key objectives:

1 *Increase and share knowledge about current developments in group analytic psychotherapy across European countries, examining how this approach is adapted to local conditions, including cultural influences, and to today's rising mental health needs.*
2 *Examine the status of research in group analytic psychotherapy within local clinical communities and explore potential future developments in the method.*

Group psychotherapy has been shown to be more cost-effective than individual psychotherapy, yet it remains underutilized and requires greater visibility through increased publications and awareness of its benefits (Whittingham et al., 2023). According to Whittingham and colleagues (2023), a 10% nationwide increase in group therapy, particularly in private practices and primary care, could improve access for over 3.5 million people in the United States, reduce the demand for additional therapists, and generate substantial cost savings. They also emphasize the importance of routine evaluation in practice, accounting for potential biases, such as overlooking clients who may deteriorate or drop out prematurely (Lambert & Harmon, 2018).

Group analytic psychotherapy, grounded in group analytic theory, emphasizes the role of social contexts and interpersonal relationships in understanding and resolving psychological difficulties. Its aim is to enhance emotional well-being and interpersonal functioning through group interactions, fostering insight, support, and personal growth in a safe environment. Group feedback – coming not only from the therapist but also from peers – enriches the therapeutic process by providing multiple perspectives. These interpersonal dynamics are particularly important in Europe today, given rising loneliness and the isolating effects of social media (Jakubowska et al., 2023; Okruszek et al., 2020; Neumann & McCormick, 2025; Schnepf et al., 2024).

The COVID-19 pandemic and contemporary social conditions have highlighted the importance of creating groups that hold a sense of "*we*". Emotional loneliness, compared to social loneliness, is particularly severe and closely associated with psychopathology (Walsh et al., 2025). Group analysis, as envisioned by Foulkes 80 years ago, addresses both *we-ness* and emotional connection, offering potential support for the growing number of lonely individuals.

Despite the demonstrated benefits of group therapy, it is not often the first choice for patients. Resistance to group methods – anticipated even by Foulkes in his early lectures – emerges across several chapters in this volume. Cultural, social, historical, and practical barriers contribute to reluctance: stigma, fear of emotional exposure, limited therapist training, and structural or administrative obstacles. Examples include cultural scepticism in Greece, historical-political legacies in the former Yugoslav region (Croatia), or practical hindrances in Germany. In some contexts, group therapy is perceived as emotionally overwhelming (Slovakia) or met with "surprise, scepticism, and fear" (Sweden).

Group analytic psychotherapy is widely practised worldwide, including in almost all European countries (see European Federation for Psychoanalytic Psychotherapy).[1] However, each country brings its own unique cultural perspectives, which can influence not only the implementation of group psychotherapy but also its research methodologies and openness to evaluation. Cultural nuances likely affect what is considered the appropriate therapeutic frame – such as session length, frequency, and payment – as well as the setting, whether public, private, inpatient, or outpatient. Additionally, cultural factors may shape the techniques and interventions considered essential, along with leadership styles within the group. A key question arises: *To what extent do group therapists in different European countries recognize the link between their national culture and the way prevailing theories of group analytic psychotherapy are applied and interpreted?*

Culture and social context also significantly shape how therapists perceive and respond to evolving clinical needs. Originally, group analytic psychotherapy did not specifically target patients with personality disorders. Today, however, more individuals with complex relational and comorbid difficulties are seeking mental health services, both in Western countries and globally (Shadid et al., 2025; Zajenkowska et al., 2024). Other group-based therapies, such as CBT, DBT, MBT and schema therapy groups, as well as psychoeducational groups, currently serve as alternative approaches. These shifts – driven by increasing attention to personality and dimensional approaches to diagnosis, as well as the availability of new evidence-based psychotherapies – raise several important questions: *How are group analysts practising group analytic psychotherapy in Europe today in response to these changes? How do they integrate evidence-based treatment principles while remaining faithful to the theoretical foundations of group analysis?*

Cultural Values and Group Processes

Foulkes' concept of the matrix (1975) and later formulations of the social unconscious (Hopper, 2003, 2009) emphasize that individuals enter groups already shaped by social forces, power relations, and shared meanings. Cultural values – shared ideas of what is desirable, legitimate, or threatening – can thus be understood as part of the background conditions of group life. Schwartz's theory of cultural values (2006) offers a useful heuristic here, particularly the dimensions of hierarchy versus egalitarianism, embeddedness versus autonomy, and mastery versus harmony. These value orientations do not determine group behaviour, but they may make certain patterns of relating more available, strengthening them under specific conditions – for example, in situations of heightened anxiety due to social, political, or economic factors.

In this sense, cultural values can be understood as resonating with Bion's basic assumptions (1961), that is, unconscious group states that emerge under conditions of increased anxiety and compromise the capacity for reflective work. Culture impacts not only how patients have been socialized and how they function within the context of group psychotherapy, but also how psychotherapists practise their work and how professional groups surrounding group analytic psychotherapy operate and develop their findings.

Authority, Hierarchy, and Dependency

Several authors of this book writing from contexts shaped by socialist or post-socialist histories describe how authority has traditionally been experienced as something that should not be questioned. In such settings, hierarchical structures were legitimized and sustained over long periods of time, and compliance often functioned as a means of psychological and social survival. These experiences may to some extent continue to influence how authority is perceived in psychotherapeutic groups – is the psychotherapist more a facilitator, conductor, or the curer? In group analytic work, this may resonate with the basic assumption of dependency, in which the group unconsciously seeks an omnipotent, strong leader who will provide care, certainty, and protection. Idealization of the conductor, fear of disagreement, hesitation to speak openly, or anxiety about responsibility may perhaps appear stronger in groups described by authors from post-Soviet contexts, including those with Polish, Ukrainian, Lithuanian, or post-Yugoslav cultural backgrounds. At the same time, several chapters describe tensions between inherited patterns of dependency – for example, on the crown in the UK, or in Finland, where historical subjugation under Swedish and later Russian rule is particularly significant, as demonstrated by the importance of teaching group analysis in Finnish – and contemporary movements toward autonomy, pluralism, and psychological self-expression.

Embeddedness, Autonomy, and Social Transition

The polarity between embeddedness and autonomy becomes particularly visible in societies undergoing rapid social and economic transformation, like for example Greece. Embeddedness emphasizes belonging, tradition, and loyalty to the in-group, while autonomy values individual choice, self-expression, and personal meaning. Shifts along this dimension may provoke considerable group anxiety. In Greece, marked by a strong agrarian heritage, rapid urbanization and economic restructuring within a few generations have altered social bonds and expectations. In such contexts, groups may struggle to establish a stable work-group mentality while negotiating losses associated with declining traditional structures and uncertainties linked to emerging forms of autonomy. These tensions may generate oscillations between embeddedness and autonomy, reflected in the fight/flight basic assumption, in which the group unconsciously splits into "fighters" and "runners" in response to perceived threat, as groups struggle to negotiate safety and responsibility in changing social environments.

Mastery, Individualism, Hope, and the Future

In other chapters, written from more individualistic cultural contexts such as Sweden, Norway, or Germany, different challenges emerge. Strong emphases on achievement, market values, and competition may undermine the social legitimacy of group-based treatments. In these settings, group analysis may be perceived as inefficient, risky, or insufficiently evidence-based when compared to individual approaches.

The basic assumption of pairing may become particularly salient in such contexts. Here, hope for change is unconsciously projected onto a dyad – often between two members or between a member and a leader – or onto future developments, such as new theories and therapies, influential figures, or research outcomes, rather than being invested in sustained collective work. Research outcomes may function as symbolic forms of pairing, carrying the group's hope that group analytic psychotherapy will gain greater recognition and stronger empirical support in the future.

Trauma, Incohesion, and Theoretical Plurality

Earl Hopper's concept of incohesion (2003, 2009) provides an important framework for understanding groups shaped by collective trauma. The incohesion basic assumption, expressed through aggregation or massification, is rooted in helplessness, shame, and annihilation anxiety rather than envy. Cultural histories marked by large-scale trauma may predispose groups to oscillate between hostile fragmentation (aggregation) and excessive fusion (massification).

Contemporary political events, such as the Russia–Ukraine war, influence not only how group analytic treatment is practised but also who seeks and receives treatment. These circumstances raise important questions about the role of group analysis in countries where reflective functioning may be under pressure or disrupted by conflict. At the same time, bringing together authors from countries on opposing sides of a conflict – particularly where one country is the perpetrator – is especially poignant and highlights the potential of group analytic approaches to foster understanding, dialogue, and resilience across divided communities, and potentially to prevent aggregation.

Culture, Research, and the Work Group

Across chapters, a recurring theme concerns the challenge of sustaining a Work group mentality (Bion, 1961) within contemporary mental health systems. A Work group requires the capacity to think, tolerate uncertainty, test hypotheses, and remain oriented toward external reality rather than unconscious phantasy. Cultural anxieties – whether related to authority, individuality, trauma, or legitimacy – may pull groups toward basic assumption functioning and away from reflective work.

We hope that the book itself can be understood as a Work group: a matrix in which group analysts from 16 different cultural contexts engage with a shared task while bringing their own histories, assumptions, and values. Integrating research, evidence-based practice, and clinical tradition inevitably introduces change – and contact with difference changes us. Several authors, like those from Norway, the UK, or Poland emphasize that strengthening research in group analysis is not merely a technical requirement, but a cultural challenge that touches professional identity, training, and values.

Rather than resolving cultural tensions, this volume aims to make them thinkable. By placing diverse voices in dialogue, it invites reflection on how cultural values, historical legacies, and unconscious group processes shape group analytic practice – not only with patients but also within groups of practitioners – and how awareness of these processes can support more flexible, reflective, and ethically grounded work with groups.

Diverse voices represent the unique situations and group analytic psychotherapy practices of 16[2] countries, addressing three key questions. The authors of each chapter respond to these questions in their own idiosyncratic ways, partially shaped by their specific cultural, social, and clinical contexts:

1 *Do group therapists in various European countries see the link between their home country's culture and how the prevailing theories of group analytic psychotherapy are executed and interpreted?*
2 *How do group analysts practise group analytic psychotherapy these days in various European countries, addressing the aforementioned changes and factors?*
3 *How do group analysts address the need for evidence-based treatment?*

We conclude the book with three chapters: The first focuses on the social applications of group analysis, exemplified by reflective citizens' workshops; the second addresses recent developments in modern group analysis; and the third explores an integrative approach to research in group analytic psychotherapy.

We hope that group analytic psychotherapy can become a central force in promoting mental health and supporting effective personality-focused treatment, particularly given the large numbers of individuals affected by these issues

(Shadid et al., 2025; Zajenkowska et al., 2024). This approach facilitates integration both within each patient and among individuals, creating a supportive environment that fosters personal growth and collective well-being.

The challenge that group analysts are facing is balancing embeddedness in traditional analytic theories with a simultaneous striving for autonomy and development, as seen in the incorporation of, for instance, mentalization-based treatments. While remaining rooted in classical group analytic theory, the approach continues to evolve to meet contemporary clinical and social needs. In Sweden, for example, various adaptations have been developed, like short-term interventions, or summer camps for children with mental health or social challenges, often involving their parents. In Ukraine, despite the challenges posed by ongoing conflict and social disruption, there is growing recognition of the value of group analysis in processing collective trauma and fostering community resilience. In Poland, historical traumas and social factors have shaped innovative social applications of group analysis, reflecting the country's specific context. In Russia, group analytic work sometimes includes specialized groups for children and adolescents, such as "mom–baby" groups for mothers with children from birth to three or four years, adapted to developmental needs. In Norway, the integration of mentalization-based therapy with group analytic approaches illustrates how traditional frameworks are being expanded to respond to contemporary clinical demands. Overall, while deeply embedded in classical group analytic theory, these examples demonstrate how the method continues to evolve, adapting to cultural, developmental, and clinical contexts across Europe.

Notes

1 See https://efpp.org/
2 Fourteen chapters describe situations in individual countries, while the post-Yugoslav countries – Croatia, Bosnia and Herzegovina, and Serbia – co-authored a chapter together.

References

Bion, W.R. (1961). *Experiences in Groups.* London: Tavistock Publications.

Council of the European Union. (2024). *Mental Health Policies.* See www.consilium.europa.eu/en/policies/mental-health/.

Foulkes, S.H. (1975). *Group Analytic Psychotherapy: Methods and Principles.* London: Gordon & Breach.

Foulkes, S.H. (1946/1990). *Selected Papers: Psychoanalysis and Group Analysis,* 1st edition. London: Routledge. doi:10.4324/9780429479847.

Gelb, A., & Goldstein, K. (1920). *Psychologische Analysen hirnpathologischer Fälle* (Vol. 1). Oxford: Barth.

Hopper, E. (2003). Aspects of aggression in groups characterized by incohesion: Aggregation/massification or (BA) I:A/M. *Psychodynamic Practice: Individuals, Groups and Organisations*, 9(3), 335–352.

Hopper, E. (2009). The theory of the basic assumption of incohesion: Aggregation/massification or (BA) I:A/M. *British Journal of Psychotherapy*, 25(2), 214–229.

Jakubowska, A., Zajenkowska, A., Kaźmierczak, I., Zarazińska, A., Olechowska, A., Molińska, W., & Pinkham, A.E. (2023). Anger sensitivity and relatedness frustration as predictors of depression. *Personality and Individual Differences*, 215, 112379.

Karterud, S. (2024). *Group Analysis: A Modern Synthesis.* London: Taylor & Francis.

Lambert, M.J., & Harmon, K.L. (2018). The merits of implementing routine outcome monitoring in clinical practice. *Clinical Psychology: Science and Practice*, 25(4), 60.

Lorentzen, S. (2013). *Group Analytic Psychotherapy: Working with Affective, Anxiety and Personality Disorders.* Oxford: Routledge.

Lorentzen, S. (2022). *Focused Group Analytic Psychotherapy: An Integration of Clinical Experience and Research.* Oxford: Routledge.

Lorentzen, S. (2025). Research in group analysis: What works for whom? *Group Analysis*, 58(3), 299–316.

Neumann, T., & McCormick, B.P. (2025). Loneliness among adults with serious mental illness. In T. Nelson (Ed.), *The Handbook of Loneliness* (pp. 281–302). Berlin: Springer Nature.

Okruszek, Ł., Aniszewska-Stańczuk, A., Piejka, A., Wiśniewska, M., & Żurek, K. (2020). Safe but lonely? Loneliness, anxiety, and depression symptoms and COVID-19. *Frontiers in Psychology*, 11, 579181.

Radjuni, A.J. (2021). Glocalization: An emerging approach in teacher education. *Open Access Indonesia Journal of Social Sciences*, 4(4), 416–422.

Rosendahl, J., Alldredge, C. T., Burlingame, G.M., & Strauss, B. (2021). Recent developments in group psychotherapy research. *American Journal of Psychotherapy*, 74(2), 123–145.

Schnepf, S.V., d'Hombres, B., & Mauri, C. (2024). *Loneliness in Europe: Determinants, Risks and Interventions* (p. 176). Berlin:Springer Nature.

Schwartz, S.H. (2006). A theory of cultural value orientations: Explication and applications. *Comparative Sociology*, 5(2), 137–182.

Shadid, J., Ferrari, A.J., Bach, B., Sellbom, M., Sharp, C., Hutsebaut, J., d'Huart, D., Santomauro, D.F., & Chanen, A. (2025). The global epidemiology of personality disorder: a systematic review and meta-regression. *The Lancet Psychiatry*, 12(12), 932–946.

Walsh, B.E., Rottenberg, J., & Schlauch, R.C. (2025). Why loneliness requires a multidimensional approach: a critical narrative review. *Nature Mental Health*, 3(2), 175–184.

Weinberg, H., Rolnick, A., & Leighton, A. (Eds.). (2023). *The Virtual Group Therapy Circle: Advances in Online Group Theory and Practice.* London: Routledge.

Whittingham, J., Sparre, M., Pfrommer, C., & Pakmor, R. (2023). The impact of magnetic fields on cosmological galaxy mergers–II. Modified angular momentum transport and feedback. *Monthly Notices of the Royal Astronomical Society*, 526(1), 224–245.

World Health Organization. (2024). *Implementation Manual for Psychological Interventions: Integrating Evidence-Based Psychological Interventions into Existing Services.* See www.who.int/publications/i/item/9789240087149 (accessed May 28, 2026).

Yalom, I.D. (1975). *The Theory and Practice of Group Psychotherapy*, 2nd edition. New York: Basic Books.

Zajenkowska, A., Czajkowska-Łukasiewicz, K., Włodarska, A., Chrzczonowicz-Stępień, A., Nowakowska, I., Cieciuch, J., … Niezgoda, E. (2024). Factors related to the level of personality functioning and implications for the mental health care system in Poland. *Psychiatria, Psychologia Kliniczna*, 24, 14–27.

Chapter 2

Group Analysis in Ukraine

Development and Practice in a Time of War

Taras Levin[1] *and Iryna Frankova*

Introduction

Ukraine, one of the largest countries in Europe, is located in Eastern Europe and shares borders with Poland, Slovakia, Hungary, Romania, Moldova, Belarus, and Russia. With a Human Development Index of 0.779 (The World Bank Group, 2022), it ranks in the lower-middle income group among European and Central Asian countries. Limited resources, bureaucratic inefficiencies, and systemic distrust continue to hinder the development and integration of mental health services, creating substantial barriers for both professionals and those seeking help (Frankova et al., 2024). Ukraine faces high levels of poverty, inequality, and corruption, with a pensioner dependency ratio of 45% (Markina, 2022). One-third of families with children experience material deprivation, leading to widespread distrust of institutions, including health care and mental health services (Frankova et al., 2024).

Ukraine's collective identity, help-seeking behaviour, and attitudes toward psychotherapy are deeply shaped by its traumatic history – a dynamic that has also influenced the forms and reception of group psychotherapeutic approaches across the country (Gornostai, 2019, Frankova et al., 2023). From medieval occupations to 20th-century totalitarian regimes, Ukraine has endured multiple layers of historical trauma (Kappeler, 2014). Events such as the Holodomor famine (1932–33), the Second World War and Nazi occupation, Soviet repression, the Chornobyl disaster, and post-independence political upheavals have left a significant imprint on national consciousness (Bezo & Maggi, 2015; Gorbunova & Klymchuk, 2020). The fragmentation of historical memory, compounded by Russian propaganda and historical revisionism, has made identity formation a complex and politically charged process. Since gaining independence in 1991, Ukraine has been reclaiming its historical narrative, culminating in the 2014 Revolution of Dignity and ongoing resistance against Russian aggression since the 2022 full-scale invasion.

DOI: 10.4324/9781003597674-2

Theoretical Foundations and Cultural Links in Group Analytic Psychotherapy

In Ukraine, cultural perceptions of the self and mental health have long been shaped by Soviet ideology (Power & Suvalo, 2021). This system neglected concepts like soul, spirit, and individual needs. Mental health issues were heavily stigmatized, and individuals with psychological difficulties were often hidden from public view. Soviet psychiatry emphasized biological models and used psychiatric institutions to suppress dissent (Ougrin et al., 2006). As a result, Ukrainians today still harbour fear and distrust toward psychiatry and psychotherapy, fearing disclosure, stigmatization, or involuntary hospitalization (Keukens et al., 2019).

However, this legacy of totalitarian ideology rooted in decades of Soviet rule and, more broadly, in two centuries of Russian imperial influence stands in tension with Ukraine's deeper historical trajectory. The country has a rich and resilient tradition of statehood, civic autonomy, and cultural continuity, stretching back over a millennium (Kudlenko, 2023). From the democratic assemblies of Kyivan Rus (the early East Slavic polity) and the educational heritage of the Kyiv-Mohyla Academy (a major 17th-century centre of humanist education) to the self-governance of the Zaporizhian Sich (a Cossack self-governing republic), Ukraine has preserved enduring values of collective agency, intellectual inquiry, and national identity. Despite systematic efforts by imperial regimes to erase or marginalize these traditions, the latter have shown remarkable vitality and continue to shape modern Ukrainian consciousness, including in the field of psychotherapy.

Modern Ukrainian psychotherapy began to emerge only after independence. Although psychoanalysis briefly flourished in the early 20th century, with active psychoanalytic groups and communities in Odesa, Kharkiv, and Kyiv, it was later suppressed under Stalinism (Pustovoyt, 2018; Velykodna & Yakushko, 2025). It wasn't until the late 1980s and early 1990s, with the fall of the Iron Curtain, that Western approaches, including group analysis, reached Ukraine (Romanov & Pushkareva 2000). Key initiatives such as the Truskavets project (1994), supported by foreign analysts, established group analysis as a tool for supporting democratic values, pluralism, and respectful communication, and were among the early efforts to establish a group analytic culture (Pritz & Vykoukal, 2006). As Mahler-Büngers (1999) noted, "the tradition of psychotherapy was scarce, and the openness for emotional experience was still hindered by years of totalitarian repression" (Mahler-Bungers, 1999). Mahler-Büngers also emphasized the importance of cultural sensitivity and mutual learning in early cross-national group analytic efforts, observing that "therapists and participants alike were challenged to confront differences in communication styles, expectations, and emotional expression".

For a long time in Ukraine, where systematic exposure to contemporary European psychotherapy only began in the mid-1990s, one component of the standard tripartite model of group analytic education (personal group experience, theoretical training, and supervised practice) significantly outpaced the others. Students often received extensive personal analytic experience, sometimes exceeding that found in many Western institutions, while lacking sufficient theoretical instruction and practical application within therapeutic groups. Supervision frequently focused on individual cases, reflecting a broader pattern of theoretical and institutional asymmetry. As noted in an early Ukrainian-language textbook on group psychoanalysis, "the issue of theoretical preparation in this project was consciously sacrificed to more important matters: personal practical experience and the construction of a proper project structure … Despite the fact that Ukrainian group analysts mastered the practical models of work well, the theoretical deficit increasingly made itself felt, and this disproportion, like any other significant imbalance, began to hinder further development of the work" (Filts et al., 2004).

This practical–theoretical imbalance was not merely logistical but echoed deeper cultural patterns shaped by history and collective experience. Several cultural and historical factors also shaped early preferences for individual over group formats, contributing to broader difficulties in implementing group analytic models in Ukraine. One deeply rooted belief in the post-Soviet mentality holds that sincere disclosure of personal suffering, feelings, and hopes is only possible in a confidential one-on-one setting, with a professionally authoritative listener. Group settings, where communication might flow laterally among participants, were historically structured in a directive model: the leader issued exercises or interventions, and individuals passively complied. This model dominated in the 1980s and 1990s, when group autogenic training and group hypnosis – directive, suggestion-based interventions characteristic of late Soviet psychotherapy – were common (Ivanov, 1961; Ougrin et al., 2006).

By contrast, the notion of a non-directive therapeutic group, where healing arises from interpersonal communication among equally suffering and competent members, was alien to the prevailing cultural matrix and required gradual transformation. With the fall of the Iron Curtain, individual psychoanalytic therapy initially attracted greater interest than group-based approaches (Velykodna & Yakushko, 2025). Most early literature translations and training initiatives focused on psychoanalysis, reinforcing individual modalities. For many Ukrainian practitioners, group work was not viewed as a distinct method but rather as a means of accessing psychoanalytic experience despite a shortage of qualified individual analysts. The term "group psychoanalysis" was often preferred over "group analysis", even though most trainers and supervisors came from Foulkesian traditions.

In this context, the dyadic pattern persisted even in group analytic settings, with communication often unfolding along the vertical axis between participant and conductor(s), rather than horizontally among group members. This was reinforced by the fact that all early group conductors were foreign professionals from Austria, Germany, Israel, Norway, Switzerland, and the UK, whose presence, while essential, introduced further dynamics of distance and idealization (Filts et al., 2019). Their role was mediated through translation, limiting full integration into the group matrix (Mahler-Bungers, 1999). Idealization of these "bearers of new knowledge" from perceived better societies was accompanied by latent ambivalence or resentment that could rarely be expressed openly due to the perceived preciousness and fragility of the contact (Filts et al., 2019).

As a result, several generations of Ukrainian graduates from group analytic training in the 1990s and 2000s received long but limited experiences of actual group analytic processes. Many retained uncertainty about their capacity to conduct analytic groups, despite strong psychoanalytic theoretical grounding. In some cases, they were unfamiliar with core texts by S. H. Foulkes and foundational principles of group analytic theory. Those who remained in practice often gravitated toward individual therapy. Institutional structures also hindered development: the Ukrainian mental health system was resistant to implementing group analysis, and its application in public settings remained limited to isolated efforts by individual enthusiasts facing systemic opposition during the early post-independence decades.

Although the situation has gradually changed, these foundational challenges continue to shape group analysis in Ukraine. The method still remains excluded from national training and health care systems. Relevant literature is slowly becoming more available, though its volume remains small. However, there are signs of cultural evolution: societal values are shifting toward greater democratic sensibility, civic dignity, and horizontal cooperation (Friedman, 2023). As group analytic thinking becomes more embedded in local practice, trust in group processes is growing, and the number of Ukrainian training group analysts has increased. New generations of practitioners are moving beyond the image of the silent, distant psychoanalyst who intervenes with enigmatic interpretations, toward a more facilitative role aimed at supporting genuine communication and mutual engagement among group participants.

One important contribution to understanding this shift comes from a 2019 study conducted within the framework of a psychotherapeutic educational project in Truskavets (Filts et al., 2019), where a large group of 150 participants from various Ukrainian regions gathered for five days. The key psychosocial themes identified through this group process included: Traditions vs. Change, Autonomy vs. Connections, Chaos vs. Order, Anxiety vs. Security, Uncertainty, Confidence, War, Trust vs. Distrust, and Justice vs. Injustice. Initially, participants exhibited a schizoid-paranoid position marked by mistrust and defensive behaviour rooted in collective trauma. Over time, this dynamic evolved toward a more cohesive and trusting group atmosphere, culminating in a shared narrative space where painful experiences could be processed, and a stronger group identity could emerge. The transition from social mistrust to maximal trust captured in this study not only illustrates the evolving group dynamics observed in Ukrainian practice but also reflects the broader increase in trust toward group processes discussed above. It highlights the potential of group analytic work to transform collective trauma into resilience and shared meaning.

The demand for group analytic therapy has been steadily increasing, both in quantity and in qualitative depth. While in earlier years analytic groups were composed mainly of mental health professionals, psychologists, and psychotherapists, motivated primarily by training goals, today they increasingly include individuals from diverse professional backgrounds seeking help for personal therapeutic concerns.

This broadening of the participant base reflects a maturation of the field. A growing number of participants now consciously choose group analysis as a method in its own right, rather than viewing it as a less costly or more accessible alternative to individual psychotherapy. These participants tend to be more psychologically literate, articulate in their expectations, and capable of critical reflection on the therapeutic process and the competence of professionals. There has been a noticeable rise in participants' capacity for spontaneous emotional expression within the group, greater contact with their own affective states, and a foundational trust in the group as a potentially safe and supportive space.

Since the onset of the war, the significance of the group analytic setting has grown exponentially. With its potential to foster belonging, process emotional trauma, generate mirroring and resonance, and provide powerful interpersonal support, group analysis has become not only a tool for personal growth but, in many cases, a vital resource for psychological survival amid conditions of extreme uncertainty and distress. In doing so, it continues to affirm the evolving identity of Ukrainian group analysis as a practice rooted in both cultural resilience and democratic values.

Practices, Settings, and Adaptations

Current Institutional Landscape and Access to Group Analytic Psychotherapy

Mental health services in Ukraine are provided largely through a fragmented and underfunded system, with psychotherapy operating predominantly outside formal medical institutions (Frankova et al., 2024). Group analytic psychotherapy, in particular, is primarily situated within the private sector, driven by individual practitioners, training initiatives, and professional associations. Public clinics and hospitals rarely offer group analytic formats; where group-based interventions do occur, they tend to follow directive, non-analytic models.

Group analysis remains under-recognized at the national level. There is currently no formal accreditation system for group analysts, nor institutional support for the promotion or integration of group analytic approaches within the public health care infrastructure. As a result, access to such therapy remains uneven across regions and is typically limited to urban centres where private training and practice networks have taken root.

Nevertheless, recent legislative and regulatory developments suggest a growing willingness to integrate psychotherapy, group analytic modalities included, into the national mental health system (Verkhovna Rada of Ukraine, 2025). Between 2023 and 2025, significant reforms were enacted, including updates to official qualification standards. These changes formally recognized professional roles such as "psychotherapist" and "clinical psychologist", for both medical and non-medical professionals. The reforms also reflect a shift toward the European model of psychotherapy training: long-term, method-specific postgraduate education, carried out not only by academic institutions but also by professional organizations.

The 2025 Law "On the Mental Health System in Ukraine" and corresponding Ministry of Health regulations envisage an official role for civil society actors in providing psychotherapy education and services (Verkhovna Rada of Ukraine, 2025). This development opens a path for established associations, such as the Association of Psychotherapists and Psychoanalysts of Ukraine (APPU), to participate in recognized educational and service frameworks (APPU 2025). For decades APPU have implemented training aligned with European standards (e.g. EFPP, EGATIN), although this work has remained largely outside the sphere of formal state recognition. The new legislation, while still undergoing implementation, signals a cultural and structural reorientation in which psychotherapy is increasingly viewed as a distinct and necessary component of public health.

Despite the lack of systemic support, access to group analysis has steadily expanded. While initially concentrated in L'viv and Kyiv, practice and training initiatives have since taken root in Ivano-Frankivsk, Khmelnitsky, Vinnitsa, Chernivtsi, Odesa, Chernihiv, Dnipro, and Poltava. These developments are largely the result of bottom-up initiatives by dedicated professionals and small-scale training communities.

The ongoing war has dramatically intensified both the demand for psychological support and the urgency of institutional reform (Pinchuk et al. 2024; Singh et al. 2021). Though group analysis remains under-integrated in formal health care, its relevance has become increasingly apparent. Practitioners have launched trauma-informed groups, peer-based initiatives, and online interventions for internally displaced persons and others impacted by collective trauma (Bogdanov et al., 2021; Nguyen et al., 2023). These efforts have provided not only emergency psychological support, but also a broader demonstration of group analysis as a framework for sustaining mental health at both individual and communal levels.

This evolving wartime role of group analytic work is the focus of the next section, which addresses how Ukrainian institutions and practitioners have adapted their methods, settings, and priorities in response to the challenges of war and displacement.

Training Programmes and Institutional Development

Psychotherapeutic training in Ukraine reflects the fragmented and under-regulated nature of the broader mental health system, resulting in uneven standards, significant regional variation, and inconsistent quality in the delivery of group analytic education and supervision. Formal educational routes for psychotherapists, particularly for those with medical backgrounds, often involve brief, four-month survey courses focused on diagnostics and theoretical models, with limited emphasis on experiential learning or supervised clinical practice (Shalak, 2023). Despite some gradual improvement in postgraduate psychology education, there remains no unified national standard for psychotherapeutic training or certification.

In contrast to many Western countries, where insurance systems and legal frameworks heavily influence the shape and delivery of psychotherapeutic services, Ukraine's underdeveloped health insurance infrastructure and lack of regulation have created a paradoxical context in which the absence of rigid institutional frameworks has, in some respects, benefited psychodynamic approaches. Without strong pressure to conform to short-term, manualized methods often required by insurance systems in the West, traditions like psychoanalysis and group analysis have found greater freedom to develop organically, particularly within the private sector. Psychodynamic approaches, including psychoanalysis and group analysis, retain significant appeal and relevance (Velykodna & Yakushko, 2025).

Long-term training programmes in group analysis are currently offered within several professional associations, including the Association of Psychotherapists and Psychoanalysts of Ukraine (APPU), the Ukrainian Umbrella Association for Psychotherapy (UUAP), and the Ukrainian Confederation for Psychoanalytic Psychotherapy (UCPP). The absence of legal regulation of psychotherapy in Ukraine leads to a paradoxical situation: most training is conducted outside the formal education system, often with high quality, but remains unrecognized at the state level (Pritz & Vykoukal 2006).

The first educational project to introduce group analysis in Ukraine was the Truskavets School of Psychotherapy (1994), organized by the UUAP (Mahler-Bungers, 1999). While this programme provided an introduction to a variety of modalities, including client-centred therapy, psychodrama, gestalt, systemic family therapy, Adlerian analysis, and others – it played a pioneering role in exposing Ukrainian therapists to group analytic thinking. Since then, both UUAP and UCPP have worked to develop and promote the European Association of Psychotherapy (EAP)-endorsed model of psychotherapy training in Ukraine. Meanwhile, the APPU has maintained international affiliation with EFPP and, specifically for group analysis, has aligned its standards with those of EFPP and EGATIN.

One of the most sustained efforts in the development of group analytic training in Ukraine has been carried out by the Section for Group Analytic Psychotherapy of the APPU, founded in 2003. Its roots lie in the convergence of several formative training initiatives, including the Kyiv-based five-year project organized by the Internationale Arbeitsgemeinschaft für Gruppenanalyse (led by Josef Shaked, Alice Ricciardi, and Michael Hayne), the Truskavets School, and the Austrian training programme in Altaussee (APPU, 2025). These programmes produced the first generation of Ukrainian group analysts, many of whom would later become trainers and supervisors, significantly shaping the landscape of group analytic education in Ukraine.

The history of the APPU Section reflects broader trends in Ukrainian psychotherapy: initial waves of enthusiasm and idealization of Western mentors gave way to periods of disillusionment, internal growth, and increasingly self-sustaining development. For many Ukrainian therapists, group analysis represented a profound shift away from rigid diagnostic models and toward experiential, meaning-oriented approaches rooted in authentic interpersonal connection. This shift inspired a group of early adopters to formalize their efforts within the APPU and build a professional community committed to developing and transmitting group analytic practice.

Over time, the Section created a structured training curriculum in accordance with EGATIN guidelines, incorporating personal experiential groups, theoretical seminars, and supervised clinical practice. Ukrainian professionals have increasingly assumed the roles of trainers and supervisors, and the programme now welcomes not only students but also experienced clinicians and community leaders. While institutional and financial constraints remain, the Section has succeeded in training multiple cohorts of group analysts and in cultivating a resilient, ethically grounded, and internationally connected professional community.

Current Practice and Adaptation

The Ukrainian community has also remained active in the international professional arena, particularly through collaborative conferences. A foundational moment in this regard was the 2016 EFPP conference in Kyiv, titled "Bridge Over Troubled Water: Professional Identity of a Psychoanalytic Psychotherapist in a Changing World", which marked the first official gathering of the Ukrainian EFPP National Network. The event addressed questions of psychoanalytic identity and institutional development amid post-Soviet transitions.

Further milestones include the 2020 international conference "Psychotherapy – the Modern Science of Man" and the 2021 event "Between Body and Soul". These events provided vital platforms for exploring the intersections of psychoanalysis and contemporary Ukrainian realities, strengthening the visibility and cohesion of local practitioners.

The outbreak of full-scale war in 2022 marked a turning point in the landscape of group analytic practice in Ukraine. Amid mass displacement, loss, and trauma, group-based approaches gained new significance, not only as therapeutic interventions, but as means of psychological survival, social connection, and professional solidarity. Ukrainian practitioners had to quickly adapt their work to unstable and often dangerous conditions, including remote facilitation, interrupted infrastructure, and personal exposure to trauma (Dorozhkin, 2023; Velykodna et al., 2024). Yet the war also galvanized an unprecedented wave of cooperation, innovation, and collective resilience.

One of the first structured responses to this crisis was the launch of the "Walking Together Through Difficult Times" project (also known as the "sandwich project"), initiated in early 2022 by Robi Friedman and the Israeli Institute of Group Analysis (IIGA), in partnership with Ukrainian group analysts (Levin et al., 2024). Designed specifically for therapists, psychologists, and social workers working under wartime conditions, the project offers alternating large and small group formats that support psychological containment and analytic reflection. As of mid-2025, 40 blocks have been completed, all on a volunteer basis and with APPU serving as the principal national organizer, in close collaboration with UUAP and Ukrainian School of Group Analysis (USGA). Demonstrating the potential of group analytic practice for mutual recognition and narrative repair in crisis, the project also embodies Friedman's concept of the "soldier's matrix", a group container for humanization under conditions of violence and dehumanization (Friedman, 2015, 2018, 2023).

Another sustained effort is the weekly online group facilitated by John Schlapobersky for board members of APPU since March 2022. Consisting of 14 senior professionals from across Ukraine, this group has provided continuity, strategic thinking, and collective containment for Ukrainian leadership in the psychotherapeutic field. The group's work has contributed to institutional resilience and informed national-level decision making within the community of Ukrainian group analysts. Schlapobersky's theoretical contributions, such as viewing the group as a site where survivors "regain their voice, reclaim their history, and restore their capacity to relate", have resonated deeply with Ukrainian colleagues navigating the moral and existential dilemmas of war (Schlapobersky, 2024). In a 2023 Kyiv seminar, he remarked that "in the traumatic field of war, defences adapt and survive by becoming invisible (Schlapobersky, 2018). The work of psychotherapy begins by making them seen again, not to dismantle them, but to honour how they helped us live, and how they can now help us live differently".

Most recently, in 2024, the online conference "Thoughts and Dreams. Psychology and Psychopathology of Wartime" brought together over 30 international participants and around 100 Ukrainian clinicians, creating a truly resonant space for shared reflection. A post-conference article published in a German journal noted: "It was important for us to speak, in our own words, about our experiences. Even on screen, the shared presence created a real group, one that transcended geography and offered a space to be seen, heard, and held" (Levin et al., 2024).

In his keynote address during the 2024 conference, Robi Friedman reflected on the evolving dynamics of large groups in Ukraine. He observed a noticeable shift in the group's relationship with authority, describing a process of "weaning", whereby participants move away from excessive deference toward leadership and instead foster greater autonomy and democratic interaction. "The leadership within the large group is perceived as non-dictatorial", Friedman noted, "fostering an environment where members are encouraged to express their voices and take part in collective decision-making" (Friedman, 2025).

He also addressed the role of 'patriotic unity' in shaping the group's identity during wartime. This unity, forged in response to existential threat, supports emotional bonding, strengthens group resilience, and fosters a shared Ukrainian identity that includes a rejection of Russian cultural and linguistic influence. While this cohesion enhances solidarity, Friedman also cautioned about the challenges of bridging this experience with perspectives of outsiders who may not fully grasp its existential urgency.

This symbolic role of the group as a container of collective experience is also mirrored in recent empirical work. A study of dream-sharing during the war revealed that dreams served as a "shared language for emotional containment and symbolic transformation in the midst of existential threat" (Kaźmierczak et al., 2024). The study highlights how collective dreaming processes offered not only a reflection of psychic suffering but also a creative way of restoring meaning and social bonds, resonating with the core tenets of group analysis in times of collective trauma.

These developments demonstrate how, even in extreme adversity, group analytic work continues to foster meaning-making, emotional resonance, and mutual recognition. The war has catalysed the emergence of new models of practice, deepened existing international ties, and encouraged a redefinition of the group analytic role in conditions of mass trauma. As Brian Martindale has observed, the experience of Ukrainian psychotherapy reflects both the legacy of post-Soviet fragmentation and a remarkable acceleration of professional integration (Martindale, 2023). He notes that "the war has paradoxically accelerated the professionalization and international integration of Ukrainian psychotherapy by exposing its practitioners to new forms of cooperation, peer exchange, and solidarity".

Together, these efforts represent not just responses to crisis but affirmations of a psychoanalytic worldview rooted in dignity, interdependence, and the transformative power of the group.

Challenges and Evidence-Based Practice

The chronic trauma of war affects not only patients but also therapists, many of whom are working under conditions of emotional exhaustion, existential threat, and personal loss. The blurring of boundaries between professional and personal suffering creates unique challenges for analytic neutrality and reflective capacity (Dorozhkin, 2023). Nonetheless, this proximity to trauma has also intensified the urgency and relevance of group analytic work, as therapists search for spaces of resonance, containment, and relational repair.

At the same time, the emotional burden is shaped by broader cultural narratives. As articulated in a recent professional reflection: "There is pressure to be strong, to show resilience, and yet it is just as important to be able to acknowledge our pain, fear, and fatigue." This paradox reflects a deeper tension: between survival and subjectivity, between collective endurance and individual vulnerability.

Group analytic psychotherapy in Ukraine faces several interrelated challenges:

- **Structural and legal barriers**: The lack of formal recognition for psychotherapists trained outside the narrow state framework discourages institutional development. There is no legal differentiation between short-term courses and rigorous long-term training.
- **Economic and political instability**: Recurrent crises, from the 1990s economic collapse to the 2022 full-scale war, have disrupted both training and practice. Many therapists operate in precarious conditions.
- **Cultural stigma and medical dominance**: Despite improvements, stigma remains high, and the dominance of biologically oriented psychiatry limits the integration of psychodynamic approaches within public services.
- **Evidence base**: While there are isolated initiatives—such as clinical case studies, exploratory outcome monitoring in training groups, and informal practice-based evidence—systematic research is lacking. A recent literature review examining the empirical evidence for the effectiveness of group analysis was published in Ukrainian, aiming to raise awareness within the mental health community in Ukraine (Velykodna, 2017). However, none of the articles included in the literature review were based on research conducted in Ukraine. Empirical studies on the effectiveness of group analytic psychotherapy, or it's implementation in the country, are limited. While some qualitative studies do offer valuable insights into the dynamics of large groups, their methodologies are often poorly described (Filts et al., 2019). Key information regarding the research framework, type of analysis, transcription procedures, ethical approval, and study limitations is frequently missing. Additionally, there is a notable absence of scientific publications by Ukrainian group analysts in English on this topic.
- **Potential future directions**: Research capacity could be developed through collaboration with European institutions and participation in international networks (e.g., EFPP, EGATIN). Areas for investigation include group therapy with trauma-exposed populations, online group processes, and the impact of cultural-historical trauma on group dynamics.

Despite formidable challenges, group analytic psychotherapy in Ukraine continues to develop. The current crisis has reinforced the relevance of group analytic thinking, especially in contexts of collective trauma, displacement, and social fragmentation. Ukrainian therapists are demonstrating resilience and commitment, seeking ways to integrate evidence-informed practices without losing the richness of psychoanalytic traditions.

Furthermore, many Ukrainian practitioners view the psychoanalytic approach not only as a therapeutic method but as a worldview grounded in human dignity, freedom, and responsibility. In the face of both authoritarian legacies and reductive models of care, psychoanalysis offers a symbolic counterweight – a way of thinking that resists dehumanization and sustains meaning-making amid uncertainty. As articulated in professional reflections, defending psychoanalytic values today is inseparable from defending the conditions in which they can meaningfully exist.

I want to believe there will still be Ukraine, and we will have the strength to speak in our own voice. That we will not dissolve into cultural anonymity but will remain present, traumatized, but alive, thinking, and speaking.

Note

1 Corresponding author: Taras Levin (taraslevin@gmail.com).

References

APPU. (2025). *Milestones of Section of Group Psychoanalytical Psychotherapy, Association of Psychotherapists and Psychoanalysts of Ukraine.* Available at: https://groupanalysis.com.ua/en/elementor-1393/%d0%bf%d1%80%d0%be%d1%81%d0%b5%d0%ba%d1%86%d1%96%d1%8e/%d0%b5%d1%82%d0%b0%d0%bf%d0%b8/.

Bezo, B., & Maggi, S. (2015). Living in "survival mode": Intergenerational transmission of trauma from the Holodomor genocide of 1932–1933 in Ukraine. *Social Science & Medicine*, 134, 87–94. doi:10.1016/j.socscimed.2015.04.009.

Bogdanov, S., Augustinavicius, J., Bass, J.K., Metz, K., Skavenski, S., Singh, N. S., Moore, Q., Haroz, E. E., Kane, J., Doty, B., Murray, L., & Bolton, P. (2021). A randomized-controlled trial of community-based transdiagnostic psychotherapy for veterans and internally displaced persons in Ukraine. *Global Mental Health*, 8, e32. doi:10.1017/gmh.2021.27.

Dorozhkin, V. (2023). Therapeutic relationships in wartime Ukraine. *Psychoanalytic Psychology*, 40(4), 247. doi:10.1037/pap0000482.

Filts, O., Haubl, R., & Lamott, F. (2004). *Group Psychoanalysis.* Lviv. VNTL – Classics.

Filts, O., Sedykh, K., & Turetska, N. (2019). Big psychanalytical group as an instrument of analysis of psychosocial processes in Ukraine. *Psychology and Personality*, 2, 185–202. doi:10.33989/2226-4078.2019.2.177356.

Frankova, I., Bahmad Leigh, M., Goloktionova, G., Suvalo, O., Khyzhniak, K., & Power, T. (2024). Mental health and psychosocial support in Ukraine: Coping, help-seeking and health systems strengthening in times of war. *Amsterdam. ARQ International*, 71. https://arq.org/en/publications/mhpss-ukraine.

Frankova, I., Chaban, O., Petrenko, G., & Tokarchuk, A. (2023). Collective trauma in Ukraine: Realities and prospects of the multigenerational legacies research. *Psychosomatic Medicine and General Practice*, 8(3). doi:10.26766/pmgp.v8i3.442.

Friedman, R. (2015). A soldier's matrix: A group analytic view of societies in war. *Group Analysis*, 48(3), 239–257. doi:10.1177/0533316415588253.

Friedman, R. (2018). Beyond rejection, glory and the Soldier's Matrix: The heart of my group analysis. *Group Analysis*, 51(4), 389–405. doi:10.1177/0533316418792487.

Friedman, R. (2023). Group Analytic Therapy and the online groups: Some principles of the group analytic approach to Online group therapy. *The Virtual Group Therapy Circle*, 101–111.

Friedman, R. (2025). Reviewing the group analytic approach to Large Groups' therapeutic potential – learning from a three-year monthly sandwich with a Ukrainian community. *Group Analysis*, 58(4), 499–517. doi:10.1177/05333164251394902

Gorbunova, V., & Klymchuk, V. (2020). The psychological consequences of the Holodomor in Ukraine. *East/West: Journal of Ukrainian Studies*, 7(2), 33–68. doi:10.21226/ewjus609.

Gornostai, P. (2019). Awareness experience, social and psychological tools to overcome collective traumas. *Issues of Political Psychology*, 89–114. doi:10.33120/popp-Vol22-Year2019-27.

Ivanov, N. (1961). A Soviet view of group therapy. *Soviet Review*, 2(3), 13–27. doi:10.2753/RSS1061-1428020313.

Kappeler, A. (2014). Ukraine and Russia: Legacies of the imperial past and competing memories. *Journal of Eurasian Studies*, 5(2), 107–115. doi:10.1016/j.euras.2014.05.005.

Kaźmierczak, I., Zajenkowska, A., Bodecka-Zych, M., Jasielska, D., Olechowska, A., Molińska, W., & Moniuszko, K. (2024). Exploring the emotional and thematic matrix of dreams during war: The role of anxiety and depression. *Current Psychology*, 43 (14), 12558–12566. doi:10.1007/s12144-023-05339-w.

Keukens, R., Sartorius, N., Thornicroft, G., & Baks, J. (2019). Inside Ukrainian social care homes. *Lancet*, 394(10216). doi:10.1016/S0140-6736(19)32528–0.

Kudlenko, A. (2023). Roots of Ukrainian resilience and the agency of Ukrainian society before and after Russia's full-scale invasion. *Contemporary Security Policy*, 44(4), 513–529. doi:10.1080/13523260.2023.2258620.

Levin, T., Kustor, B., & Keval, S. (2024). Taras Levin aus der Ukraine im Gespräch mit Beatrice Kustor und Susanna Keval. *Gruppenanalyse*, 34(2), 77–92. doi:10.30820/0939-4273-2024-2-77.

Mahler-Bungers, A. (1999). Group analysis in the Ukraine. *Group Analysis*, 32(2), 195–206. doi:10.1177/05333169922076662.

Markina, O. (2022). Taxation, inequality, and poverty: Evidence from Ukraine. *Central European Economic Journal*, 9(56), 1–18.

Martindale, B. (2023). Changes in psychoanalytic therapy in Europe over three decades: Then and now. *Psychoanalytic Psychotherapy*, 36(4), 101–154. doi:10.1080/02668734.2022.2124534.

Nguyen, A. J., Russell, T., Skavenski, S., Bogdanov, S., Lomakina, K., Ivaniuk, I., Aldridge, L.R., Bolton, P., Murray, L., & Bass, J. (2023). Development and piloting of a mental health prevention and referral program for veterans and their families in Ukraine. *Global Health: Science and Practice*, 11(3). doi:10.9745/GHSP-D-22-00488.

Ougrin, D., Gluzman, S., & Dratcu, L. (2006). Psychiatry in post-communist Ukraine: dismantling the past, paving the way for the future. *Psychiatric Bulletin*, 30(12), 456–459. doi:10.1192/pb.30.12.456.

Pinchuk, I., Leventhal, B.L., Ladyk-Bryzghalova, A., Lien, L., Yachnik, Y., Casanova Dias, M., Virchenko, V., Szatmari, P., Protsenko, O., Chaimowitz, G.A., Chisholm,

D., Kolokolova, V., Guerrero, A.P.S., Chumak, S., Myshakivska, O., Robertson, P. G., Hanson, M.D., Yee Liu, H., De Picker, L.J., Kupchik, M., Pinto da Costa, M., Scott, J.G., Leonard Wainberg, M., Shevaga, L., Weintraub Brendel, R., van Voren, R., Feldman, I., Mihalopoulos, C., Kaminska, S., & Skokauskas, N. (2024). The Lancet Psychiatry Commission on mental health in Ukraine. *The Lancet Psychiatry*, 11(11), 910–933.

Power, T., & Suvalo, O. (2021). Developing a capacity-building programme to support a mental health service modernisation pilot project in Lviv region of Western Ukraine. *BJPsych International*, 18(2), 40–42. doi:10.1192/bji.2020.23.

Pritz, A., & Vykoukal, E. (2006). *Group Psychoanalysis: Theory, Technique, Application*. Lviv: Astrolabe Publishing.

Pustovoyt, M. (2018). Psychoanalyse in Odessa. Auf der Suche nach der verlorenen Freiheit. In *Zwischen Hoffnung und Verzweiflung* (pp. 279–290). Giessen: Psychosozial-Verlag doi:10.30820/9783837974140-279

Romanov, I., & Pushkareva, T. (2000). On the history of psychoanalysis in Ukraine. How to practice psychoanalytic psychotherapy during periods of social instability. The 8th East European Psychoanalytical Conference (Kyiv, 28 April–1 May 2000). Available at: https://psychoanalysiskharkov.com/к-истёрии-психёанализа-в-украине/

Schlapobersky, J. (2018). Group analysis on war and peace. In *A Bridge Over Troubled Water* (pp. 19–50). London: Routledge. doi:10.4324/9780429471223

Schlapobersky, J. (2024). From toxic bonds to healing relationships. A journey through group analytic theory and practice. *Group Analysis*, 57(2), 129–160. doi:10.1177/05333164241245904.

Shalak, K. (2023). Survey on psychotherapy training in Ukraine, and its importance in the current war. *European Psychiatry*, 66(S1), S56–S56. doi:10.1192/j.eurpsy.2023.204.

Singh, N. S., Bogdanov, S., Doty, B., Haroz, E., Girnyk, A., Chernobrovkina, V., Murray, L.K., Bass, J.K., & Bolton, P. A. (2021). Experiences of mental health and functioning among conflict-affected populations: A qualitative study with military veterans and displaced persons in Ukraine. *American Journal of Orthopsychiatry*, 91(4), 499. doi:10.1037/ort0000537.

The World Bank Group. (2022). *GPD per Capita, PPP – Ukraine*. Available at: https://data.worldbank.org/indicator/NY.GDP.PCAP.PP.CD?locations=UA.

Velykodna, M. (2017). Group analysis in the 21st century: Empirical studies of effectiveness. *International Psychotherapeutic, Psychiatric and Psychoanalytic Journal*, 10(1–2), 79–84. doi:10.31812/123456789/3876.

Velykodna, M., Nalyvaiko, N., Pavlovska, O., Arshevska-Guérin, O., & Butsykin, Y. (2024). Ethical challenges in psychoanalytic practice in wartime: conference report, Kyiv, Ukraine, 2023. *Psychodynamic Practice*, 30(1), 49–66. doi:10.1080/14753634.2023.2258036.

Velykodna, M., & Yakushko, O. (2025). Prologue: Psychoanalysis and psychotherapy in wartime: Ukraine – The impossibilities and possibilities of psychoanalysis in Ukraine facing war. *Psychoanalytic Inquiry*, 45(4), 333–339. doi:10.1080/07351690.2025.2484993.

Verkhovna Rada of Ukraine. (2025). *On the Mental Health System in Ukraine. 4223-IX*. Available at: https://reliefweb.int/report/ukraine/law-ukraine-mental-health-system-ukraine?_gl=1*3mywq7*_ga*MjEyOTQ3NTMxNi4xNzQ4MzU2MTU0*_ga_E60ZNX2F68*czE3NTE0NzgwMTYkbzckZzEkdDE3NTE0NzgzMjkkajYwJGwwJGgw.

Chapter 3

Why Are Group Analytic Psychotherapies Not More Prominent in Britain?

A Discussion

Susanne Vosmer

Introduction

Foulkes' (1973, 1984) theoretical conceptualisations hold that everybody is affected via the matrix, the invisible network of relationships and communication. Additionally, people are influenced by the representation of social forces and power relations in the psyche, i.e., the social unconscious (Dalal, 2001). Whilst every person has unique experiences and own perceptions of reality, these have socio-cultural dimensions (Bacha, 2025). In other words, researchers, clinicians, and clients are also moulded by power relations and socio-cultural practices. Schwartz (2006) defined culture as the rich system of meanings, beliefs, practices, symbols, norms, and values, which are prevalent amongst people in a society. Values tend to be the most central feature of a culture, shaping the beliefs and behaviour of individuals/groups (p. 138).

Statistics show an increase in ill mental health in Britain (Priory, 2025). Even though Papanastassiou (2021) advocates that group analytic psychotherapy should be viewed as the treatment of choice for people in distress, and studies have demonstrated the effectiveness of psychodynamic psychotherapy for several disorders (Leichsenring et al., 2024), these approaches are rarely recommended by the National Institute for Health and Care Excellence (NICE). Depression is one notable exception. Overall, due to prioritising evidence from randomised controlled trials (RCTs), NICE recommends cognitive behaviour therapy (CBT). And so does the World Health Organization.[1] CBT is the dominant treatment in Britain (Clark, 2018), where most clinicians are trained as individual psychotherapists. Hence, although clients prefer depth in therapy (Li et al., 2024), Bionian/Tavistock and Foulkesian group analytic psychotherapies are seldom offered. Psychoanalytic group psychotherapies address unconscious conflicts and motivations, defences, transferences, and dysfunctional patterns in relationships or behaviour (Kaklauskas & Olson, 2020, p. 13). Even though the existing Balint (1979) groups also use an analytic approach to explore the emotional aspect of the doctor–patient relationships, they are not psychotherapy groups.

DOI: 10.4324/9781003597674-3

In this chapter, I will discuss why group analytic psychotherapies are not more prominent in Britain. Following a brief outline of the Bionian/Tavistock and Foulkesian approaches, I will describe a typical analytic psychotherapy group. Then I will elucidate the British context by focusing on values and research, additionally discussing obstacles. My discussion will conclude with suggestions for research and ideas about how to shift away from individual psychotherapy.

Bionian/Tavistock and Foulkesian Approaches

Bion (1961) applied Kleinian psychoanalytic thinking to the group. His approach led to the Tavistock model (Beveridge, 2023). Focusing on the group-as-a-whole, this group psychotherapy model adopts systemic thinking. Bion (1961) postulated that groups operate at both rational and *unconscious basic assumptions* levels. Shared basic assumptions (psychic defences) can destroy the capacity for thinking in groups. Then groups behave as if certain assumptions and behaviours were true and vital to their survival (Banet & Hayden, 1977, p. 15).

In the 'dependency' basic assumption, group members want leaders to fulfil all their needs (Bion, 1962). Two people form a bond in the 'pairing' assumption. Other members expect them to offer solutions to difficulties. Members may be hostile in 'fight' mode, or leave the group when it functions in 'flight' mode. Although people gradually gain insight into these defensive processes, they may never be entirely free of them (Bion, 1961).

The psychotherapist is viewed as the sole group leader and the only source of higher-level functioning, interpretation, and knowledge, Ezquerro and Cañete (2024) write. Delving into unconscious dynamics, s/he attempts to create a more 'task' oriented group mentality, particularly, through transference interpretations of unconscious hostility. Transference means something is transferred from important childhood figures to people/groups in the present.

Using Bion's (1962) 'learning from experience' methodology, the Tavistock favours transdisciplinary working to produce knowledge. This includes 14-day experiential learning events that provide a space to reflect on leadership within an international cohort.[2] It teaches psychotherapists to examine the how, what, and why of unconscious processes in groups, institutions, and organisations (Ehrlich, 2023). Its Institute of Human Relations is responsible for research.

Some group psychotherapists integrate Bionian and Foulkesian approaches. However, this is unusual. The Institute of Group Analysis (IGA) describes Foulkes' group analysis as a form of psychotherapy by and of the group, including its conductor (group therapist). Achieving healthier integrations in individuals and in their relationships is one aim of therapy (Lumsden, 2023, p. 310). Interpretation is an important technique to understand defences and other unconscious processes (Schermer, 2011), such as the workings of the social unconscious. Locating disturbances and making these conscious (translation) are crucial to treatment (Schlapobersky, 2016).

Analytic Psychotherapy Groups

Evidence suggests that group analytic psychotherapies can improve psychological functioning (e.g., Ashton et al., 2025; Lorentzen, 2020). Heterogenous/homogenous groups are delivered online and face-to-face. Different types of clients (forensic, prison population, refugees/asylum seekers, children, the elderly, people with disabilities) have received psychoanalytic group psychotherapy.

Analytic groups do not have an explicit agenda. A typical group consists of up to eight clients and one therapist. Most groups are of mixed gender. Members will have a range of psychological issues. Everyone uses the group differently. Some join a group, because they would like to learn more about themselves (Millar, 2006). Typically, a group analytic session lasts for 90 minutes and clients attend at least for six months. Ideally, a benevolent group process develops from which all group members benefit. Although unhelpful patterns tend to emerge, they enable members to see themselves through the eyes of others. In this way, they gain insight into how they relate to others. The psychotherapist aims to develop nurturing and trusting atmospheres. Nevertheless, a group member, including the psychotherapist, may feel threatened, distressed, anxious, or uncertain towards other members at different times during therapy (Beazley, 2023). To maintain confidentiality, group members should not discuss the group outside. They are expected not to meet up privately, because this could affect group processes.

Analytic Psychotherapy Groups, Systems, and Research in Britain

Group psychotherapy is efficient, effective, and equivalent to individual therapy in outcomes (Burlingame et al., 2024). However, most clients prefer individual psychotherapy. Fear of appearing emotionally vulnerable in front of others, the risk of being shamed, and having to 'compete' for the psychotherapist's attention are some obstacles to joining therapy groups (Shay, 2021). But groups have many positive aspects: the instillation of hope when group members see others getting better; development of compassion; gaining insight into own behaviour, feelings, and social interactions; formation of attachments; learning from each other (Yalom & Leszcz, 2020).

The Group Analytic Society International (GASI) was established in 1952 and the IGA in 1971. Not immune to discriminating against others (Vosmer, 2022, 2024), the IGA is the dominant Foulkesian training organisation in Britain. It is involved in establishing adult training programmes globally. After completing the 1-year Introductory and the 1-year Diploma course, trainees attend the 3-year Qualifying Course. Following successful completion, group analysts can register with the United Kingdom Council for Psychotherapy (UKCP).

Ironically, they become part of the Council for Psychoanalysis and Jungian Analysis, comprising individual and organisational members, who all share a psychoanalytic philosophy of psychotherapy.

Group analysts work in private practice, for private hospitals/organisations, or for the National Health Service (NHS).[3] Established in 1948, the NHS offers free health care. Some people have extra private health insurance.

Ten organisations regulate health professionals in England by law.[4] No statutory regulation exists for psychotherapists, but group analysts must be registered with the UKCP when they work for the NHS or other organisations. Services are regulated at national and local levels. The independent Professional Standards Authority for Health and Social Care oversees the statutory bodies that regulate health care professionals across the UK. Its statutory remit ensures the safety of service users and protection of the public from poor practice.[5] Furthermore, the Care Quality Commission is involved in the implementation of health care standards.[6]

In line with neoliberal policies, NICE[7] emphasises value for money. It offers guidance on what kind of treatment should be offered. Its recommendations ensure that 'Best Practice' is followed. Group analytic psychotherapists are expected to adhere to NICE guidelines and other policies/regulations. As Foucault (2019) highlights, policy always has a target, a group that it seeks to regulate.

Group analytic researchers and psychotherapists are also 'unofficially regulated' in Britain. Many services and organisations expect that researchers provide quantitative evidence for the efficacy/effectiveness of psychotherapies, because NICE predominantly follows the 'pyramid model of evidence'. It prioritises meta-analyses, systemic reviews, and RTCs (Murad et al., 2016).

Potter noted in 2011 that group analytic psychotherapy was not recommended by NICE. This has not changed much due to the dearth of robust (effectiveness) research (Stocks et al., 2020). Although NICE nowadays acknowledges the benefit of real-world research, it nevertheless favours RCTs. So, robust group analytic research is needed to influence future decisions about the provision of psychotherapy. Currently, individual CBT features prominently in the psychological therapies programme for severe mental health problems (NHS England, 2024).

Many psychotherapists tend to use the Clinical Outcomes in Routine Evaluation (CORE) questionnaire to gather data on how much clients improve during treatment. Other than this, most group analytic psychotherapists do not research psychoanalytic groups. If they did, studies would not be lacking. This raises questions about the group analytic postulate that people's practices are *moulded by the dominant culture* (Foulkes, 1948; de Maré et al., 1991). Britain has a strong research culture in the social/natural sciences and other fields. Considering that many studies of individual CBT exist, why have group analytic, or other researchers, not carried out more group analytic research? Could the answer be found in the wider British culture?

It must be noted that the term 'British' refers to social and political matters (e.g., passport). Most Scots, English, Welsh (I would add the Irish), do not think of themselves as 'British', Şchiopu (2023) explains. Due to England's power in the past, the usage of 'England'/'English' prevailed over the term 'British' for a long time, and 'English' is a highly emotive word.

British' Culture, Values, De/colonisation, and Group Analytic Psychotherapies

Power structures and historical contexts un/consciously influence social systems and people (Dalal, 2001). Britain is a capitalist country. Therefore, one would expect that capitalist values, i.e., individualism and the notion of a separate, autonomous, independent Self (Fishbane, 2001), would mould British attitudes towards groups, psychotherapy, and research. However, to understand people, practices, and values in contemporary Britain, one must also look at its history (Tăbăcaru-Stoian, 2023). Unsurprisingly, certain values are related to imperialism, the monarchy (Johnson, 2003), and paternalism. Imperialism and colonialism involve practices of domination. Many natives (e.g., Africa, Asia, Australia/New Zealand) were subjugated by the English/British. Paternalism overrides people's decisions in the name of safety and well-being, interfering with freedom and autonomy (Shiffrin, 2000), and paternalistic psychiatric care is hard to eradicate (Lepping et al., 2016).

The monarchy may strengthen the class system and wealth inequality, although members of the Royal Family provide funding for mental health problems (Clancy, 2021). It also plays a significant role in trying to promote Britishness as a collective identity (Nakić & Vištica, 2023). Ironically, although capitalism favours individuals over the community, it can devalue the experience of individuals (Skaife & Martyn, 2022).

According to Schwartz' (2006) theory of cultural value orientation, egalitarianism and intellectual autonomy usually appear together in Western European societies. Hence, one would expect to also encounter these values in Britain. Indeed, when the NHS was created, it was based on the egalitarian notion that all people should receive the same quality of free care, irrespective of where they live. However, access to health care depends on the so-called postcode lottery (Redhead & Lynch, 2024). Some view this as proof that universalism is impossible and as justification for NHS reforms. Economic inequality and geographic disparities in health/social care (Redhead & Lynch, 2024) indicate that imperialism still echoes through British society. Hierarchical, elitist, structures are common. The monarchy could even be viewed as a symbol of hierarchy.

The British conservative tradition has given civil society a central role in socialising and moralising individuals (Maschette, 2024). Anglicanism is tied to Englishness and conservative values. Woven into the fabric of Britain is the Church of England, whose Supreme Governor is King Charles III. Due to its connection to many schools and expression of views about public matters, it is influential (West, 2022).

The UK government shifted its focus to promoting both shared values and a British national identity after the terrorist attacks in the 2000s. Minorities are expected to assimilate these values. Disconcertingly, values can sometimes form the basis of Britishness and be used to justify exclusion, Clarke (2023) found. Whereas Britishness has been promoted as a multicultural identity that incorporates a wide range of cultures and symbols (Tăbăcaru-Stoian, 2023), only 8% of the population embrace a firm commitment to multiculturalism (Harutyunyan, 2024).

The British society is not as cohesive as Eastern cultures, where the traditional family, respect for elders, and ethnic cohesion prevail (Tăbăcaru-Stoian, 2023). Wales, Scotland, Northern Ireland, and England have distinct cultures. Moreover, Brexit has deepened existing societal divisions (Pickert et al., 2022). So, Britain seems to be an incohesive country, where an overall sense of 'we' could be lacking. Additionally, it is capitalist. As Tomšič (2015) points out, capitalist socio-economic structures play a causal role in alienating the psyche from itself, and from others. All these factors could explain why *group* psychotherapies are not favoured.

Although the link between Britishness and Whiteness is rooted in Britain's imperial history, nations reproduce themselves through the embodied practices of daily life, as Clarke (2023) notes. Accents, behaviours, specific values, and dress are markers of nationhood. Sadly, accent is linked to feeling insecure (Tăbăcaru-Stoian, 2023). Certain habits and behaviours (e.g., social awkwardness, over-apologising) seem to be characteristic of Brits. Social inhibitions, humour, moderation, hypocrisy, moaning, class consciousness, etiquette, courtesy, and modesty also form part of Englishness/English behaviour (Fox, 2004). Feeling socially awkward could partly explain why groups (e.g., analytic psychotherapy groups) might be experienced as anxiety provoking. Hence, people would avoid joining them.

Patriarchal, or misogynist, views amongst British people do not make them any less British. Since Whiteness and class co-produce the normative White, middle-class, British person, people of colour face barriers to recognition. As the racialisation of White migrants from Eastern Europe shows, Whiteness is not confined to White bodies (see Clarke, 2023). This might explain why it is particularly difficult for psychotherapists of colour to feel a sense of belonging in Foulkesian and Tavistock organisations, because the profession is predominantly White.

Decolonising requires making amends for the past, recognising White privilege, fostering inclusivity and social justice, and re-evaluating racist practices. The need for decolonising group analytic models and practice has been recognised (Blackwell, 2003; Nayak, 2023), because traditional models reflect the thinking of privileged, White, European, middle-class, and predominantly male professionals. Almost no attention is being paid to decolonising research. That quantitative methodologies are underpinned by racist Western philosophies (Vosmer, 2026) seems irrelevant to 'RCT enthusiasts'. Such avoidance of decolonisation is disheartening, considering that many group analysts originate from other countries.

Disconcertingly, although the main parties are Labour and the Conservatives, the right-wing party founded by Nigel Farage swept into office in the latest election (Hendrix, 2025). Right-wing thinking makes decolonisation impossible. It may adversely affect analytic organisations and perceptions of groups. Under conditions of perceived politico-cultural threats, even institutions can regress. Then primitive defences prevail. Splitting ('us'/'them') occurs. This could strengthen a separation between the individual and the group.

Societal regression may happen due to existential fears. Britain is affected by the implementation of past neoliberal policies, which includes reduced investment in public services, privatisation, market-driven decisions, and managerialism. When the wealthiest ten percent hold approximately half the wealth of Britain (ONS, 2021), many ordinary citizens struggle to make a living and have existential anxieties.

Social stressors adversely affect mental health, and since the British stiff upper lip has given way to emotional openness (Blackwell, 2011), more people may seek and need therapy. Sadly, the provision of psychotherapy is insufficient (NAO, 2023). Few clients can join once weekly analytic groups on the NHS. Thus, it is not uncommon that clients pay to join privately run groups, where psychotherapists set the fees. Inevitably, poorer clients lose out.

However, group analysts could offer more online groups at a lower cost. They could do cost analyses to increase funding for analytic group psychotherapies. Since NICE emphasises value for money, labour and financial impact analyses (see Whittingham et al., 2023) would be useful. If cost cutting results were demonstrated, these could be presented to policymakers and funders.

Obstacles to Research and to the Availability of Group Analytic Psychotherapies

To be widely and freely available, the effectiveness of group analytic psychotherapies must be established robustly. Then NICE would recommend them. However, RCTs and a more recent systematic review are lacking. In comparison to Scandinavia, Germany, and America, little group analytic research is carried out in Britain. Notable recent exceptions include Ashton et al.'s (2025) pilot study of a patient-reported outcome measure to capture the therapeutic outcomes of group analysis, Story et al. (2024) using the CORE to support the effectiveness of group analytic psychotherapy, Jackson et al.'s (2024) study of group members' experience of 'survive & thrive', and Stocks et al.'s (2020) research to identify areas of 'recovery' specific to group analytic psychotherapy.[8]

Unfortunately, group analytic psychotherapies are divided (Hutchinson, 2017). Fragmentation may impede the development of a group analytic (professional) identity and research culture, If group analytic psychotherapists cannot identify themselves with one profession that is united, they may see little need to conduct research to advance their therapies, or to engage with other researchers, and to contribute to studies. Currently, an attempt is made by the IGA to develop a research strategy. *Case Studies in Group Work*, an e-Journal, has been launched in 2025. Whether this will increase group analysts' interest and engagement in research remains to be seen.

Other obstacles exist. Although NICE does encourage qualitative research, RCTs are the gold standard in psychotherapy research (Philips & Falkenstrő́m, 2021). Hence, evidence-based power hierarchies directly dictate which research methodologies should be chosen. However, neoliberalist policies have resulted in less available funding. For group analysts, who do not hold academic posts or have links to research centres, it is impossible to conduct high-quality studies. Whilst many clinicians carry out audits, designing a robust quantitative study is more demanding. Making sense of complex research designs, statistics, data analyses, and the philosophical underpinnings of methodologies requires expertise. But contemporary adult psychotherapists are only expected to be taught *basic* research methodology and methods, as part of their psychotherapy training, by the UKCP (2017, p. 6). Expectations that therapists should engage in research activities and know several methodologies (Vossler & Moller, 2014), are at odds with UKCP requirements.

Due to the limited number of research seminars on professional training programmes in Britian, the onus is on the individual to become more knowledgeable. So, individualism even prevails in group analytic organisations. Margaret Thatcher's famous declaration that there is no such thing as a society, but only individuals (Maschette, 2024), is hard to contradict in contemporary Britain. This may explain why individual psychotherapy research seems more common (OpenAI, 2025).

Suggestions for Research

Bionian and Foulkesian psychotherapists could work together with researchers. To demonstrate the effectiveness/efficacy/benefit of analytic groups, clinicians and researchers could jointly carry out projects. Group analysts could routinely gather data that researchers could pool together by creating a national database and analysing results. If all analytic groups were routinely evaluated, every clinician collected such data, and uploaded them on a national database, then these data would not be lost (for methods see Vosmer, 2026). At the very least, the usefulness of group analytic psychotherapy could be demonstrated and areas of improvement identified. Clients would feel more reassured about the benefit of analytic groups.

Training organisations could integrate more diverse methods into their curricula and offer more research seminars to group analytic trainees, who could routinely research their training groups and do empirical dissertations. In this way, students would be socialised into doing research and a nurturing decolonising research culture could develop that counters past complacency (see Blackmore et al. 2009). The future generations of groups analysts would have more research experience.

More specifically, how much the workings of the social unconscious in Britain affect values, and attitudes towards groups and group analytic treatment could be researched. Additionally, what impact British norms and values have on the practice of group analysts, particularly those originating from other countries/cultures, would be good to know. What happens if their personal values clash with the dominant British norms/values? Furthermore, do all group analysts experience 'neoliberalist fragmentation' and 'disempowerment' (Skaife & Martyn, 2022)? Importantly, diversity (e.g., whether clients from different ethnic backgrounds 'get better' in analytic groups) could be researched.

Summary and Conclusion

In addition to outlining Bionian and Foulkesian approaches, I have discussed these group analytic psychotherapies by focusing on culture, values, and research to provide possible reasons as to why they are not more prominent in Britain. There seems to be a preference for both individual psychotherapy and individual research practices. My discussion suggests that the prevailing individualism, which is linked to capitalist values, free market ideologies, and elite entrepreneurialism, could partly explain this preference. Furthermore, sociopolitico conservative, hierarchical elitist power structures, Royal patronage, paternalism, economic inequalities, inner fragmentation of Britain, and lack of decolonisation may contribute to the preference for individual therapy. The lack of effectiveness and other group analytic research, possibly due to group analysts' missing research expertise, professional unity, research culture, and lack of opportunity, could further explain why group analytic therapies are not recommended and funded. Unsurprisingly, they are less common, and I have made some research suggestions how to change this. Fears and other cultural characteristics (e.g., feeling socially awkward) could additionally explain why groups might be experienced as anxiety provoking. Ultimately, there are a plethora of reasons as to why individual psychotherapy is favoured over group psychotherapy and multidisciplinary research is needed to identify the most determining reasons. However, it seems clear that a cultural shift away from the individual towards the group cannot be achieved by research alone. Alleviating fears about groups and group therapy could be an important step in the instigation of an attitudinal and cultural change that psychotherapists could take.

Notes

1 See www.who.int/news-room/fact-sheets/detail/depression
2 See www.tavinstitute.org/professional-development/the-leicester-conference
3 See www.nhs.uk/

4 See www.professionalstandards.org.uk/
5 See www.professionalstandards.org.uk/
6 See www.cqc.org.uk/
7 See www.nice.org.uk/
8 For reviews on groups and the effectiveness of group treatment see Blackmore et al. (2012), Barkowski et al. (2020), Rosendahl et al. (2021) and Schwartze et al. (2019).

References

Ashton, A., Chadwick, H., & Panteliou, E. (2025). Asking the right questions: Developing a patient-reported outcome measure (PROM) specific to group analytic psychotherapy. *Group Analysis*. doi:10.1177/05333164251335881.

Bacha, C.S. (2025). *The Group Dimension*. London: Karnac.

Balint, E. (1979). The Balint Group approach. *Journal of the Royal Society of Medicine*, 72(6), 469–471.

Banet, A.G., & Hayden, C. (1977). The Tavistock primer. In J.E. Jones & J.W. Pfeiffer (Eds.), *The 1977 Annual Handbook for Group Facilitators* (pp. 15–20). London: University Associates.

Barkowski, S., Schwartze, D., Strauss, B., Burlingame, G.M., & Rosendahl, J. (2020). Efficacy of group psychotherapy for anxiety disorders: A systematic review and meta-analysis. *Psychotherapy Research*, 30(8), 965–982.

Beazley, A. (2023). My first experience of group analysis. *Group Analysis*, 56(4), 527–540.

Beveridge, A. (2023). An historical overview of psychodynamic psychotherapy. In P. Graham (Series Ed.), *Cambridge Guide to Psychodynamic Psychotherapy* (pp. 1–17). Cambridge Guides to the Psychological Therapies. Cambridge: Cambridge University Press.

Bion, W.R. (1961). *Experiences in Groups: And Other Papers*. London: Tavistock Publications.

Bion, W.R. (1962). *Learning from Experience*. Hamburg: Heinemann.

Blackmore, C., Beecroft, C., Parry, G., Booth, A., Tantam, D., Chambers, E., Simpson, E., Roberts, E., & Saxon, D. (2009). *A Systematic Review of the Efficacy and the Effectiveness of Group Analysis/Group Analytic Psychotherapy*. Sheffield: University of Sheffield.

Blackmore, C., Tantam, D., Parry, G., & Chambers, E. (2012). Report on a systematic review of the efficacy and clinical effectiveness of group analysis and analytic/dynamic group psychotherapy. *Group Analysis*, 45(1), 46–69.

Blackwell, D. (2003). Colonialism and globalization: A group-analytic perspective. *Group Analysis*, 36(4), 445–463.

Blackwell, D. (2011). Ships in the night: The 'Open Group' for clients on the waiting list. *Group Analysis*, 44(3), 247–265.

Burlingame, G.M., Strauss, B.M., & Clayton, D. (2024). The complexity of becoming an evidence-based group clinician: Introducing an evidence-based group treatment website. *Group Dynamics: Theory, Research, and Practice*, 28(3), 121–131.

Clancy, L. (2021). The corporate power of the British monarchy: Capital(ism), wealth and power in contemporary Britain. *The Sociological Review*, 69(2), 330–347.

Clark, D.M. (2018). Realizing the mass public benefit of evidence-based psychological therapies: The IAPT program. *Annual Review of Clinical Psychology*, 14(1), 159–183.

Clarke, A. (2023). Recognising British bodies: The significance of race and whiteness in 'post-racial' Britain. *Sociological Research Online*, 28(1), 279–295.

Dalal, F. (2001). The social unconscious a post-Foulkesian perspective. *Group Analysis*, 34(4), 539–555.

de Maré, P.B., Piper, R., & Tompson, S. (1991). *Koinonia: From Hate, Through Dialogue, to Culture in the Large Group*. London: Karnac.

Ehrlich, S. (2023). Unbounded worlds: A challenge for group relations? In C. Archer, R. Kelly, G. Strauss & J. Triest (Eds.), *The Ecosystem of Group Relations. Culture, Gender and Identity in Groups and Organizations. The Group Relations Conferences Series* (pp. 7–18). London: Routledge.

Ezquerro, A., & Cañete, M. (2024). Genesis and development of group-analytic therapy in Great Britain: Bion, Bowlby, Foulkes, and the relevance of group attachment. In S.G. Taukeni, M. Mollaoglu, & S. Mollaoglu (Eds.), *The Theory and Practice of Group Therapy*. IntechOpen.doi:10.5772/intechopen.111826.

Fishbane, M. (2001). Relational narratives of the self. *Family Process*, 40(3), 273–291.

Foucault, M. (2019). *Power: The Essential Works of Michael Foucault, 1954–1984*. London: Penguin.

Foulkes, S.H. (1948). *Introduction to Group Analytic Psychotherapy*. London: Karnac.

Foulkes, S.H. (1973). The group as matrix of the individual's mental life. In L.R. Wolberg & E.K. Schwartz (Eds.), *Group Therapy: An Overview* (pp. 211–220). New York: Intercontinental Medical Book Corporation.

Foulkes, S.H. (1984). *Therapeutic Group Analysis*. London: Karnac.

Fox, K. (2004). *Watching the English: The Hidden Rules of English Behaviour*. London: Hodder & Stoughton.

Harutyunyan, N. (2024). Multiculturalism as a trojan horse of Britishness. *Armenian Folia Anglistika*, 20(1), 115–128.

Hendrix, S. (2025). A political 'tipping point' in Britain? Right-wing Reform UK gains clout. *The Washington Post*, May 14. Available at: www.washingtonpost.com/world/2025/05/14/britain-reform-uk-farage/.

Hutchinson, S. (2017). Group analytic identity. *Group Analysis*, 50(4), 419–435.

Jackson, L., Power, K., Mitchell, S., Duncan, K., Graham, L., & Wilson, K. (2024). Understanding female survivors of interpersonal trauma and their experience of the 'Survive and Thrive' course. *Group Analysis*, 54(1), 23–49.

Johnson, R. (2003). *British Imperialism: Histories and Controversies*. Basingstoke: Palgrave.

Kaklauskas, F.J., & Olson, E.A. (2020). History and developments. In F.J. Kaklauskas & L.R. Greene (Eds.), *Core Principles of Group Psychotherapy: An Integrated Theory, Research, and Practice Training Manual* (pp. 3–24). London: Routledge.

Leichsenring, F., Abbass, A., Fonagy, P., Levy, K.N., Lilliengren, P., Luyten, P., Midgley, N., Milrod, B., & Steinert, C. (2024). WHO Treatment guideline for mental disorders. *The Lancet Psychiatry*, 11(9), 676–677.

Lepping, P, Palmstierna, T., & Raveesh, B. (2016). Paternalism versus autonomy – are we barking up the wrong tree? *British Journal of Psychiatry*, 209(2), 95–96.

Li, E., Kealy, D., Aafjes-van Doorn, K., McCollum, J., Curtis, J. T., Luo, X., & Silberschatz, G. (2024). 'It felt like I was being tailored to the treatment rather than the treatment being tailored to me': Patient experiences of helpful and unhelpful psychotherapy. *Psychotherapy, Research*, 35(5). doi:10.1080/10503307.2024.2360448.

Lorentzen, S. (2020). Short-term focused group-analytic psychotherapy (SFGAP): An integrative approach to change based on research. *Group Analysis*, 50(3), 243–360.

Lumsden, A. (2023). Group Analysis and its application. In P. Graham (Series Ed.), *Cambridge Guide to Psychodynamic Psychotherapy: Cambridge Guides to the Psychological Therapies* (pp. 310–321). Cambridge: Cambridge University Press.

Maschette, L.C. (2024). Was Margaret Thatcher a conservative? Thatcherism and society. *Journal of Political Ideologies*, 31(1), 160–182. doi:10.1080/13569317.2024.2395821.

Millar, D. (2006). The adolescent experience: From omnipotence to delinquency. *Group Analysis*, 39(1), 37–49.

Murad, M.H., Asi, N., Alsawas, M., & Alahdab, F. (2016). New evidence pyramid. *British Medical Journal*, 21(4), 125–127.

Nakić, M., & Vištica, O. (2023). Collective identity as a tool of cultural diplomacy: The case of Britishness. *Annals of Disaster Risk Sciences*, 6(1–2). doi:10.51381/adrs.v6i1-2.65.

NAO. (2023). Progress in improving mental health services in England. *National Audit Office*, May 9. Available at: www.nao.org.uk/press-releases/progress-in-improving-mental-health-services-in-england/.

Nayak, S. (2023). *Decolonising the Curriculum of Group Analysis (Phase 1)*. Report on Findings. December 2023. Institute of Group Analysis. September 8, 2024. Available at: www.iga.co.uk.

NHS England. (2024). *Implementation Guidance 2024. Psychological Therapies for Severe Mental Health Problems.* Available at: www.england.nhs.uk/long-read/implementation-guidance-2024-psychological-therapies-for-severe-mental-health-problems/ (accessed July 4, 2025).

ONS. (2021). *Distribution of Individual Total Wealth by Characteristic in Great Britain: April 2018 to March 2020*. Release date January 7, 2022. Available at: www.ons.gov.uk/peoplepopulationandcommunity/personalandhouseholdfinances/incomeandwealth/bulletins/distributionofindividualtotalwealthbycharacteristicingreatbritain/april2018tomarch2020.

OpenAI. (2025, November 19). *Response to 'Is Individual Psychotherapy Research More Prevalent Than Group Research in Britain?'* ChatGPT (GPT-5.1 model). Available at: https://chat.openai.com/.

Papanastassiou, M. (2021). Group analytic psychotherapy and the group analytic model: A clinician's guide. In R. Gibbons, & J. O'Reilly (Eds.), *Seminars in the Psychotherapies* (2nd Edition), College Seminar Series (pp. 135–146). Cambridge: Cambridge University Press.

Philips, B., & Falkenström, F. (2021). What research evidence is valid in psychotherapy research? *Frontiers in Psychiatry, 11*. doi:10.3389/fpsyt.2020.625380.

Pickert, H., Bove, V., & Efthyvoulou, G. (2022). You (Bre)exit, I stay: The effect of the Brexit vote on internal migration. *Political Geography*, 95. doi:10.1016/j.polgeo.2121.102576.

Potter, J. (2011). Research in group analysis: Commissioning the systematic review. *Group Analysis*, 45(1), 3–14.

Priory. (2025). *Mental Health Statistics UK 2025*. Available at: www.priorygroup.com/mental-health/mental-health-statistics (accessed May 6, 2025).

Redhead, G., & Lynch, R. (2024). The unfairness of place: A cultural history of the UK's 'postcode lottery'. *Health & Place*, 90. doi:10.1016/j.healthplace.2024.103301.

Rosendahl, J., Alldredge, C.T., Burlingame, G.M., & Strauss, B. (2021). Recent developments in group psychotherapy research. *American Journal of Psychotherapy*, 74(2), 52–59.

Schermer, V.L. (2011). Interpreting psychoanalytic interpretation: A fourfold perspective. *The Psychoanalytic Review*, 98(6), 817–842.

Şchiopu, L. (2023). Connotation and translation of Englishness/Britishness. *ACROSS*, 7(4), 54–64.

Schlapobersky, J.R. (2016). *From the Couch to the Circle: Group-Analytic Psychotherapy in Practice*. London: Routledge.

Schwartz, S. (2006). A theory of cultural value orientations: Explication and applications. *Comparative Sociology*, 5(2–3), 137–182.

Schwartze, D., Barkowski, S., Strauss, B., Knaevelsrud, C., & Rosendahl, J. (2019). Efficacy of group psychotherapy for posttraumatic stress disorder: Systematic review and meta-analysis of randomized controlled trials. *Psychotherapy Research*, 29(4), 415–431.

Shay, J. (2021). Terrified of group therapy: Investigating obstacles to entering or leading groups. *American Journal of Psychotherapy*, 74(2), 71–75.

Shiffrin, V. (2000). Paternalism, unconscionability doctrine, and accommodation. *Philosophy & Public Affairs*, 29(3), 205–250.

Skaife, S., & Martyn, J. (Eds.) (2022). *Art Psychotherapy Groups in the Hostile Environment of Neoliberalism: Collusion or Resistance?*London: Routledge.

Stocks, H., Kyriakopoulos, A., & Ashton, T. (2020). Measuring meaningful markers of change. *Group Analysis*, 53(2), 177–193.

Story, G., Dalton, F., Selway, A., Caparrotta, L., O'Reilly, J., Colam, A., Larney, A., Ritchie, S., & Hillen, T. (2024). Effectiveness of group analytic and psychodynamic psychotherapy in routine secondary-care practice. *Group Analysis*, 57(4), 480–496.

Tăbăcaru-Stoian, G. (2023). Scottishness and Englishness versus Britishness: Major identity concerns. *Linguistic and Literary Broad Research and Innovation*, 12(1), 24–30.

Tomšič, S. (2015). *The Capitalist Unconscious: Marx and Lacan*. London: Verso.

UKCP. (2017). *Standards of Education and Training: The Minimum Core Criteria – Psychotherapy with Adults*. London: UK Council for Psychotherapy. Available at: www.psychotherapy.org.uk/ukcp-members/standards-guidance-and-policies/.

Vosmer, S. (2022). How (non)discriminatory are the Institute of Group Analysis and group analysis? An institutional ethnography study. *Group Analysis*, 55(2), 233–252.

Vosmer, S. (2024). Lived experiences of diversity in group analytic training and as a qualified group analyst: an autoethnographic study. *Group Analysis*, 57(2), 223–240.

Vosmer, S. (2026). *A New Pluralistic Paradigm for Research: Diverse Methods for Researching Analytic and Other Groups*. London: Routledge.

Vossler, A., & Moller, N. (2014). Attitudes to and perceptions of research. In A. Vossler & N. Moller (Eds.), *The Counselling and Psychotherapy Research Handbook* (pp. 17–30). Thousand Oaks, CA: Sage.

West, E. (2022). Britain as the only left-wing theocracy in history. *Blog by Ed West – Wrong Side of History*, April 19. Available at: www.edwest.co.uk/p/britain-as-the-only-left-wing-theocracy.

Whittingham, M., Marmarosh, C. L., Mallow, P., & Scherer, M. (2023). Mental health care equity and access: A group therapy solution. *American Psychologist*, 78(2), 119–133.

Yalom, I., & Leszcz, M. (2020). *The Theory and Practice of Group Psychotherapy*. 6th edition. New York: Basic Books.

Chapter 4

Slovakia

Becoming a Group: The Slovak Path Toward Group Analysis

Daniela Březnová

Introduction

A paradox may be observed in the Slovak context: despite a long-standing tradition of group psychotherapy and group-based training, group analysis is practiced only to a limited extent. Group work takes place predominantly within institutional settings – in hospitals, psychiatric wards, and day-care centers. Outside these structures, it is found only rarely, usually taking the form of short-term, problem-focused groups. Long-term, analytically oriented groups continue to be the exception rather than the norm. Both therapists and patients tend to prefer individual work: clinicians often perceive group therapy as particularly demanding, while patients may find it emotionally overwhelming or excessively exposing. In this respect, the group carries a certain stigma – as a space associated with uncertainty, loss of control, or unwanted self-disclosure. These clinical preferences reflect the broader structure of mental health services in Slovakia, where inpatient and outpatient psychiatric departments remain the dominant providers of care, while community-based and group modalities are significantly underdeveloped. As recent data indicate, this imbalance is further reinforced by chronic underfunding, a lack of adequately trained therapists, limited mental health literacy, and enduring stigma toward psychological treatment (OECD & European Observatory on Health Systems and Policies, 2023).

Several factors have contributed to this situation. Among the practical obstacles, the system of funding plays a key role: health insurance provides minimal compensation for group therapy – approximately €7–9 per participant per session, for up to 25 refunded sessions, which significantly limits accessibility and diminishes therapists' motivation to pursue this modality (Všeobecná zdravotná poisťovňa, 2024). Equally important, however, are the historical and cultural specificities that have shaped the collective relationship to the group. These factors reveal the deeper layers influencing the perception and practice of group analysis.

At the core of group analysis lies the principle of thinking about the individual within the context of the group and the broader social matrix. In this sense, group analysis is more than a psychotherapeutic technique. It provides

DOI: 10.4324/9781003597674-4

a framework for exploring how national history and unconscious social dynamics are enacted within group processes. The Slovak experience is shaped by totalitarianism, latent structures of power, dependency on authority, fear of authenticity, and a simultaneous longing for transformation.

This chapter follows the trajectory of group psychoanalytic psychotherapy in Slovakia through the lens of *three generations of practitioners.* The first generation trained and worked under conditions of restricted freedom, when psychotherapy did not officially exist, and groups were formed in the shadow of the system, outside state supervision and within an atmosphere of underground solidarity. The second generation, to which I belong, was trained in the post-totalitarian period, yet within a framework in which the group functioned largely as a setting for individual therapeutic work. Only the third generation – today's candidates – is beginning to form groups in which group processes themselves can become therapeutic.

This chapter explores the historical, cultural, and psychological factors underlying why, in Slovakia, the group has long remained a framework rather than a therapeutic instrument, and how it is now evolving into a space capable of bearing difference, frustration, and the hope for transformation.

Terminological Distinction

The focus here is exclusively on therapeutic (clinical) groups – those whose primary aim is the psychological transformation of the individual through work within the interpersonal field. These are distinguished from so-called natural or social groups, which emerge spontaneously in families, schools, workplaces, or communities, and whose purpose is not psychotherapeutic.

A therapeutic group is conducted by a trained professional, held within a stable setting, and allows for work with either or both conscious and unconscious dynamics. It provides a distinct space in which the individual's subjectivity can emerge and evolve within the context of relational experience. To better understand the historical development and current challenges of group psychotherapy in Slovakia, it is useful to distinguish three key forms of analytically oriented group work, each of which has taken root in the Slovak context to varying degrees. Based on clinical experience and informal conversations with Slovak colleagues, these modalities are typically practiced in a way that reflects their theoretical distinctions:

- *Psychodynamic groups* are primarily focused on supporting ego functions, alleviating symptoms, and enhancing the individual's capacity to manage external reality. They acknowledge the impact of past experiences on present functioning, but involve limited interpretation of unconscious processes and place less emphasis on *the group-as-a-whole.* They are often short term or stabilizing in nature, co-led by two therapists, and oriented toward individual change within a shared group setting.

- *Group psychoanalytic psychotherapy* refers to psychoanalytically oriented group work in which one or two therapists occupy a dominant role as interpretive authorities. They set the tempo, construct meaning, and work through the content of interactions. The focus remains on individual narratives and their interpretation. Transference is primarily vertical, with participants relating mainly to the therapist rather than to each other. The group functions largely as a setting for serial individual therapy, where interpersonal connections are mediated by the therapist. It is thus *therapy in the group*: while the therapeutic potential of both therapist and members is acknowledged, the group itself does not become the active agent of change.
- *Group analysis*, rooted in the work of S.H. Foulkes and W.R. Bion, views the group as a living entity – a "group-as-a-whole" system in which members mutually influence each other and construct new meanings. Central to this approach is the here-and-now experience, the exploration of shared unconscious processes, and the group matrix as the foundational structure underpinning communication and relationships. The therapist does not act as the primary agent of change but facilitates the emergence of a therapeutic group process. Transference is primarily horizontal – between members and toward the group itself. The group is thus an active medium of transformation: it is *therapy by the group* (Foulkes, 1975).

Historical and Political Background

Group psychotherapy in Slovakia has a long-standing and institutionally embedded history, with its roots dating back to 1919. In psychiatric hospital wards, regular community meetings were introduced in which patients could comment on ward functioning, share emotional responses, or request individual consultations. These 30–45-minute sessions became a routine element of hospital practice. However, they were primarily structured as discussions focused on social functioning and institutional regulation, rather than on unconscious dynamics or affective meaning. From today's perspective, they may be viewed as *socially oriented groups with therapeutic potential*, but not as fully psychotherapeutic groups.

Throughout the 20th century, *psychodynamic group psychotherapy* gradually evolved and was primarily utilized with patients suffering from anxiety disorders, mild to moderate depressive conditions, or personality disorders. After 2000, in specialized inpatient wards with a focus on psychotherapy and psychosomatic care, the frequency of group sessions increased to two or three times per week. These groups placed greater emphasis on personal experience, relational processes, and reflection on the hospital environment. Their main function was to support and stabilize patients within the treatment context. This model of group work remains in use to this day.

In the private sector, the development of group therapy has progressed more slowly. Unlike in institutional settings, where group work became a natural part of the ward routine, it has remained peripheral in outpatient practice. Many therapists remain hesitant to offer group therapy – due to limited compensation by health insurance or uncertainty about how to effectively initiate, sustain, and facilitate such work. Patients, too, often avoid group treatment, perceiving it as overly exposing, less secure, or less effective than individual therapy. These attitudes – typically unspoken – reflect deeper cultural patterns that shape the collective relationship to groups, beyond their function as therapeutic tools. Their roots, at least in part, lie in the legacy of collectivization during the communist regime, when groups tended to function more as mechanisms of control than as spaces of trust.

Training Culture: From SUR to Hybrid Models

During the communist era in Czechoslovakia (1948–89), psychotherapy was not recognized as an autonomous discipline (Gjuričová, 2017). The prevailing ideology viewed the psyche as a biological function of the body, with psychological disturbances treated as medical conditions requiring mostly pharmacotherapy. Psychotherapy was granted only marginal legitimacy and, when practiced, typically functioned as an addition to psychiatry or psychology, offered by clinicians with no formal psychotherapeutic training.

In the 1970s, however, the first structured program in dynamic psychotherapy was established: *the SUR training program* (Skála, Urban, and Rubeš). It combined experiential work in small groups with large community meetings, conducted "behind the doors" of state institutions. The entire program operated informally, in the shadows of the official system.

Paradoxically, it was this very lack of freedom that fostered an exceptionally intense and personally transformative training experience. Beyond the acquisition of therapeutic skills, SUR offered participants the lived reality of an underground community, one in which they could experience a sense of distinction from the ideologically uniform world outside. As Gjuričová (2017) observes, the training group became a refuge in which a unique language, culture, and internal relational world could evolve, along with a distinctive form of outward communication. Participants were encouraged to reflect on group atmosphere and interactions, and to assertively claim space for freedom and initiative both within their professional environments and interpersonal relationships. Among the few psychotherapeutic texts available at the time, Foulkes' work circulated informally in *samizdat* form, passed hand to hand as a source on group work (personal communication, J. Hašto, September 2025).

From a group analytic perspective, these training communities were not immune to unconscious group dynamics. Bion's concept of *the basic assumption* is particularly relevant here: a state in which the group, under the pressure of unconscious anxiety, adopts a defensive stance. In particular, *the fight–flight assumption* (Bion, 1961) is not guided by rational thought but by a need to defend against perceived external or internal threats. While SUR communities offered psychological safety and cohesion, they also tended to reproduce a collective culture of suspicion and defensive solidarity in the face of a perceived external enemy.

In Slovakia, the SUR model was primarily carried forward by J. Hašto, J. Štúrová, and J. Kožnar, who had themselves completed the training and, beginning in the 1980s, conducted community-based programs following a similar format. Although SUR shaped the education of nearly all senior Slovak psychotherapists, an initiative by P. Breier and J. Hašto in the 1980s to establish a group psychotherapy section within the Psychiatric Association did not receive institutional support (Morovicsová et al., 2017).

In 2000, the Institute of Psychodynamic Psychotherapy was established.[1] Although its training model was oriented toward the development of individual psychotherapists, it combined work in small groups with larger community-based groups. This format became prevalent across most therapeutic training programs and remains in place today.

In these training settings, the group primarily serves as a structural container: participants are physically present in the group but focus mainly on individual material. One person assumes the role of "patient," while others either observe the therapist's interventions or engage as secondary therapists. Group dynamics – such as emotional resonance, tensions, and alliances – typically emerge outside the formal group space, during breaks. When these dynamics are brought back into the session, they are usually processed through an individual lens. As a result, the capacity to reflect on the here-and-now of the group process often remains underdeveloped.

From a group analytic perspective, these groups often exhibit characteristics of what E. Hopper (2003) describes as *the fourth basic assumption: aggregation/massification*. Although the group may exist structurally, members do not genuinely engage with each other – functioning either as isolated individuals focused solely on their own experience (aggregation), or merging into normative group pressure, with little differentiation or authentic participation (massification). This dynamic blocks the development of the group-as-a-whole, a thinking entity capable of reflecting on its own processes.

This so-called hybrid model – individual therapy conducted within a group framework – remained, until 2023, as the only officially recognized form of experiential training for certified psychotherapists. Within this model, experiential group participation was mandatory, yet served primarily as a self-experience component in the training of therapists who would go on to work with individual clients. Only a minimal requirement of 100 hours of individual therapy was in place, and supervision was focused exclusively on work with individual patients. There was no training pathway dedicated to the development of group therapists as such. In practice, therapeutic groups – when offered – were typically led by individual psychotherapists without specific training in group dynamics, with the group serving more as a structural setting than as an active therapeutic agent.

While individual narratives and participation in the training community created conditions for unconscious group processes to emerge, these dynamics unfolded primarily outside the formal framework. In the backstage of the group, unconscious processes came alive but remained unspoken. As a result, the group's therapeutic potential was left unused: the therapist, not the group, served as the primary therapeutic instrument. This model effectively reduced the group to a logistical structure for organizing meetings, stripping it of its relevance as a modality of treatment. Consequently, group psychotherapy has remained, in practice, at the margins of professional engagement.

The Social Unconscious and Backstage Groups

To understand why therapeutic groups in Slovakia often function more as formal structures than as active therapeutic instruments, it is essential to consider the unconscious processes that shape our cultural patterns. The concept of the *social unconscious* refers to the shared, co-created unconscious of members of a social system – whether a society, community, or nation. It encompasses anxieties, fantasies, defenses, myths, and collective memories that shape what can be felt, thought, or spoken (Weinberg, 2007).

As E. Hopper (2001) emphasizes, engaging with the social unconscious is crucial for understanding how groups unconsciously and repeatedly recreate aspects of past social trauma. Within this framework, certain questions arise: Why does the Slovak training model emphasize group meetings without activating group dynamics? Why are hierarchically led groups preferred, while authentic group life unfolds outside formal training spaces? And why does group therapy remain marginal in clinical practice, while individual formats continue to dominate?

Slovak cultural identity has historically been shaped by adaptation to external authority – emerging in the shadow of larger powers and often defined in relation to others. Until the 19th century, many inhabitants of present-day Slovakia lacked a clear national consciousness; language, cultural identity, and collective belonging were not part of everyday experience. Slovak identity developed largely as a response to prolonged external pressures – most notably from Hungarian assimilationist policies (Hudek, 2011). In such a historical context, the group is not experienced as a safe space of belonging, but rather as an external structure governed by authority, to which one must adapt.

Formal groups thus came to be experienced as spaces of conformity, emotional suppression, and surveillance. Under these conditions, informal, backstage groups developed as the only spaces where emotional life and a sense of authenticity could be experienced, hidden from the gaze of official structures. These two types of groups – one visible and controlled, the other intimate yet hidden – proved equally functional under communism. Václav

Havel[2](1978/2024) famously described life under ideology as a "life in lies": individuals outwardly complied with the system while remaining inwardly detached. He writes: "An individual ... does not have to accept the lie. It is enough to have accepted life with it and in it. By this very fact, he confirms the system, fulfills it, makes it, is it." In a totalitarian society, it is common for anyone to be a potential informant and to be punished for difference. Under such conditions, it becomes safer not to feel, not to speak, and to say only what is expected. Helena Klímová[3] (2011) observed that under totalitarian regimes, the false collective Self tends to emerge through identification with the aggressor – mirroring the development of the false Self in individuals. Traumatized groups often submit to authority in the hope of gaining protection.

In the language of group analysis, one might say that the cultural unconscious in Slovakia has long been organized around Bion's *basic assumption of dependency* (Bion, 1961) – the unconscious expectation that a group can function only under the leadership of a strong figure who possesses the answers, ensures safety, and protects against anxiety. Such a group does not operate as a space for thinking, but rather as a formation dependent on its leader, defensively structured to ward off uncertainty and emotional complexity. This dynamic is carried into therapeutic and training groups, where leadership is not only accepted but actively sought.

These cultural residues – fear of authentic sharing, the longing for a leader, paranoia about exposure, as well as deprivation – have penetrated deeply into the development of group psychotherapy in Slovakia. What once functioned as a necessary strategy for survival has been unconsciously carried into the present, shaping both training and clinical practice. The group becomes a compulsory framework, but not a therapeutic one. Its emotional and relational life tends to unfold backstage: in corridors and during coffee breaks.

The shift from therapy-in-the-group to therapy-by-the-group is therefore more than a professional change. It is deeply connected to a psycho-cultural movement away from totalitarian modes of relating, toward a group mind capable of thinking, bearing difference, and tolerating uncertainty.

Formal Group Analytic Training in Slovakia

A more formal training in group psychoanalytic psychotherapy became available only after the fall of the totalitarian regime in 1989. In 1990, IPA psychoanalyst Jiří Kocourek – then a leading authority in the Czech psychoanalytic community – founded the Institute of Applied Psychoanalysis (IAPSA) in the Czech Republic, with the aim of offering systematic education in psychoanalytic work with groups. The training program was rooted in the SUR model, enriched with psychoanalytic theory, elements of Yalom's interpersonal approach, and the German interactional method developed by H. Argelander. It was Argelander's strong emphasis on the scenic events of the here-and-now and his view of the group as a dynamic whole, rather than a sum of individuals, that brought the training closer to the Foulkesian concept of group analysis.

In addition to theoretical seminars and supervision, the IAPSA training included a five-year experiential component in the form of intensive week-long retreats held annually. Over the next three decades, 55 training groups were completed, with more than 100 graduates from Slovakia. Of the 80 fully certified therapists, at least 25 were Slovak (Institut aplikované psychoanalýzy, n.d.). The majority of them, however, do not currently work with groups. Nevertheless, the training constituted a significant step toward the systematic education of Slovak psychoanalytic therapists.

Although a considerable number of Slovak therapists completed training in group psychoanalytic psychotherapy through the IAPSA, there was no professional society in Slovakia to represent or support this orientation. To address this gap, the Slovak Society for Psychoanalytic Psychotherapy (SSPAP)[4] was founded in 2011, with the aim of promoting training and establishing a national professional platform. In its early years, however, progress was gradual due to limited organizational structures, financial resources, and a small member base.

A significant turning point came in 2016, when the society underwent a comprehensive restructuring. Initially, SSPAP had drawn on the methodology of IAPSA, but growing interest in group analysis gradually led to a shift in theoretical orientation. In 2017, SSPAP became a member of the European Federation for Psychoanalytic Psychotherapy (EFPP), enabling more intensive international collaboration – particularly with Israeli group analyst Uri Levin. In the same year, the first training program accredited by the Slovak Ministry of Health was launched. The experiential group led by Luděk Vrba from the Prague Institute for Group Analysis (IGA Praha), marked the first historical step toward systematic education in group analysis in Slovakia.

In 2023–24, SSPAP applied for accreditation of two new training programs – one of which was devoted exclusively to group analysis. Its approval in 2024 marked a historic milestone: the launch of the first officially accredited training in group psychotherapy in Slovakia. The program fulfills the requirements of Slovak legislation as well as the standards of the EFPP and European Group-Analytic Training Institutions Network (EGATIN).

With regard to the professional group component, the training includes 350 hours of experiential group work (delivered in five block meetings per year over four years); 300 hours of theoretical–clinical seminars (held as full-day meetings once a month); 200 hours of supervision of one's own therapeutic group within a supervision group; and a minimum of 150 hours of individual psychoanalytic psychotherapy, undertaken before or during the training (program standards as of 2025; subject to periodic revision in line with EFPP/EGATIN guidance).

This overview reflects only the core group analytic elements of the program. Additional requirements – such as clinical practice and institutional placements – are outlined separately. The program concludes with a final examination and the presentation of clinical work with a group.

By 2025, three cohorts had completed the experiential component, with a fourth having started in autumn. Until that point, these groups had consisted exclusively of candidates enrolled in the full training program. In 2025, however, a shift was introduced: a new group was opened to professionals from the broader helping professions who may not wish to pursue full training but are interested in gaining experiential exposure to group analysis. This shift was motivated both by the limited number of applicants for full training and by the need to create a more natural group setting – one that better reflects real therapeutic conditions, as opposed to a closed circle of therapists.

The SSPAP training is grounded in the group analytic concepts of S.H. Foulkes and W. Bion. Emphasis is placed on working with the group-as-a-whole, cultivating a group language, and fostering the capacity to think within the matrix rather than focusing solely on individual narratives. The therapist is not perceived as an authoritative figure, but as a conductor – one who facilitates awareness of group processes and supports the emergence of a shared reflective space. The training thus aims to develop both a sense of belonging within the group and an appreciation of each participant's individuality.

As of 2025, we are witnessing the very early stages of group analytic work emerging in clinical practice. Candidates in the SSPAP training program are gradually beginning to open their own analytic groups, grounded in the principles of group analysis as defined earlier in this chapter. These groups are still few in number, operating in private settings, and reflect a significant shift from previous models in which the group functioned only as a structural frame for individual therapy. We are, quite literally, present at the birth of group analytic clinical work in Slovakia – a development that brings theoretical training into contact with the lived reality of therapeutic practice.

It is essential to recognize, however, that the social unconscious inevitably shapes the way we implement theory. We are not immune to the formative influences of our cultural and historical context. Group analytic concepts as formulated by Foulkes and Bion emerged in Western Europe, where values such as individuality, openness, and pluralism have long been embedded in the society. While the conductor is understood in that context as a facilitator of shared reflection, within the Slovak setting – shaped by experiences of unfreedom, collectivism, and conformity – the role may be perceived as passive or ambiguous, potentially evoking uncertainty or frustration. The figure of the therapist as authority continues to emerge, not from theoretical misunderstanding, but from an unconscious need for clarity and control. Similarly, the notion of the group-as-a-whole may be grasped intellectually, yet not fully experienced, as the felt experience of a living, thinking group is often unfamiliar and emotionally challenging.

Implications and Future Directions

This chapter does not seek to argue for the superiority of one therapeutic modality over another. Rather, its aim is to outline how the Slovak context – shaped by specific historical, cultural, and psychological forces – has long provided little space for open professional dialogue regarding different modes of practice. Obedience to authority and the parallel existence of "backstage groups" became so deep-rooted that, for many years, they constituted the only conceivable framework for both training and clinical work.

As J. Kocourek remarked in a personal communication (email, December 1, 2023) in response to my inquiry about the strong interest among Slovak therapists in training with IAPSA: "I too asked myself about the motives … I think they do not wish to share their *privatissima* with familiar colleagues in Slovakia." This observation highlights how unconscious anxieties about exposure within one's immediate professional environment can inhibit open reflection. Despite the long-standing presence of group psychotherapy, we are, in many ways, still at the beginning of working with the group as a therapeutic entity.

From the perspective of group analysis, we may be regarded today as a "*second generation*" – professionals educated after 1989, trained within IAPSA, and simultaneously shaped by growing connections with European institutions such as the EFPP and EGATIN. Our aim is to cultivate a deeper understanding of the distinction between therapy in the group and therapy by the group – not only at the level of theoretical formulation but also within clinical and training practice. Our candidates are encouraged to perceive the group as a subject in its own right, with its own internal dynamics, rather than merely as a container for individual narratives.

The "*third generation*" – today's candidates – are entering a professional space still marked by historical mistrust and entrenched authority, but also possessing potential for transformation. Unlike previous generations, they have access to internationally recognized training standards, the reflective language of group analysis, and opportunities to participate in thinking groups. It is this generation that may become capable of creating groups in which dynamics no longer unfold "behind closed doors" but within the room itself – groups in which the therapist no longer acts as a leader but as a facilitator of shared awareness.

Our belief that the group can be experienced not as a threat but as a therapeutic instrument is grounded in our own clinical experience and in ongoing international collaboration. At the same time, we recognize that the broader social context employs opposing forces: current political and cultural developments in Slovakia reveal that regression toward authoritarian structures, the weakening of pluralism, and the intensification of "us versus them" divisions are not merely residues of the past, but immediate and pressing challenges.

In this context, the ambition to develop a group analytic practice in which therapeutic groups function as spaces that can endure difference, tolerate uncertainty, and sustain cohesion without an omnipotent leader becomes both clinically demanding and potentially transformative in the broader social and cultural context.

Such transformation, however, is not possible without maintaining high standards of training. In addition to experiential group work, individual experience remains essential. Group analytic work requires more than theoretical knowledge or participation in a group setting – it demands the internal capacity to engage with one's own unconscious processes, including transference and countertransference. Individual psychoanalytic psychotherapy is therefore regarded as fundamental to the development of the candidate's reflective capacity and their ability to contain and sustain the group process.

For these reasons, our training includes a mandatory requirement of at least two years of individual psychoanalytic psychotherapy, with a minimum frequency of twice weekly. For those preparing to become training analysts, the standard is higher – at least 350 hours of analytic experience on the couch. We believe that only a therapist who has engaged in sustained, in-depth inner work is capable of containing the complex unconscious dynamics of the group and of upholding the quality of both clinical work and training.

One of the key challenges facing group analysis in Slovakia is the complete absence of research on its clinical effectiveness or real-world application. Given the small number of trained group analysts, the limited availability of functioning groups outside training structures, and the general lack of institutional support for research in dynamic therapies, no systematic studies are currently available. Clinical practice remains based primarily in experiential knowledge, supervision, and international exchange.

Although group analytic training is gradually traction ground within the Slovak professional community, group analysis remains rarely practiced in everyday clinical work. The foremost challenge for the coming years will therefore be the ability to establish a sufficiently broad clinical base from which meaningful research can later emerge. Developing research frameworks that reflect the specificities of group analytic work within the Slovak cultural and institutional context is a logical and necessary next step. In contrast to countries such as the UK, Israel, or Germany – where group analysis is more firmly embedded within mental health care and clinical services – the Slovak context remains in an early stage of development. Group analytic work continues to emerge primarily within training structures, and its integration into mainstream clinical practice is still in its infancy.

Notes

1 It builds on the traditions of SUR training and psychoanalysis in the Czech and Slovak contexts, and its founders were J. Hašto, P. Černák, Ľ. Juráš, and M. Chylík.

2 Václav Havel (1936–2011) was a Czech playwright, essayist, and dissident who became one of the leading figures of the anti-communist movement Charter 77.

After the fall of the totalitarian regime, he was elected president of Czechoslovakia in 1989, and later of the Czech Republic. His essays and plays are characterized by a philosophical engagement with themes of identity, truth, power, and the responsibility of the individual within an unfree system. His essay, *The Power of the Powerless*, was one of the key texts that helped the West to grasp what was actually happening behind the Iron Curtain.

3 Helena Klímová (b. 1938) is a Czech psychoanalyst and group analyst. In both her therapeutic and publicist work, she explores the mechanisms of collective silence, guilt, identification with the aggressor, and the strategies of survival under a totalitarian regime.

4 Founding members of the society: M. Babík, D. Březnová, Z. Michlerová, E. Mlejnková, A. Nagajová, S. Nürnberger, A. Strečko, and P. Zámečník.

References

Bion, W.R. (1961). Experiences in groups. In W.R. Bion, *Experiences in Groups and Other Papers* (pp. 1–22). London: Tavistock.

Foulkes, S.H. (1975). *Group Analytic Psychotherapy: Methods and Principles*. London: Gordon & Breach.

Gjuričová, A. (2017). Bohatství pod neviditelným pláštěm? K psychoterapii v Československu po roce 1968. *Soudobé dějiny*, 24(3), 311–334.

Havel, V. (2024). *Moc bezmocných a jiné eseje*. Prague: Knihovna Václava Havla.

Hopper, E. (2001). The social unconscious: Theoretical considerations. *Group Analysis*, 34(1), 9–27.

Hopper, E. (2003). Incohesion: Aggregation/massification: the fourth basic assumption in the unconscious life of groups and group-like social systems. *Group Analysis*, 36(1), 57–111.

Hudek, A. (2011). Between Czechs and Hungarians: Constructing the Slovak national identity from the 19th century to the present. *History Compass*, 9(4), 257–268. doi:10.1111/j.1478-0542.2010.00759.x.

Institut aplikované psychoanalýzy. (n.d.). *Sebezkušenost*. IAPSA. Available at: www.iapsa.cz/sebezkusenost/institut/sebezkusenost (accessed May 2026).

Klímová, H. (2011). The false we – the false collective self: A dynamic part of the social unconscious. In E. Hopper & H. Weinberg (Eds.), *The Social Unconscious in Persons, Groups and Societies, Volume 1: Mainly Theory* (pp. 187–208). London: Karnac.

Morovicsová, E., Heretik, A. Sr., Heretik, A. Jr., & Škodáček, I. (2017). History of psychotherapy in Slovakia. *European Journal of Mental Health*, 12(1), 88–103. doi:10.5708/EJMH.12.2017.1.6.

OECD and European Observatory on Health Systems and Policies. (2023). *Slovakia: Country Health Profile 2023 (State of Health in the EU)*. Paris: OECD Publishing.

Všeobecná zdravotná poisťovňa. (2024). *Katalóg výkonov – psychoterapia (skupinová a individuálna forma)*. VšZP. www.vszp.sk (accessed October 2025).

Weinberg, H. (2007). So what is this social unconscious anyway? *Group Analysis*, 40(3), 307–322.

Chapter 5

Group Analytic Psychotherapy in Sweden

Pia Litzell Berg, Paul Benér and Christer Sandahl

Historical Background

In 1949 a Swedish psychoanalyst and psychiatrist, Torsten Sjövall, traveled to Boston where he worked for two years at an outpatient psychiatric clinic at Beth Israel Hospital. During his time there he experienced and was taught the basics of psychoanalytically oriented group psychotherapy. He was deeply influenced by what he had learned, and he brought his knowledge back to Sweden. During the following years several colleagues went both to the USA and the UK to learn how to work with psychoanalytic group psychotherapy and Group Analysis. Many were also impressed by the work at the therapeutic communities and other types of group practices in England at, for example, the Tavistock clinic and Henderson hospital. All these early group-therapists worked for the introduction of analytic group psychotherapy and Group Analysis in Sweden.

An association for group therapists was founded in Stockholm 1962. Soon thereafter associations were initiated all over the country. The National Federation for group therapy associations was created in 1975. There were about 2,500 people involved in the associations. Group analytic psychotherapy flourished. So did family therapy, which of course is another story, but many who trained as group therapists were also in family therapy training and the exchange of experiences between the two fields were frequent.

During this period there was a strong belief in groups in general, and the society at large was collectively oriented. There was a great interest in group psychotherapy and in society people got together in groups for many other reasons than therapy. Sweden has a long group tradition based in the early 20th-century labor, women's suffrage, and temperance movements.

During the 1970s and into the 1980s, various forms of group treatment and therapeutic communities were common in psychiatry and social work. Enthusiasm was high but the level of education among therapists was low. A wild flora of experience-based methods spread, which contributed to the association of group treatment as frivolous. However, in this rich variety there were also many professionals who worked with group analysis in both long-

DOI: 10.4324/9781003597674-5

term and short-term formats. For them, it was obvious that education at an academic level was necessary if group therapy was not to fall into disrepute.

The group analytic tradition was introduced in Sweden in the 1970s through accredited training programs at the Institute for Psychotherapy, under the leadership of psychologists Hans Gordon, Lars Lorentzon, and Eric Steadman. The culture of these training programs was strongly influenced by Eric Steadman, who drew upon his experience at the therapeutic community of the UK's Henderson Hospital and his studies with Foulkes. The establishment of the Group Analytic Institute, Stockholm (GAI), in 1981 reflected a pressing need to strengthen both training and research in the field of group analysis. Within this network, books on group analysis were published in Swedish (Lorentzon, 1985; Widlund, 1989; 1995). Widlund's 1989 volume included, in addition to Swedish contributions, chapters authored by Hans Bosse, Caroline Garland, and Colin James. Members of GAI also contributed chapters to the 1995 volume edited by Inge Widlund. These publications were subsequently integrated into all Swedish training programs in group analysis.

In the late 1980s interest in groups decreased and individual perspective as well as individual psychotherapy was prioritized. One important reason was that a state license to practice as a psychotherapist was introduced. This was regarded as a great step forward, but most academically approved institutions which offered training to get the license only offered training in individual psychotherapy

Some of the local group therapy associations were not long-lived. In 2002 the National Federation and the Association in Stockholm was transformed into the Swedish Association for Group Psychotherapy and Group Development. At the end of 1980s the individual perspective dominated both in the Swedish society and within the psychotherapeutic field. This change might have been related to a political change from Social Democratic dominance to a more liberal and market-oriented ideology, including an emphasis on values of personal freedom and choice.

Theoretical Foundations and Cultural Links in Group Analytic Psychotherapy

Foundational Theories Guiding Group Analytic Psychotherapy Practices

This mixture of North American influences, which later came to be dominated by the Yalom interactional approach in combination with psychoanalytic group psychotherapy was introduced in Sweden in the beginning of 1960s, with inspiration also from therapeutic communities. When group analytic training started in collaboration with IGA London in Denmark and Norway in the mid-1980s, group analysis was already established in Sweden.

Representatives of IGA London were invited on several occasions to convene conferences and workshops. There was a lively exchange between IGA London and members of the Swedish network. However, the fact that IGA London did not arrange formal training in Sweden created some hesitation in parts of the English group analytic establishment. Did the training in Sweden really correspond to the criteria of the time for what was required to conduct group analytic psychotherapy? Perhaps there was reason for the hesitation, given that the training in Sweden certainly contained the standard works in Group Analysis, but also input from other orientations, such as interactional group psychotherapy, self-psychology, systems theory, and the group relations tradition.

The psychoanalytic and psychodynamic scene in general had a similar development in Sweden, that is, it was influenced by both English and British object relations theory and North American versions of psychoanalysis, self-psychology in particular. Faced with the dominance of Cognitive Behavioral Therapy (CBT), research-based and sophisticated short-term therapies with a focus on affective and emotional processing have become increasingly used in psychodynamic psychotherapy. The development of Focused Group Therapy (FGT) in Sweden took place against the same background, i.e. the need to develop evidence-based methods which could be an alternative to CBT. FGT has a deep foundation in group analysis but also has roots in self-psychology, and it is "competitive" in the sense that it is research-based and has a format that suits large parts of the patient base (see below).

Examination of How Local Culture May Affect the Interpretation and Execution of Group Analytic Psychotherapy Theories

In the World Value Survey[1] Sweden has been characterized as high on secular values, i.e. less emphasis on religion, traditional family values and authority and high on self-expression values which give high priority to environmental protection, growing tolerance of foreigners, gays and lesbians and gender equality, and rising demands for participation in decision making in economic and political life.

Analytical philosophy has for a long time been the dominant perspective in the Swedish academic world. It is characterized by its focus on logic and conceptual analysis and has strong ties to the natural science traditions. The value system measured by the World Value Survey which dominate Swedish culture, in combination with a strong belief in the natural science have influenced psychiatry in Sweden. The medical approach in psychiatry harmonizes with the natural science perspective of CBT. This in combination with the overwhelming scientific support for CBT in terms of number of publications makes it attractive for the medical professions. Today, the evidence for psychodynamic and relational approaches, including group therapy, for several patient categories is equally strong, but this has not yet influenced the authorities.

From this situation it followed that psychotherapy provided by public health care should be cost-efficient and preferably of short-term format. Today, CBT, which aims for short-term treatment, is part of the treatment guidelines for health care. Psychodynamic approaches are not recommended by the public guidelines. A general development within licensure-qualifying psychotherapy programs in Sweden has been the removal of the requirement for personal therapy in most trainings. This shift further reinforces the emphasis on research and methodology rather than on the psychotherapist's own personal and professional development. In contrast to many other countries, several professional backgrounds in Sweden may lead to licensure as a psychotherapist—not only psychologists and physicians, but also social workers, nurses, physiotherapists, and clergy. Despite the current gloomy situation, psychodynamic psychotherapy is still delivered to some degree in publicly sponsored treatments and among private practitioners both in the form of individual and group psychotherapy. Group approaches are still common in health care and social care, but they are mostly psycho-educational which offers little room for exchange and interaction.

How the Role of Group Analysts Is Perceived

The strong emphasis in Swedish culture on equality and individual freedom have resulted in low power distance plus a very negative attitude towards authoritarian expressions.

In a study of managerial leadership, authoritarianism was even shown to have negative effects on employee health in Sweden, which was not the case in an Italian comparison cohort (Nyberg, 2009). However, worst for employee health in both countries was, as expected, managerial laissez-faire style, and best a leadership style which delegates authority and encourages participation. It is not by chance that the Swedish Armed Forces has adopted a Swedish version of transformational leadership which argues that leaders should have a positive attitude that supports, encourages, and inspires their co-workers (Larsson et al., 2018)

Against this background it should be no surprise that the group analytic leadership approach fits Swedish culture well. Foulkes was very aware of the authority that comes with the role of conductor, but as a Jewish refugee he wanted to avoid the word "leader" which literally is translated as *Fuhrer* in German, with its terrible connotations. He wanted to separate the two concepts, leader and conductor, to make practitioners aware that it is a special kind of leadership to conduct a therapeutic group. The literal translation of conductor into Swedish would be referring to directing an orchestra. Most common is to use the word group psychotherapist, or group leader, which in the Swedish context would not have the negative connotations that Foulkes feared.

Training in Group Analytic Psychotherapy

The first training in group psychotherapy started in 1967 at Stockholm University. Then, other educators both at universities and within professional associations started training programs in group psychotherapy. The programs were based on a mixture of Group Analysis, interactional psychodynamic group psychotherapy and experiences from therapeutic communities. This approach was adopted by the Institute for Psychotherapy, albeit with a stronger emphasis on Group Analysis.

Based on hard work, one three-year training program in Group Analysis, in cooperation with the Group Analytic Institute (GAI), was, however, approved by the authorities in 1989. Unfortunately, the University and Higher Education Board later decided that the training in Group Analytic Psychotherapy no longer was to be approved and had to end in 2012. However, until then The Educational Institute in Stockholm Psychiatry (later The Psychotherapy Society Inc., of which Göran Ahlin was the director, succeeded by Pia Litzell Berg in 2003) examined about 100 group analysts. The decision by the board was a result of a stricter policy regarding academic requirements and a prioritization of CBT.

Since the introduction of psychotherapy licensure in Sweden, nine three-year licensure-qualifying training programs in psychodynamic group therapy and group analysis have been conducted between 1989 and 2009. Seven of these programs focused primarily on group therapy with adults, although some attention was also given to work with children and adolescents. Two of the programs were offered within Child and Adolescent Psychiatry in Stockholm and were oriented toward group therapy with children, adolescents, and parents.

Within the programs, students engaged in both long-term and short-term groups as part of their clinical training. All nine programs were grounded in the British tradition of group analysis and psychoanalytic/psychodynamic group therapy, although influences from the United States were also represented. Prominent theoretical and clinical figures included S.H. Foulkes, W. Bion, D. Stock Whitaker, and I. Yalom. Guest lecturers from England, Germany, and Norway were regularly invited to teach.

In the adult groups, the traditional British group analytic mode of working was taught. In the short-term groups, methods and research related to brief therapy were incorporated. In the children's groups, play served as the foundation for the group analytic perspective. The understanding of group processes and dynamics was based on the psychodynamic and group analytic traditions. However, interpretations were made differently than in the adult groups—often within the ongoing dialogue between co-therapists. Such interpretations were clarifying and supportive and typically remained on a manifest level. Work in adolescent groups largely followed the model applied in the adult groups.

Because these programs were part of the Swedish higher education system, their structure was regulated accordingly. One requirement was a thesis corresponding to 15 ECTS credits, with the entire program comprising 90 ECTS credits. This academic framework strengthened the emphasis on research and scientific grounding, though it also reduced the time and demands placed on clinical practice.

Following the discontinuation of the three-year program, the GAI in Stockholm conducted three two-year Diploma Programs in Group Analysis between 2017 and 2023. These programs included not only psychotherapists but also professionals working within organizational contexts. The supervised groups in the training included both clinical groups and groups based in organizational settings.

The Institute has also organized three two-year online diploma courses in Iran, which, apart from their online format, follow the same structure as those conducted in Sweden.

Two types of academic courses have been arranged by the Karolinska Institutet, a medical university in Stockholm. One was a one-year course, 15 ECTS-credit, in Focused Group Therapy, offered three times in the early 2000s. Unfortunately, it coincided with a period when employers were primarily investing in CBT training for their staff. Despite excellent evaluations, it was not possible to continue the program due to a lack of employer interest in funding the course.

The second course, also worth 15 ECTS credits, focused on methods for conducting group treatment within health care settings. It was offered between 2011 and 2023, enrolling approximately 20–25 students per year. The course attracted professionals from a range of disciplines, including physiotherapy, nursing, social work, occupational therapy, medicine, and psychology. Both courses combined lectures, seminars, supervision of training groups, and self-experiential group participation.

From time to time, practitioners in psychiatry, social work, and rehabilitation express a desire to deepen their understanding of group work and to learn how to enhance interaction and communication among patients in the groups they lead, something their patients themselves often request. Members of the Institute and the Association have responded to these needs by offering seminars, workshops, and supervision to support professionals in such contexts.

To further promote group analysis and group psychotherapy, and to provide resources for interested professionals and employers, several group analysts decided to write an introductory book on group psychotherapy. A Swedish edition was published in 2014 (Sandahl et al., 2014), followed by a revised and expanded English version in 2020 (Sandahl et al., 2020).

Current Practice and Adaptation

The review below is based on internet searches using keywords such as “group therapy,” “group treatment,” “group analysis,” and “psychological group therapy” in various combinations.

Group therapy in this context is often referred to as group discussions and is more frequently offered within public health care, typically for people of similar ages, such as adolescents or “girls’ groups,” or for patients sharing the same diagnosis, such as cancer or diabetes. Several private providers briefly mention group therapy as an alternative, but it appears to be given lower priority compared to individual therapy—both in public and private sectors. Region Skåne, for instance, collaborates with private psychotherapists who are contracted under regional health care agreements.

Among the websites reviewed, the method of group therapy is generally described in broad terms, but rarely with reference to theoretical background or methodology. Most psychotherapists are licensed, though they do not specify any training in group therapy or group analysis. One website provides more detailed educational information. Non-licensed practitioners can also be found online, stating training in counselling but not specifically in group therapy. The actual number of licensed psychotherapists offering group therapy is difficult to estimate but is likely around 30–40 practitioners.

Public health care mainly provides manual-based group treatments such as MBT (Mentalization-Based Therapy), DBT (Dialectical Behaviour Therapy), and CBT. It is, however, seldom specified which group therapy training the practitioners have. The roles of professionals within treatment teams are also often unclear, though psychologists are commonly included. In larger cities, particularly within psychiatric care, group therapy is offered at affective disorder clinics. These treatments are typically combined with individual sessions, supportive conversations, and psychoeducation, with the duration often stated as 10–12 meetings.

The Church of Sweden offers counselling and psychotherapy in various forms, individual, couples, family, and group (for example bereavement groups), but does not specify which therapeutic methods are used or what education the practitioners have. Non-profit organizations across the country also provide mental health support, sometimes through group treatment, though details regarding their methods and qualifications are rarely disclosed.

In summary, access to group therapy in Sweden remains unclear. Internet searches for "group therapy" most often return general psychotherapy results, where individual therapy, particularly CBT-oriented approaches, dominates.

Psychotherapists trained in group dynamics or group analysis are primarily based in Malmö and Stockholm in the public and private sectors. They are often members of international psychotherapy associations as the Group Analytic Society international, GASi, and the International Association for Group Psychotherapy, IAGP.

Providing group therapy in private settings in Sweden often presents challenges, particularly when recruiting members for semi-open, ongoing groups. The contemporary zeitgeist favors individual therapy. People seeking psychological help typically think of one-on-one treatment, and group therapy rarely forms part of their mental framework. When offered, it is often met with surprise, skepticism, fear, and resistance. A few actively seek group therapy out of curiosity or prior knowledge, but most clients first attend individual therapy and later become open to joining a group once a trusting alliance with the therapist has been established. For those who do join, the group often becomes a meaningful and healing experience, where one can be seen, help others, and feel less alone.

In psychology training in Sweden, personal therapy remains a requirement at a basic psychotherapeutic level. At Lund University, students can choose 20 sessions of group therapy. This experience is often rewarding and may inspire future interest in group therapy training.

Group Analytic Applications

Summer Camps

An ongoing activity in Sweden is the organization of therapeutic summer camps for children and their parents. This initiative began in 1934, when a nurse invited a group of children to spend several weeks at a summer camp in the countryside. During this time, the children were able to enjoy being away from the city while also learning and practicing social skills. The sense of group belonging and community were central aspects of the experience.

Over the following years, the activity developed and became, for many decades, an integrated part of Child and Adolescent Psychiatry in the Stockholm region. Children and adolescents who were patients in psychiatric care and had ongoing therapeutic contact could, as part of their treatment, spend several weeks at a therapeutic summer camp located on one of the islands in the Stockholm Archipelago. These were often children and teenagers who struggled with social isolation or frequent conflicts with peers.

The staff were trained to use group dynamics as a therapeutic tool, helping the children and adolescents to develop new social skills and to find more constructive ways of managing conflicts. Everyday situations in camp life were used deliberately as therapeutic opportunities.

The theoretical foundation of the therapeutic work was based on psychodynamic and group analytical theories, including individual psychotherapy, group psychotherapy, family therapy, and therapeutic community.

In 2000, decision makers determined, for economic reasons, that summer camps would no longer be a mandatory part of Child and Adolescent Psychiatry. Consequently, an independent organization—The Association for Therapeutic Summer Camps—was established to take over the activity. The Association became a specialized unit within psychiatric services.

In recent years, the summer camps have have focused on programs for children together with their parents. Knowledge of early attachment has guided the development of a one-year program designed for both children and parents. The group process and its therapeutic potential remain central components of the program. The program is grounded in psychodynamic theory, emphasizing the group as the main therapeutic agent. Staff work with the group on different levels. The program begins with preparatory meetings in Stockholm involving both parents and children—sometimes separately, sometimes together. This is followed by a one-week stay at a summer camp in the Stockholm Archipelago, where environmental therapy plays a key role in the therapeutic process.

After the camp week, follow-up sessions are held in Stockholm to help the families consolidate what they have learned and experienced during the camp.

The Association for Therapeutic Summer Camps has received financial support from the Swedish General Inheritance Fund, which has enabled it to continue this important work with children and their parents, to evaluate the methods, and to further develop them. The Association has also benefited from private donations that contribute to the continuation and sustainability of its programs. The results in follow-up studies and evaluation with children and their parents have been very positive.

Application of Group Analysis within the Context of MBT

In Stockholm County, there is a long-standing tradition of providing Mentalization-Based Treatment (MBT) for patients with substance use disorders combined with either Emotionally Unstable or Antisocial Personality Disorder. The treatment program lasts between one and one and a half years. Following an introductory phase, patients receive weekly individual psychotherapy in combination with group therapy. Strict boundaries are maintained regarding self-harm, relapses, threats, and violence.

Each group is led by two conductors who are somewhat more active than in traditional group analysis. For example, they aim to minimize silence and offer empathic support. Their interventions are brief and focused on conscious, present-moment emotions with the goal of strengthening mentalization. The conductors, in a sense, take shared responsibility for the patient's mental state, for example, by interrupting patients when necessary and involving other group members to reduce transference reactions and prevent mentalization collapse.

At the end of each session, the conductors summarize the discussion and ask participants to reflect on what they are thinking about and what has been most meaningful to them during the meeting. This approach has evolved through clinical experience over the years and has also been inspired by empirical evidence presented by Norwegian colleagues (Karterud, 2015).

Focused Group Therapy

This short-term variant of group analytic psychotherapy was developed and evaluated as part of a research project on treatment for work-related depression (burnout) (Sandahl et al., 2011; Ahlin & Sandahl, 2022). The starting point in Focused Group Therapy (FGT) is the identification of what functions well in a person's life. Prior to the start of therapy, an individualized focus is formulated together with the patient, capturing experienced obstacles to coping and problem-solving in relationships with others.

Attention is directed toward current experiences. When working with a relational focus in FGT, problems should be described in everyday language so that both the conductor and group members can recognize them when they emerge in group interaction, which invariably occurs if the identified relational problem is genuine. Thus, FGT requires both a clearly defined group focus and an individual member focus that must be explicitly stated, well understood, and evident throughout the therapeutic process.

FGT employs a here-and-now therapeutic approach. It is time-limited, with two sessions per week during the initial 8–9 meetings, followed by one session per week for another 8–10 meetings. The short-term format necessitates a structured framework and a somewhat more active therapeutic stance compared to that used in long-term group analysis (Sandahl et al., 2020; Sandahl & Lindgren, 2006).

Dialogue Groups for Professionals

Group analysis has also inspired applications in organizational and professional development, particularly for individuals in managerial or medical roles. Reflection on experienced challenges and problems is essential for professional growth and forms the foundation of experiential learning. Such reflection can take place individually, with a mentor or supervisor, or collectively with colleagues in a group facilitated by an experienced conductor.

At the Karolinska Institutet, a model for such group dialogues was initially developed for physicians (Bergman et al., 2007, 2009a) and later adapted for managers (Bergman et al., 2009b; Lornudd et al., 2016; Sandahl, 2006). The groups are composed of participants who are not in direct working relationships with one another, although they may come from the same organization. Meetings are held once a month for three hours over a period of one year or longer. Each session focuses on one member's current professional challenges and follows four structured phases:

1 Defining the problem;
2 Generating hypotheses about underlying issues;
3 Developing potential solutions; and
4 Evaluating the session.

These groups typically foster strong bonds among participants, and some choose to continue supporting each other even after the group has formally ended. Evaluations of dialogue groups for managers indicate that employees whose leaders have participated in such programs perceive their leadership as more positive and effective. Employees describe these managers as more focused on leadership tasks and more self-confident in their ability to act (Palm et al., 2015).

Challenges and Evidence-based Practice

Major Challenges Faced in Practicing Group Analytic Psychotherapy

Evidence-based practice has exerted a strong influence on all aspects of public health care in Sweden for at least the past four to five decades. Although empirical support for psychodynamic psychotherapy has increased over the past 20 years, health care authorities continue to favor Cognitive Behavioral Therapy (CBT). The natural science–oriented culture that characterizes this field has also shaped the practice of Group Analysis (GA). Traditional long-term group analytic psychotherapy has largely disappeared from public health care settings.

In response, group analytic psychotherapists have adapted to the prevailing circumstances by applying GA primarily in short-term formats, with some further adaptations within organizational psychology. While CBT maintains a strong empirical foundation in Swedish psychotherapy research, several high-quality studies on individual psychodynamic psychotherapy have also been conducted (e.g., Berg et al., 2008; Falkenström et al., 2013, 2016; Lindgren et al., 2010; Lindqvist et al., 2020; Philips et al., 2018; Sandell et al., 2000; Werbart et al., 2023, 2025).

Review of Existing Research and Treatment Outcomes

Research on Group Analysis conducted in Sweden has primarily focused on the fields of addiction and work-related depression. A few researchers—most notably Associate Professor Göran Ahlin, the first director of the Group Analytic Training Program, and Professor Christer Sandahl at the Karolinska Institute in Stockholm—have taken on the challenge of securing financial support for empirical research on Group Analysis and its applications. Their work has contributed internationally to the fields of group process research, treatment outcome research, and treatment development (Ahlin, 1996; Ahlin et al., 1996; Lindgren et al., 2008; Sandahl et al., 1998; Sandahl et al., 2000; Sandahl et al., 2004b; Sandahl et al., 2011).

Group Process Research

A central concept in Group Analysis is the matrix. The Swedish psychiatrist and group analyst Göran Ahlin has published extensively on this topic. He operationalized the concept into eight determinants that can serve as focal points for process research, enabling the examination of what occurs in group therapy both moment to moment and between sessions. The Matrix Representation Grid (MRG) was originally developed as both a clinical and research tool for studying group interactions and themes, as well as the interrelationships among emerging group themes within and across sessions in relation to the dynamic matrix. In Ahlin's work, the MRG was both theoretically elaborated and empirically validated through comparison with another observational method, the System for Analyzing Verbal Interaction (SAVI) (Ahlin, 1996; Ahlin et al., 1996).

The working alliance is a core construct in psychotherapy research. In group therapy, the alliance with the group conductor has traditionally been studied more frequently than the arguably more central aspect in relational group therapy—the alliance with the group-as-a-whole. In one study, Lindgren et al. (2008) found that this type of alliance, specific to group analytic settings, had predictive value for treatment outcomes.

In a comparative study, self-efficacy, a central construct within cognitive behavioral therapy (CBT) was measured before and after treatment. Although this construct was not explicitly targeted in short-term Group Analysis (GA) groups, a paradoxical finding emerged: patients in the GA condition demonstrated greater improvement in self-efficacy than those in the CBT groups (Sandahl et al., 2004a).

It is reasonable to assume that therapist leadership styles differ between CBT and GA groups. However, when an instrument for analyzing verbal interaction was used to assess videotaped sessions, results indicated that the therapists' communication styles were more similar than different—except that the CBT therapist spoke approximately twice as much as the GA therapists. Notably, the two most effective communicators identified by the instrument were one CBT therapist and one GA conductor (Sandahl et al., 2000).

Group Treatment Outcome Research

An early attempt to evaluate Group Analysis (GA) for patients with borderline personality disorder was conducted in the late 1980s at the University of Umeå. At that time, treatment options for personality disorders were less developed, and dropout rates were relatively high. However, patients who remained in treatment differed in background characteristics from those who discontinued, providing valuable insights for defining selection criteria for GA with this patient population (Stiwne, 1989; Stiwne, 1994).

A short-term GA treatment for patients with moderate alcohol dependence was later developed, consisting of 15 weekly sessions of 90 minutes each, and compared with group-based CBT. At the 15-month follow-up, patients in both treatment conditions showed improvement; however, those with higher scores on psychological mindedness in the GA condition demonstrated greater gains in drinking behavior and psychological well-being compared with patients in the CBT groups. Conversely, patients with low scores on measures of psychological mindedness showed better outcomes in CBT (Sandahl et al., 1998).

An adaptation of GA, Focused Group Therapy (FGT; see above), was developed for patients on long-term sick leave due to work-related depression. FGT was compared with group CBT, and at the one-year follow-up, approximately

70% of patients in both treatments showed clinically significant improvement, with no significant difference between the two approaches. Further development of FGT, adjusted to accommodate patients' motivation to return to work, also proved successful (Ahlin & Sandahl, 2022; Sandahl et al., 2011).

Group Treatment Development

Based on research findings on group treatment for alcohol dependence, which indicate that the degree of psychological mindedness can differentiate patients who benefit from either CBT or GA treatment, a stepped-care model was developed. In this model, it is recommended that a thorough psychological assessment be conducted during the initial phase of treatment, followed by allocation to one of two treatment tracks. Patients with low psychological mindedness are referred to group CBT, whereas those with high psychological mindedness are offered short-term GA. If appropriate, these short-term treatments are followed by different forms of individual support for the CBT group and long-term Group Analysis for the GA group (Sandahl et al., 2004a).

Group Analysis represents a broad theoretical school that encompasses meta psychological tensions like those found in psychoanalysis. The relational perspective appears to dominate research on short-term psychotherapy in general, particularly in studies emphasizing emotional processes. Drawing inspiration from this, Focus Group Therapy (FGT) was developed as a method for short-term group work (see above). The theoretical foundation of FGT and detailed guidelines for conducting such groups have been described elsewhere (Sandahl et al., 2020; Sandahl & Lindgren, 2006).

Future Research and Evidence-Based Practice

Resources for mental health services in Sweden are limited, creating challenges in managing patient loads and long waiting lists. Some outpatient clinics have identified group treatment as a cost-effective strategy to address these issues. However, it remains difficult to convey to clinicians and administrators that evidence-based group therapy practices are grounded in empirical research conducted by well-trained therapists skilled in interactive methods.

The younger generation of clinicians interested in group therapy often lacks personal experience with long-term Group Analysis and has only a limited theoretical understanding of its foundations. To ensure the continuation and development of GA, it is crucial that high-quality training in this field remains accessible to clinicians.

Note

1 See www.worldvaluessurvey.org/WVSContents.jsp

References

Ahlin, G. (1996). Exploring psychotherapy group cultures: Essays on group theory and the development of the Matrix Representation Grid—An observation method for studying therapeutic group processes. Doctoral dissertation. Stockholm: Karolinska Institutet.

Ahlin, G., Sandahl, C., Herlitz, K. & Brimberg, I. (1996). Developing the Matrix Representation Grid (MRG): A method for observing group processes. Findings from time limited group psychotherapy for alcohol dependent patients. *Group*, 20(2), 145–173.

Ahlin, H.N., & Sandahl, C. (2022). Focused group psychotherapy in the rehabilitation and return to work from occupational burnout and longterm sick leave. *Revista Brasileira de Psicodrama*, 30, e1022.

Berg, A.L., Sandahl, C., & Clinton, D. (2008). The relationship of treatment preferences and experiences to outcome in generalized anxiety disorder (GAD). *Psychology and Psychotherapy: Theory, Research and Practice*, 81(3), 247–259.

Bergman, D., Arnetz, B., Wahlström, R., & Sandahl, C. (2007). Effects of dialogue groups on physicians' work environment. *Journal of Health Organization and Management*, 21(1): 27–23.

Bergman, D., Stotzer, E., Wahlström, R., & Sandahl, C. (2009a). Learning from dialogue groups-physicians' perceptions of role. *Journal of Health Organization and Management*, 23(2): 225–239.

Bergman, D., Fransson-Sellgren, S., Wahlström, R., & Sandahl, C. (2009b). Healthcare leadership: Impact of short-term intensive and long-term less intensive training programmes. *Leadership in Health Services* 22(2), 161–175.

Falkenström, F., Ekeblad, A., & Holmqvist, R. (2016). Improvement of the working alliance in one treatment session predicts improvement of depressive symptoms by the next session. *Journal of Consulting and Clinical Psychology*, 84(8), 738.

Falkenström, F., Granström, F., & Holmqvist, R. (2013). Therapeutic alliance predicts symptomatic improvement session by session. *Journal of Counselling Psychology*, 60(3), 317.

Karterud, S. (2015). *Mentalization-based Group Therapy (MBT-G): A Theoretical, Clinical, and Research Manual*. Oxford: Oxford University Press.

Larsson, G., Lundin, J., & Zander, A. (2018). *The Leadership Model: The Art of Matching Individual and Organizational Characteristics*. Lund: Studentlitteratur.

Lindgren, A., Werbart, A., & Philips, B. (2010). Long-term outcome and post-treatment effects of psychoanalytic psychotherapy with young adults. *Psychology and Psychotherapy: Theory, Research and Practice*, 83(1), 27–43.

Lindgren, A., Barber, J.P., & Sandahl, C. (2008). Alliance to the group-as-a-whole as predictor of outcome in psychodynamic group therapy. *The International Journal of Group Psychotherapy*, 58, 163–184.

Lindqvist, K., Mechler, J., Carlbring, P., Lilliengren, P., Falkenström, F., Andersson, G., … & Philips, B. (2020). Affect-focused psychodynamic internet-based therapy for adolescent depression: randomized controlled trial. *Journal of Medical Internet Research*, 22(3), e18047.

Lorentzon, L. (1985). *Gruppen – skeenden och föreställningar* [*The Group – Events and Imaginations*]. Stockholm: Rabén och Sjögren.

Lornudd, C., Bergman, D., Sandahl, C., & von Thiele Schwarz, U. (2016). A randomised study of leadership interventions for healthcare managers. *Leadership in Health Services*, 29(4), 358–376.

Nyberg, A. (2009). The impact of managerial leadership on stress and health among employees. Dissertation, Stockholm: Karolinska Institutet.

Palm, K., Ullström, S., Sandahl, C., & Bergman, D. (2015). Employee perceptions of managers' leadership over time. *Leadership in Health Services*, 28(4), 266–280.

Philips, B., Wennberg, P., Konradsson, P., & Franck, J. (2018). Mentalization-based treatment for concurrent borderline personality disorder and substance use disorder: a randomized controlled feasibility study. *European Addiction Research*, 24(1), 1–8.

Sandahl, C. (2006). Group supervision for managers: Preliminary findings from a research project. *Forum – Journal of the Association for Group Psychotherapy and Group Processes*, 1.

Sandahl, C., Ahlin, H. N., Asklin-Westerdahl, C., Björling, M., Saracino, A. M., Wennlund, L., … & Örhammar, A. (2020). *Why Group Therapy Works and How to Do It: A Guide for Health and Social Care Professionals.* Oxford: Routledge.

Sandahl, C., Ahlin, H. N., Asklin-Westerdahl, C., Björling, M., Saracino, A. M., Wennlund, L., … & Örhammar, A. (2014). *Gruppens potential. Att leda och utveckla gruppbehandling*. Stockholm: Natur och Kultur.

Sandahl, C., Lundberg, U., Lindgren, A., Rylander, G., Herlofsson, J., Nygren, Å., & Åsberg, M. (2011). Two forms of group therapy and individual treatment for work-related depression: A one-year follow-up study. *International Journal of Group Psychotherapy*, 61(4), 539–555.

Sandahl, C., & Lindgren, A. (2006). Integrative focused group psychotherapy. *Journal of Contemporary Psychotherapy*, 36, 113–119.

Sandahl, C., Gerge, A., & Herlitz, K. (2004a). Does treatment focus on self-efficacy result in better coping? Paradoxical findings from psychodynamic and cognitive behavioural group treatment of moderately alcohol dependent patients. *Psychotherapy Research*, 14(3), 388–397.

Sandahl, C., Busch, M., Skarbrandt, E., & Wennberg, P. (2004b). Matching group therapy to patient needs. In B. Reading & M. Weegman (Eds.), *Group Psychotherapy and Addiction*, pp. 42–58. London: Whurr Publishers.

Sandahl, C., Lindgren, A., & Herlitz, K. (2000). Does the group conductor make a difference? communication patterns in group-analytically and cognitive-behaviourally oriented therapy groups. *Group Analysis*, 33(3), 333–351. https://doi.org/doi:10.1177/05333160022077380

Sandahl, C., Herlitz, K., Ahlin, G., & Rönnberg, S. (1998). Time-limited group psychotherapy for moderately alcohol dependent patients: A randomized controlled clinical trial. *Psychotherapy Research*, 8, 361–378.

Sandell, R., Blomberg, J., Lazar, A., Carlsson, J., Broberg, J., & Schubert, J. (2000). Varieties of long-term outcome among patients in psychoanalysis and long-term psychotherapy: A review of findings in the Stockholm outcome of psychoanalysis and psychotherapy project (Stoppp). *The International Journal of Psychoanalysis*, 81(5), 921.

Stiwne, D. (1994). Group psychotherapy with borderline patients: Contrasting remainers and dropouts. *Group*, 18(1), 37–45.

Stiwne, D. (1989). Borderline patients in group psychotherapy: Studies in process and outcome. Doctoral dissertation, Umeå universitet.

Werbart, A., Gråke, E., & Klingborg, F. (2023). Deadlock in psychotherapy: A phenomenological study of eight psychodynamic therapists' experiences. In *Therapeutic Failures in Psychotherapy* (pp. 28–46). Oxford: Routledge.

Werbart, A., Broby, M., & Carlsson, L. (2025). Obstructive silence in work with adolescents: a phenomenological study of psychotherapists' experiences. *Counselling Psychology Quarterly*, 1–22.

Widlund, I. (Ed.) (1989). *Gruppanalytiska perspektiv* [Group Analytic Perspectives]. Stockholm: Natur och Kultur.

Widlund, I. (Ed.) (1995). *Den Analytiska Gruppen, Gruppanalys i teori och praktik* [*The analytic group: Group analysis in theory and practice*]. Stockholm: Natur och Kultur.

Chapter 6

Group Analytic Psychotherapy in Russia

Assessment of the Current Situation and Prospects for Development

Darina Ilyanina, Nadezhda Mitryashkina, Andrey Sklizkov, Galina Stepanova, Maria Tvorogova, Anna Tsapenko and Zoya Shargalina

In the 1990s group analytic psychotherapy appeared in Moscow and St. Petersburg, and then in other cities of Russia. Currently, the basis of the professional group analytic community in Russia is made up of group analysis training institutions that prepare specialists in accordance with EGATIN,[1] and EFPP[2] standards. Among them are two in St. Petersburg,[3] three in Moscow,[4] one in Novosibirsk,[5] and two in Stavropol.[6] In addition, there are separate non-standard programs offering different forms of insight into group analysis and its variations.

The chapter presents the general situation in the field of group analytic psychotherapy in Russia, describing in detail the experience of three organizations: the Group Analysis Society (SGA, St. Petersburg),[7] the Moscow Institute of Group Analysis (MIGA, Moscow),[8] the Group Analysis Section of the Association for the Development of Psychotherapy and Psychoanalysis (ADPP, Stavropol),[9] whose representatives have teamed up to co-write this work. Attention is paid to the characteristic features of theory, practice, and research concerning group analytic psychotherapy in Russia.

Prevailing Theoretical Approaches, Their Connection with Culture and Impact on Practice

The theoretical approach of most Russian institutions is determined by the EGATIN standards, based on the Sigmund Foulkes group analysis model, methodologically based on psychoanalytic theory, Gestalt psychology, sociology, and systems theory. Both the approaches underlying group analytic psychotherapy and Foulkes' group analytic model itself, which involves not only the therapy of an individual in the group, but also a "form of group psychotherapy by the group, including its conductor" (Foulkes, 1975), seem to meet the cultural code, mentality, and needs of Russians.

DOI: 10.4324/9781003597674-6

Proximity of the Group Analysis Concept to Russian Culture

Foulkes' ideas about the social nature of the individual's psyche determined by family and society, about the group as the main psychological unit, about the group matrix as a network of relationships, about the group as a whole, not reducible to the sum of its parts, as well as about treatment by communication, are deeply consonant with Russian history, literature, as well as with its scientific and philosophical thought.

Living in groups, thinking in the logic of groups is understandable and familiar to Russians. Most of the country's history is somehow connected with collectivism. First, pre-industrial pre-revolutionary communities, then collective farms, communist, and socialist ideology.

Russian classical literature immanently contains the ideas of a group as an integrity that is not reducible to the sum of its parts, a matrix as a network of relationships, the role of a leader as a member of a group, though with special functions.

Thus, the works of Leo Tolstoy (1828–1910) describe the "spirit" of the people, the "spirit" of the troops that determine the course of history from the logic of the whole, where individuals and historical figures are part of the whole, united by unconscious connections. In the epic novel *War and Peace*, L.N. Tolstoy tells about Kutuzov before the battle with Napoleon in the Patriotic War of 1812:

> He knew from long-term military experience and understood with his elder's mind that it was impossible for one person to lead hundreds of thousands of people, struggling with death, and knew that the fate of the battle was not decided by the orders of the commander-in-chief, not by the place where the troops were standing, not by the number of guns and people killed, but by that elusive force, called the spirit of the army, and he followed this force and conducted it, as much as it was in his power.
>
> (Tolstoy, 1980)

In the work of another great Russian writer, F.M. Dostoevsky (1821–81), the polyphonic principle of artistic thinking discovered by him and the new genre of polyphonic novel for Russian and European novels (in contrast to the monological novel), largely echo the group analytic view of the group and psyche. Dostoevsky, in his works, creates a polyphonic pluralistic world, where in a single space and time there exist many equal voices of heroes, each of which has a separate consciousness and worldview. Dostoevsky's polyphony means a fundamentally new relationship both between the heroes of the book themselves and between the author and the heroes. In the famous literary study *Problems of Dostoevsky's Poetics* (Bakhtin, 1972), M.M. Bakhtin (1895–1975) writes about this as follows:

> The hero's words about himself and about the world are as full-fledged as the usual author's words; they are not subordinate to the object image of the hero as one of his characteristics, nor do they serve as the mouthpiece of the author's voice. They own exceptional independence in the structure of the work, they sound as if next to the author's words and in a special way, combining with them and with the full-fledged voices of other heroes.

The interaction between the heroes' different consciousnesses creates the polyphonic whole of the novel. The space of Dostoevsky's polyphonic novel resembles the multiplicity of voices in a group analytic group and the interaction between them in the process of group dynamics. The author's position is comparable to that of a group analyst.

Maria Rohde (Munich) spoke about M.M. Bakhtin, his literary study of Dostoevsky's work, the study of the problem of the relationship between the "I" and the "Other," which, according to Bakhtin, arises "on the border of interaction," in the context of the group analytic roots of the Russian basic matrix, at the opening of a training project in Moscow in 1999. She also quoted his own experience of discussion in a group with like-minded people, which delighted her by the affinity with group analytic thinking: "In the end, I cannot attribute any verbal manifestation to any single speaker – they were in fact the product of an exchange between the speakers!"

Another intersection point between the ideas of the group analytic concept and Russian culture is the philosophical direction of "Russian cosmism" at the turn of the 19th and 20th centuries. Its followers – K. Tsiolkovsky, N. Fedorov, V. Vernadsky, A. Chizhevsky, V. Solovyov, N. Berdyaev, S. Bulgakov, P. Florensky, and other famous Russian thinkers – developed the doctrine of *sobornost* (collegiality), disclosing the principles of social integration, communication in society, mechanisms of interaction between individual and collective consciousness, universal interconnection in space and on Earth, proportionality of macrocosm and microcosm, which had a great influence on the development of humanitarian knowledge (Barmashova & Lomanov, 2020) and on the theory of systems in modern sociology, one of the methodological foundations of group analysis, in particular.

The psychoanalytic theory, which is one of the roots of group analytic psychotherapy, aroused great interest and has been widespread in Russia since its creation by Freud. Before and after the revolution, until the end of the 1920s, the works of Freud and other psychoanalysts were published in Russia; the Russian Psychoanalytic Society was created and Russian psychoanalysts made up a significant part of the members of the International Psychoanalytic Association. In the 1930s psychoanalysis was banned and repressed for ideological reasons. Freud and Jung treated Russian patients, and well-known works were written on the basis of their treatment (e.g., the case of the "wolf-man," described by Sigmund Freud, Sergei Pankeev; Sabine Shpielrein is also well known – she was analyzed by Jung and later became a psychoanalyst and contributed to the development of psychoanalysis).

In the late 1970s access to psychoanalysis began to open up, and in the early 1990s the revival of psychoanalysis in Russia began. Currently, psychoanalytic psychotherapy occupies an authoritative place among other methods of psychological assistance. For Russian culture, literature, character, it is common to turn to the inner world of a person and their study; therefore, psychoanalytic psychotherapy is close and understandable to Russians. In addition, the fundamentality and elaboration of psychoanalytic theory is appreciated by professionals.

In conclusion it can be noted, concerning the topic of proximity of the group analytic concept to Russian culture, that Russia, a multinational state inhabited by more than 193 ethnic groups that speak 270 languages, is a cultural and linguistic polyphony, where there is place for the identity of each nation, while at the same time there is a sense of belonging to a single whole culture, not reduced to the sum of its parts.

General Features of Theoretical and Practical Approaches

As described above, the prevailing theoretical approach in Russia is the Foulkes model of group analytic psychotherapy. Most of the power is delegated to the group, work is under way to ensure that the group itself becomes an active therapeutic factor. The proportion of the roles of conductor and therapist in the position of the leader is determined by the stage the group is at, the dynamic situation, and the individual style of the specialist.

The social upheavals and changes that Russia has gone through many times seem to determine the specific features of Russian group analytic psychotherapists: special attention, sensitivity, and the desire to be aware of the aspect of power. The individual style of group analytic therapists can vary on a continuum from a more directive approach to the difficulties of applying the necessary power of the conductor for fear of turning into a totalitarian object. In general, in the structure of group analytic education, opportunities are already laid for students to gain a conscious approach and develop their own style in relation to power in working with the group. Not only the conductor, but the groups contribute as well.

Since most of the first Russian group analysts had practiced individual psychoanalytic psychotherapy before joining group analysis, great importance is attached to the application of psychoanalytic concepts to the individual and the group. The formation of the group analytic identity is based on the development of the students' ability to deal with the unconscious: to create a group space in which the group unconscious manifests itself, observes its manifestations and phenomena, describes them, and understands the meaning.

Specificity of Institutional Approaches

The theoretical base of most Russian institutions is determined by the standards of EGATIN and EFPP, which is a similarity that gives a common language to Russian group analysts. Differences in institutional approaches are determined by where the training took place, who trained (the educational matrix of the organizations that trained the first graduates), and who was trained (the specifics of basic education and the experience of the students). We will tell you in more detail about the institutions represented by the authors of this chapter; this will be a more targeted introduction to the state of affairs in group analytic organizations at present.

Society for Group Analysis (SGA), St. Petersburg

SGA is one of the oldest professional associations in Russia. For more than 35 years it has been training specialists in the field of group analysis, publishing collections of articles, holding conferences for students and group analysts, energetically conducting educational, scientific, and social activities, uniting psychiatrists, psychotherapists, clinical psychologists, and psychoanalysts. Membership is available starting from the end of the Introductory Course on Group Analysis in one of the institutions of Russia. The educational standard in the field of group analysis corresponds to EGATIN. In 2019, the GASI Winter School was held in St. Petersburg, bringing together about 100 specialists from Russia, Great Britain, Norway, Kazakhstan, Ukraine, Germany, Israel, and other countries.

Throughout the first years of the organization's existence, training was carried out by representatives of the London Institute of Group Analysis: Raymond Blake, David Kennard, Jeff Roberts, Barbara Elliot, and later a Qualification Course was conducted, led by Sue Einhorn with the participation of Sheila Ernst, Harry Wright, Robert Harris, and many other colleagues; later Sheila Ritchie took part in the first Supervision Course. It is difficult to overestimate the huge contribution of foreign colleagues who have been supporting SGA for many years.

SGA members turn to group analysis in private practice, in public hospitals, neuropsychiatric dispensaries, research institutes (V.M. Bekhterev Institute, V. A. Almazov FSBI National Medical Research Center), and conduct lectures on group analysis in public and private institutes; for example, the first Introductory Course on group analysis was read and accredited in 1996 at the East European Institute of Psychoanalysis (with small groups) and has continued there all these years in a theoretical version (without small and large groups). According to rough estimates, over the years there have been more than 2,000 students on the Introductory (orientation) Course. Some of them then went on to study the full Qualification Training Course in Group Analysis.

Moscow Institute of Group Analysis (MIGA), Moscow

MIGA was officially registered as a legal entity on March 11, 2016; on April 24, 2016 it became a member of EGATIN; on July 2, 2019 it received an unlimited license for educational activities issued by the Moscow Department of Education.

MIGA is an institute of additional vocational education and provides professional retraining, as well as advanced training for specialists with higher psychological or medical education. Two group analysis training programs are conducted: Introductory course (1 year) and Qualification course (5 years). There are weekly and block forms of education. Specialists from Moscow, St. Petersburg, Tver', Ivanovo, Novosibirsk, Krasnoyarsk, Tyumen, Blagoveshchensk, Israel, Bulgaria, and other cities of Russia and from abroad study at MIGA. Currently, more than 50 students study at the institute, almost all on the Qualification Course. During the work of the institute more than 80 people completed the Introductory course. Graduates and senior students, working under supervision, actively practice group analytic psychotherapy.

Studies at MIGA are carried out by a team of group analysts. Currently, the staff of MIGA includes Andrey Sklizkov, Galina Stepanova, Dina Shanaeva, Maria Tvorogova, Alexandra Beniaminova, Anna Markevich, Gennady Bershatsky, Ekaterina Dubovskaya, and Anna Tsapenko. Invited lecturers are Mikhail Yerish, Elena Shuvarikova, Nadezhda Mitryashkina, Zoya Shargalina, Ella Stolper, and other colleagues.

Let us briefly dwell on the essential characteristics of group analytic psychotherapy studies at MIGA. These include a holistic approach to learning (simultaneous studies in the three main aspects – theory, supervision, and group analytic psychotherapy; a structured five-year theoretical program; availability of developed training tasks for each academic year, assistance in their timely implementation, with regard to recruitment, conducting, and descriptions of the test group analytic group in particular; no double relations – the leader of the small group does not conduct theory and supervision with members of their small group; understanding psychotherapy as treatment by relationships rather than by mechanistic techniques; full-time training format), with a focus on collegiality and dialogue in resolving issues.

Also, the specificity of teaching group analytic psychotherapy in MIGA is determined by the factors of basic and group analytic education of the MIGA teachers. MIGA employees have a fundamental academic psychological or medical education (Lomonosov Moscow State University and other leading universities of the country), and experience in research institutes and clinical practice in the field of mental health. This allows them to integrate the theory and practice of group analytic psychotherapy with fundamental knowledge of the psyche, development, society, and to conduct research in the field of group analytic psychotherapy, introducing group analytic psychotherapy in various applied fields, for instance in helping people with mental illnesses and their families.

Alma Mater in the field of group analytic psychotherapy is a joint Russian-German-Austrian-Swiss project for the training of group analysts according to EGATIN standards, carried out by the Center for European Psychotherapeutic Education jointly with the Group Analysis Section of the Austrian Association for Group Psychotherapy and Group Dynamics (FS GPA of

ÖAGG), in which MIGA teachers received their education or taught (Andrey Sklizkov). As to invited foreign lecturers, training is provided by Maria Rode and Christiana Schlossarek (Germany), Ingrid Kraft-Ebbing and Irmgard Eisenbachstangel (Austria), Hans-Peter Stutz and Bianca Gueye (Switzerland). This determines the influence of German-speaking continental group analysis schools on group analytic psychotherapy in MIGA. Also, the experience of managing small groups by two co-therapists was adopted from the educational matrix of the project. Currently, MIGA has small groups that are led by one or two therapists. This provides greater stability of the educational and therapeutic process.

From the Russian side, teaching is provided by Andrei Sklizkov and Vladimir Tsapov, psychiatrists by their first education, which determined the importance of focusing specifically on therapeutic aspects, on providing assistance. They also introduced the London model of group analysis, which underlies their group analytic education.

The theory and practice of supervision was influenced by the training of MIGA teachers in the supervision course for supervisors conducted by the London Institute for Group Analysis at the invitation of the SGA. With deep gratitude and warmth we would like to note that for many years the work of MIGA teachers has been supported by the supervision of Sue Einhorn (LIGA), which is a source of constant professional development and assistance in organizing training for group analytic psychotherapy at MIGA.

Group Analysis Section of the Association for the Development of Psychotherapy and Psychoanalysis (ADPP, Stavropol)

ADPP was created in 1999, combining specialists from several psychotherapeutic areas: individual psychoanalytic psychotherapy and psychoanalysis with adults, group analysis, the Gestalt approach, and psychodrama. To date, ADPP has 24 members who implement the following activities: providing psychological assistance to children, parents, families in individual, family and group forms of work; conducting seminars, conferences, and other professional events aimed at promoting psychoanalysis and psychotherapy; popularization of psychoanalysis, group analysis, and psychotherapy. One of the psychotherapeutic directions of ADPP is group analysis.

The history of group analysis in ADPP goes back to the early 2000s, when members of the ADPP Psychoanalysis Section (V.V. Enin, M.V. Kovalenko, N.V. Mitryashkina) received group analytic education (UUAP,[10] DAGG)[11] and began working with groups. The experience of the ADPP Group Analysis Section members is represented in their work with groups of unemployed, combatants, refugees, and the internally displaced, dependent and co-dependent, the disabled, mentally ill and their relatives, children who have experienced violence, acknowledged victims in criminal proceedings, 3–5 year-olds, adolescents in prepuberty and puberty having behavioral, emotional or personal difficulties, etc.

The beginning of the new generations training process of group analysts in ADPP is connected with the Russian–Ukrainian project on group analysis (M.A. Gavrilenko, KHRPS (Kharkov Regional Psychoanalytic Society)), within the framework of which an Introductory (2002) and then a Qualification Course (2003–6) took place. Later, in 2008 and 2009, three training seminars were held within the framework of cooperation between SGA analytic groups (A.A. Sklizkov) and ADPP. Educational projects on group analysis continue to be one of the ADPP's activities and are carried out according to international standards for training group analysts.

Under the auspices of the ADPP, cooperation is carried out between specialists interested in group analysis, including psychologists of educational organizations (nursery schools, secondary schools, a psychological center), social organizations (a social shelter, a center for family and children's aid), the penitentiary system, as well as certified group analysts.

Group analytic activity, which began for ADPP specialists in the early 2000s and has continued all these years, by January 2020 was presented in a new status – the creation of a new section in the ADPP structure – the Group Analysis Section, which on 28 January 2022 became part of the EFPP group section.

Group Analytic Psychotherapy Practice in Russia

Currently, group analytic psychotherapy is not allocated as a separate professional activity in state regulation. Therefore, the scope of application is primarily determined by the preferences and place of work of group analytic psychotherapists who implement the method locally.

The most common application of group analytic psychotherapy is in private practice, where groups are aimed at helping with solving psychological problems. These are mainly groups for adults in a standard group analytic setting (slow-open or closed groups with weekly 90-minute sessions, not exceeding 12 people in composition, lasting from several months to several years, with or without an end date). Sometimes group analytic groups are held for children and adolescents, "mom–baby" groups (for mothers with children from birth to 3–4 years of age), which have certain modifications that take into account the age of the children.

Group analytic psychotherapy is also used in public and state organizations, as a rule, as part of comprehensive treatment, socio-psychological adaptation of various categories of the population.

An example of group analytic psychotherapy in the public sector is the more than 20-year-long activity of MIGA employees and students in the Regional Charitable Public Organization Center for Socio-Psychological and Information Support "Family and Mental Health." Outside the walls of the medical institution in the city library premises, group analytic psychotherapy is carried out for people suffering from mental illness and their relatives. A standard group analytic setting with a slight modification of the method is used: a deviation from the withdrawal rule between participants outside psychotherapeutic sessions is allowed – they communicate in other classes of the organization working on the principle of a therapeutic community. The duration of the groups is 2 years, the groups are conducted by two co-therapists. This experience is presented in numerous publications and guidelines (Tsapenko, 2015; Solokhina et al., 2010).

In state institutions the application of group analytic psychotherapy is carried out within the framework of socio-psychological assistance regulated by legislation. For example, members of the ADPP analytic section conducted analytic psychotherapy groups for socially vulnerable categories of the population in state organizations subordinate to the Ministry of Labor and Social Protection. In hospitals the psychotherapeutic assistance is usually carried out in short-term groups (while the patient is in the hospital) with a session frequency from 2 to 5 per week. In general, in state institutions, the use of group analytic psychotherapy mostly depends on the framework of a particular organization. This determines the particular importance of dynamic administration, and agreement of conditions with the management and all participants in the assistance process.

Thus, group analytic psychotherapy aimed at helping the population is becoming more common and in demand. Groups are held mainly face-to-face, less often online. In addition, group analysis is increasingly used in work with organizations. Also, various group analytic formats are used widely, mainly online, for professional support within the psychological community in the form of medium and large analytic groups, group analytic supervision, intervision groups, and the matrix of social dreams.

Studies of Group Analytic Psychotherapy

Studies of group analytic psychotherapy in Russia are sparse. Of the studies known to the authors of this chapter, the main one is a long-term study (Tsapenko, 2015; Solokhina et al., 2010) of the effectiveness of group analytic psychotherapy for people suffering from mental illness (schizophrenia and similar disorders), as well as for their family members, conducted from 2003 to the present time by MIGA specialists on the basis of the Russian Social and Psychological and Information Support Center "Family and Mental Health." Approximately 150 patients and 20 relatives were tested before and after the completion of the two-year group analytic psychotherapy.

The study showed that the patients have improved social functioning, stress associated with interpersonal problems has reduced, and the number and severity of mental and somatic symptoms has decreased.

Group analytic psychotherapy was carried out for relatives of patients (mentally healthy mothers of adult patients with schizophrenia) who sought psychological help about the problems of communicating with an ill family member, as well as their own mental suffering. After a two-year course of group analytic psychotherapy, for most of them general distress associated with problems of social adaptation has decreased, while adaptation in their family has improved. Distress from problems in interpersonal communication related to diffidence and lack of self-confidence has also decreased.

Thus, the study showed the effectiveness of long-term group analytic psychotherapy in helping people suffering from schizophrenia and similar disorders, as well as their relatives.

Currently, SGA, in collaboration with government agencies in the field of mental health, is planning a study of the effectiveness of group analysis for the prevention of burnout and vicarious trauma in specialists of helping professions.

The topic of applying group analysis in clinics, in particular, to help the staff of psychiatric institutions, was developed earlier and presented in the publications of MIGA employees in collaboration with the Scientific Center for Mental Health of the Russian Academy of Medical Sciences and other state organizations in the field of mental health (Tsapenko, 2008; Tsapenko, 2009; Solokhina et al., 2011).

Challenges and Development Prospects of Group Analytic Psychotherapy

Currently, in our opinion, the main challenge for European countries, and for Russia in particular, is the preservation of the model of group analytic psychotherapy as such. Conflicts and contradictions have intensified in international group analytic organizations; there is both a desire to cope with them within the framework of group analysis (keeping within the boundaries of the method, creating and maintaining space for discussion, comprehension, containment), and a tendency towards collapse of the reflective space and acting out. Obviously, the tension is associated with the context of the basic matrix – with world changes, crisis processes, and military conflicts. An example is the exclusion of Russian member organizations from EGATIN, their transfer to the status of corresponding institutions. The dynamics of splitting to opposing sides easily arise in different groups at this stage.

Our Russian experience shows it is possible to cope with this from the position of neutrality to conflict, recognition of the complexity of life and challenges, a reminder of everyone's interest in a common cause – maintaining the model of group analytic psychotherapy and training. Particular attention is paid to maintaining the boundaries of the group analytic setting (it helps to remember the rules of the method, the difference between words and actions, the psychological approach and any other, the purpose of group work as psychotherapeutic and not political or legal, the need for confidentiality, and the inadmissibility of discrimination on any basis). At the same time, it is important to understand which anxieties at this stage of therapy or training express themselves in this way, and which developmental injuries contribute. When the parties to the conflict return their own projections, dialogue becomes possible.

The second challenge for the development of analytic psychotherapy groups, which is also universal for different countries, is the need for institutionalizing it. This topic has not been sufficiently developed by Russian group analysts. There is no conceptual vision and legal study of the model of institutionalization which would contribute to the development of analytic psychotherapy groups. In general, there is an understanding of the importance of integrating professional standards of group analytic education and legal norms, recognition and acceptance of the method by the health care and social protection system, and singling out the specialty of a group analytic psychotherapist.

Traditionally, the task is to preserve the standards of group analytic training (EGATIN and EFPP). Currently, there is an apparent need to create a professional all-Russian community that would carry out legally significant regulation of group analytic education and practice, as well as support professional standards.

At present, the Russian analytic community is developing quite well, new graduates appearing every year. Continuity in passing on the method is important, as well as attracting graduates to teaching. It is also useful to comprehend which community model will contribute to the prevention of splitting, to cooperation, finding their own place, and professional growth prospects for each group analytic psychotherapist.

Group analysts should develop both connections and processes within the community and external relations with the state and society. Further studies of group analytic psychotherapy are necessary, as well as cooperation with specialists of related specialties. The leading group analytic institutions providing high-quality education are faced with the task of reaching a new and more mature conceptual and organizational level of development.

Notes

1 EGATIN – European Group Analytic Training Institutions Network.
2 EFPP – European Federation for Psychoanalytic Psychotherapy.
3 Society for Group Analysis (SGA), Training Center of Group Analysis (TCGA).
4 Moscow Institute of Group Analysis (MIGA), Moscow Society for Group Analysis (MOGA) International School of Group Psychoanalysis (MSGA).
5 Novosibirsk Institute of Group Analysis (NIGRA).
6 Group Analysis Section of the Association for the Development of Psychotherapy and Psychoanalysis (ADPP), Group Analysis Section of the Stavropol Regional Psychoanalytic Association (SRPA).
7 See https://groupanalysis.net
8 See iga.msk.ru
9 See vk.com/club181433925
10 UUAP (Ukrainian Umbrella Association of Psychotherapy).
11 DAGG (Deutscher Arbeitskreis fur Gruppenpsychotherapie und Gruppendynamik – German Association for Group Psychotherapy and Group Dynamics).

References

Bakhtin M.M. (1972). *Problems of Dostoevsky's Poetics.* Moscow: Khudozhestvennaya literatura.

Barmashova, T. I. & Lomanov, P. V. (2020). The concept of "sobornost" in Russian philosophy. *Bulletin of Buryat State University – Philosophy,* 1, 73–80.

Foulkes, S.H. (1975). *Group-Analytic Psychotherapy: Method and Principles.* London: Gordon & Breach.

Solokhina, T.A., Yastrebov, V.S., Tsapenko, A.I., Shevchenko, L.S., & Bukreeva, N.D. (2010). *Organization of Social and Psychological Assistance to relatives of Mentally Ill Patients: Guidelines.* Moscow: Scientific center for mental health, RAMS.

Solokhina, T.A., Yastrebov, V.S., Shevchenko, L.S., Tsapenko, A.I., Aliyeva, L.M., Anokhina, V.V., Gracheva, N.S., Marushkevich, N.V., Bukreeva, N.D., & Tyumenkova, G.V. (2011). *Group Psychological Work with Medical Workers Providing Assistance to People with Mental Disorders in Medical/Psychiatric Institutions: Guidelines.* Moscow: Scientific Center for Mental Health of the Russian Academy of Medical Sciences, Ministry of Health and Social Development of Russia.

Tolstoy, L.N. (1980). *Collected Works in 22 Volumes, Vol. VI: War and Peace.* Moscow: Khudozhestvennaya literatura.

Tsapenko, A.I. (2008). *Master Class "Group Analysis: The Possibilities of Applying in Psychiatry": The Patient and His Family, from a Psychiatric Education to Social Inclusion: Organizational and Methodical Manual for Professionals Working in the Field of Mental Health* (pp. 66–69). Edited by Professor V.S. Yastrebov. Moscow: MAKS Press, 2008.

Tsapenko, A.I. (2009). *Topicality, organizational and methodological aspects of theory supervision course "Group-analytic psychotherapy: basic theoretical concepts. Group-analytic supervision." Collection: Social and Clinical Psychiatry and Narcology of the Moscow region in modern conditions (Achievements. Problems. Prospects)* (pp. 166–172). Proceedings of the Scientific-Practical Conference of Psychiatrists and Psychiatrists-Narcologists of the Moscow region. Edited by V.Y. Semenov. Orehovo-Zuevo.

Tsapenko, A.I. (2015). Experience in organizing group-analytic psychotherapy for people with mental health problems and their relatives. *Yearbook of Psychotherapy and Psychoanalysis,* 11, 43–65.

Chapter 7

Group Analytic Psychotherapy in Poland

Between Tradition, Cultural Tensions, and Contemporary Research

Agnieszka Chrzczonowicz-Stępień, Katarzyna Czajkowska-Łukasiewicz, Rafał Styła, Tomasz Wyrzykowski and Anna Zajenkowska

Introduction

We may say that Poland is an in-between country, shaped by both Western and Eastern cultural influences and balancing traditional and modern approaches. This position was also reflected in our own process of writing this chapter, as we found ourselves struggling to integrate its different parts. We have sought to combine a traditional historical perspective with contemporary research, and we hope that this patchwork description conveys the distinctive character of group analytic therapy in Poland. In this chapter, we outline the cultural background, provide a brief historical overview, describe current practices in both private and public health care, and present the results of a survey on analytic practice together with emerging directions in research.

Theoretical Foundations and Cultural Links in Group Analytic Psychotherapy

We may observe that throughout the development of group analysis in Poland, two perspectives or approaches to therapeutic work have intersected. They can be associated with the traditions of Foulkes (1975) and Bion (1961), with the former being more focused on the interpersonal, systemic, and social dimensions, viewing the group as a social matrix, and the latter emphasizing the intrapsychic, psychoanalytic level, with a particular focus on unconscious forces that are often destructive. Although Karterud (2024) described the therapist's role in Foulkesian group analysis as that of a conductor rather than a leader, we may still say that the therapist's position in this model is more relational – a participant within the group rather than an external observer and interpreter, as in the Bionian approach. These two approaches have intersected at different times, and in certain periods they have coexisted simultaneously within Polish group analytic practice.

DOI: 10.4324/9781003597674-7

As an example of the intersection between these two approaches, we can examine how the first group analytic center in Poland, the Institute of Group Analysis "Rasztów" (IGAR), operated. On the one hand, Bion's ideas of basic assumptions (Bion, 1961) and Klein's concept of projective identification (Klein, 1946) shaped a distinctive therapeutic perspective. A critical characteristic of this approach was its emphasis on the central role of frustration and deliberately passive stance of the group analyst. The founders of Rasztów understood frustration as the very essence of psychoanalytic therapy. As they stated: "Psychotherapy can be seen as constant frustration, the intensity of which is controlled by the psychotherapist" (Malewski, 1963, as cited in Wyrzykowski, 2021). Consequently, the group therapist was expected to remain passive. The founders further emphasized: "We strive to ensure that the role of the psychotherapist in our groups is as passive as possible, considering interpretation as essentially the only acceptable form of intervention" (Malewski et al., as cited in Wyrzykowski, 2021).

At the same time, however, various accounts (Pawlik, 1990, Wyrzykowski, 2021) suggest that the actual practice of group therapists in Rasztów was often quite active – more in a Foulkesian sense – as they engaged as participants rather than detached observers. Moreover, the functioning of the center was highly specific: psychotherapists lived alongside patients, sharing daily activities such as meals, which made them real, tangible figures in the patients' everyday lives. Perhaps this emphasis on the therapist's passivity served as a means of preserving a therapeutic stance despite such close living arrangements. Or perhaps, the other way around, this was precisely where the more Foulkesian approach emerged and intertwined with a more psychoanalytic framework.

Therefore, it seems particularly valuable to analyze the cultural factors that may have played a role in shaping this hybrid approach. Since psychotherapy can be understood as a cultural and social discourse (Józefik, 2011), the way group analysis is practiced in any given country is inevitably intertwined with its history and culture. How, then, can we link these two intersecting perspectives to the broader context of Polish culture?

Firstly, Poland seems to fall somewhere in the middle when considering cultural models and dimensions, such as the collectivism–individualism spectrum or Schwartz's model of cultural values (Schwartz, 2006; Bardi & Schwartz, 1996). From a collectivist perspective, Poles emphasize the importance of the group, interdependence, and, to some extent, community, where individuals often prioritize the needs of the group over their personal desires. However, on the other hand, individualistic values like personal autonomy, independence, and individual rights have become more prevalent, especially among younger generations. Poland, which can be considered part of both Eastern Europe and Central Europe, occupies a unique space between Western Europe and Asia – not only geographically but also culturally and regarding values. This partly explains why Poland reflects influences from both East and West, shifting depending on historical contexts on the continuum from embeddedness to autonomy and from hierarchy to egalitarianism. Embeddedness in tradition, maintaining social order, and preserving the status quo are central aspects of Polish culture, often blending with values of personal freedom, independent decision making, and self-expression. On the second continuum, the tendency towards hierarchy – where structured authority, power, and clear social roles are valued – contrasts with the principles of egalitarianism, which favors equality, participation, and shared decision making. Positioning between these two poles can create a dynamic space, allowing for integrating different values. However, during turbulent times, this middle ground can also lead to conflict and tension as these diverse values struggle to coexist.

Cultural dimensions intersect with historical events and, therefore, influence the course of societal development. Polish philosopher and psychoanalytic therapist Andrzej Leder (2014) describes how feudal relationships lie at the roots of Polish culture. The feudal system, present in Poland from the 12th century until the early 20th century, bound peasants to land owned by noble landowners, requiring them to work in exchange for protection and the right to live on the land. According to Leder, this feudal relationship persists in Poland as a particular mental structure, shaping many social and institutional dynamics. This type of relationship reflects a specific power dynamic between the stronger and the weaker that in Poland seems to be more disproportionate than the usual power dynamics. Although the Second World War and the communist "revolution" formally ended the feudal system, it appears that 50 years of communist rule subtly adapted and maintained these feudal patterns.

As a result, we might assume that therapeutic relationships, like other asymmetric relationships (e.g., between parents and children, teachers and students, bosses and their employees), may have a tendency to reflect the same hierarchical dynamic. These hierarchical relations discouraged closeness and responsiveness, fostering a tendency to frustrate patients' needs. Alternatively, analysts may have deliberately avoided replicating oppressive power dynamics – perhaps the role of leader carried too many associations with violence and abuse? We might hypothesize that the therapist simply could not assume a leadership role. Without a cultural experience of trust-based leadership, perhaps the group analyst preferred to remain a conductor rather than a leader.

Another key influence on Polish society and culture was the collective trauma of the Second World War, which remained largely unspoken. During this period, 14 million people were murdered in Polish territories. Research shows that this resulted in lower trust toward other people, authorities, and institutions, along with higher levels of negativity, pessimism, and susceptibility to conspiracy theories (Bilewicz, 2024). Bilewicz also notes that societies can work through trauma and even experience post-traumatic growth – but this requires a space to openly discuss the trauma, which was largely absent in Poland. This silence concerned also psychoanalysts and group therapists. "It seems that as Polish psychoanalysts, we don't have our own narrative about our history" (Wojciechowska, 2021). Polish psychoanalyst Ewa Głód (2021) observed: "To our astonishment, we discovered how each of us escapes from painful historical awareness and tries to stand 'outside our history.'"

On the other hand, when trying to understand the genesis of analytical groups in Poland, it is also important to acknowledge the influence of the period of communist rule in Poland. Psychoanalysis, as a product of Western thought, was considered by the communist authorities to be something foreign, hostile, and dangerous. For this reason, publications appearing in the West could not be legally imported into the country and contact with Western psychoanalysts was extremely limited. Additionally, state funding for psychotherapy was minimal. Pursuing professional work and personal development under such conditions demanded extraordinary effort, commitment, and passion. It was out of this passion that post-war psychoanalytic and analytic group traditions in Poland emerged. This phenomenon may also be linked to a broader spirit of freedom and solidarity that has long characterized Polish history – not only during the communist era, but also earlier, under the partitions. In this sense, it could be seen as resonating with a Foulkesian spirit of social engagement and collective responsibility.

Due to described cultural heritage, it appears that, even after the political system began to change in 1989, the practice of group analysis remained largely unchanged for many years. It seems that shifts – from collectivism toward individualism and from hierarchy to egalitarianism – were necessary first. Additionally, over the last 20 years, we have observed a strong trend toward revisiting and analyzing past traumas, with numerous conferences and publications focused on this topic. As a result, the last 10–20 years have seen gradual changes in group analysis. The therapist's role has shifted from passive and frustrating to more active and warm, from conductor to leader. Interestingly, similar processes occurred earlier in Western countries like the USA and Norway (McWilliams, 2004, Karterud, 2024). Perhaps, given Poland's historical context, this transformation arrived later.

Current Practice and Adaptation

Beginnings and Therapy in Public Health Care

The beginnings of analytical group psychotherapy in Poland date back to the first half of the 1960s when Jan Malewski and his collaborators established a therapeutic center in the village of Rasztów near Warsaw. The theoretical foundations of first groups referred to both Freudian psychoanalysis and the work of therapists from the Tavistock Clinic (Bion, Ezriel, Whitaker) as well as French psychoanalysis (Anzieu, Kaes) (Wyrzykowski, 2021). As described above, the therapist's stance was seen as withdrawn, aiming to evoke transference feelings and frustration, which was understood as a developmental factor. A special place was to be given to the emotional relationship between the patients and the psychotherapist and the therapist to the group. The interpretation should be based on the overall behavior of the patient and the group as a whole, prioritizing what is happening here and now.

After the center was opened, adapting the method to the prevailing therapeutic conditions, new assumptions were added, based on interpersonal approaches and the therapeutic community. Non-verbal techniques as well as psychodrama derived from French psychoanalysis were added. After consultations in Warsaw, patients would be admitted to the center for 8–10 week stays. They participated in daily group therapy sessions (1–2 sessions daily, up to two hours each) and other communal activities, performed housekeeping tasks, and worked in the garden (Pawlik, 1990, 1993).

As the center developed, the thinking about groups expanded and specialized. The division between outpatient groups conducted in the clinic (as a continuation of treatment or a separate form of therapy) and short-term, intensive groups conducted in Rasztów became increasingly clear. The ideas of focal conflict and current conflict became particularly useful for short-term groups (Pawlik, 1993). When contact with the West became possible, several people from Rasztów underwent training in classical group analysis in Heidelberg, and finally opened a local Institute of Group Analysis in Poland in 1992. Around the same time, the center in Rasztów was closed, and intensive therapy was moved to Warsaw, where it has been conducted in a day hospital setting ever since. Over more than 30 years, therapy in this form has become extremely popular in Poland. Today, there are several day units in Warsaw alone, and dozens across the country.

This development intensified significantly from 2018, related to the reform process that psychiatric treatment in Poland has been undergoing. The main directions of this reform were deinstitutionalization and an emphasis on outpatient treatment at the expense of inpatient treatment. The goal became community-based treatment and the building of patients' social networks. Local mental health centers (one per 100,000 inhabitants) were established, consisting of mental health clinics, reporting and consultation points, day units, community treatment teams, and inpatient units. In clinics and community treatment teams, it is now possible to conduct psychotherapy both individually and in groups (usually once a week for 90 minutes). Participation in a group for a single patient can last from several months to several years. Outpatient groups typically have 6–10 patients. These conditions allow for therapy based on analytical assumptions.

Group analysts have been involved in the reform from its inception at various levels: from shaping changes to implementing them in local centers. According to the research by Styła et al. (2024), about 40% of therapists associated with IGAR declare employment in public health care. As practice would indicate in many such places, there is a predominance of people starting their careers, so the number of group analysts who have passed through such places may be larger.

As for the scale of treatment, according to data from the Polish Ministry of Health (2023), in 2023 there were 907,489 individual psychotherapy sessions and 44,953 group or family psychotherapy sessions in outpatient mental health clinics conducted throughout the year (the given numbers are divided into all patients). Meanwhile, 5,315 people received therapy in the day hospital for neurotic disorders treatment, 18,863 people in the general psychiatric day hospital, and 2,448 people in the psychiatric rehabilitation day hospital. However, despite the changes introduced by the reform, regular psychotherapy within the public health care system – especially outpatient and individual – remains difficult to access. Access to psychotherapy offered through psychiatric day units is considerably easier to obtain. Also, neurotic disorders units are required to provide regular therapy, while in general psychiatric units therapy can be limited or almost non-existent.

Currently, therapy conducted in day units lasts three or six months. It takes place five days a week, for several hours each day. Therapy for patients suffering from various types of psychoses, severe forms of depression, manic-depressive disorders, schizotypal disorders, or those who are deeply disorganized in life is largely based on the therapeutic community, art therapy, psychoeducation, or activities related to social activation. Talk therapy may occupy a smaller part of the program.

On the other hand, therapy dedicated to neurotic patients (diagnosed with adjustment, anxiety, and depressive disorders), as well as those with various personality disorders (functioning at a borderline level) is mainly based on talk sessions. Various additional techniques are also used, such as psychodrama, non-verbal techniques, different forms of art therapy. These are intended to help patients integrate with the group, to better understand themselves and others (mentalization), intensify the therapy process and insight, provide corrective experiences, activate the potential of the group and individual patients, and navigate crises in therapy. Patients qualified for groups should maintain a minimum level of reflective ability, be able to refrain from extreme acting-out behaviors, and define their problems in relational terms.

During the consultation process, not only is the personality of the candidates examined, but the group's rules are also presented, and achievable goals are established. These may include, for example, working on excessive aggression, the ability to replace it with words, and seeking its internal, historical, or current sources. The primary conflict and the current conflict are defined.

Group work focuses primarily on specific events happening "here and now" in the group. At the beginning of therapy, each participant introduces themselves not only spontaneously (as in classical group analysis) but also in a structured way, for example, through a written and read-out biography. However, throughout the entire period of the treatment a large part of the work is done by the group based on its spontaneous activity and free-flowing discussion. Transference interpretations occur after clarifications and confrontations and concern the group's "here and now." Therapists remain somewhat more active than in other forms of classical group analysis in Poland.

People completing this type of therapy should be able to return to normal social functioning. This means, among other things, increased tolerance for frustration and other types of tension, reduced perceived psychological pain, establishing social relationships, returning to work, studies, and other aspects of everyday lives. Another important effect is a deeper understanding of one's own problems and the problems of others (mentalization).

Therapy in Private Health Care

Due to the limited availability of psychotherapy within the public health care system, the majority of group analysts conduct therapy groups in private outpatient settings. As was found in the survey described below, most therapists (45%) lead long-term slow-open groups, in which patients join and leave at different times. They are followed in frequency by: long-term (lasting more than a year) – 12%, medium-term (between 6 and 12 months) – 10%, and short-term (up to 6 months) – 9% groups with a fixed end date.

Characteristics of Group Analysts in Poland: Survey Results

The Institute of Group Analysis "Rasztów" (IGAR) is the only association in Poland offering group analysis training. According to IGAR office data from May 2024, the association comprised a total of 438 members, including 352 women (80%) and 86 men (20%). Among them, 28 are certified supervisors and group analysts (6%), 86 are certified group analysts (20%), and 11 are certified individual and group psychotherapists (3%). The remaining 313 members (71%) do not yet hold an IGAR certificate, comprising approximately 90 individuals currently enrolled in one of the four-year training programs and others who have already completed their training at the institute but have not yet obtained certification.

The primary objective of the study was to examine the characteristics of psychotherapists trained at IGAR. The secondary objective was to determine which sociodemographic and professional factors distinguish members who primarily identify as group analysts from those whose main professional identity lies elsewhere. This question is of particular interest because it sheds light on the sociodemographic and professional factors that shape the development of a group analytical identity among psychotherapists, thereby informing training, clinical practice, and the professional profile of IGAR members.

Methods

The Scientific Committee of IGAR conducted an online survey with 29 closed and open-ended questions available to our community from March 5 to May 31, 2024. The results were presented at the annual conference of IGAR on June 15, 2024, in Warsaw (Styła et al., 2024). We sent emails to all IGAR members and posted an announcement on the IGAR Facebook group, requesting participation in the study. We received 179 responses, comprising 41% of all IGAR members, with 149 (83%) women and 30 men (17%). The participants ranged in age from 26 to 73, with a mean age of 45 (SD = 9.3).

Results

Most participants have master's degrees in psychology (n=154, 86%) or pedagogy (n=20, 11%). Other educational backgrounds included sociology, medicine, economics, Polish philology, resocialization, philosophy, international relations, management, anthropology, and law. Around 20% of the participants acknowledged two or more degrees, 9% (n=17) had a PhD, habilitation degree, or professorship, and four persons were psychiatrists (2%). Around 20% (n=35) conduct (or used to conduct) psychotherapy in a language other than Polish (mainly English, n=29, 16%).

Only 37% (n=66) of respondents work only as psychotherapists. Other frequent activities include conducting workshops (31%, n=55), didactic activity at schools or universities (30%, n=53), counseling (28%, n=51), psychological diagnosis (22%, n=39), and offering supervision (19%, n=34). We also asked about the place where the respondents offer psychotherapy in person. The vast majority (n=148, 83%) works in Masovian Voivodeship (especially in Warsaw, n=99, 55%), the most populated of the 16 administrative districts in Poland with approximately 15% of the total population.

Seventy-eight percent of participants (n=139) declared using psychodynamic techniques, 73% (n=130) group analytical, and also 73% (n=130) psychoanalytical techniques. The other mentioned techniques included systemic (21%, n=38) and cognitive (14%, n=25) techniques, psychodrama (11%, n=19), mindfulness (8%, n=15), and behavioral techniques (8%, n=15).

We asked about the primary identity of our members although participants could indicate more than one answer. It appeared that 50% (n=89) of the participants see themselves as group analysts, 43% (n=77) as psychoanalytic psychotherapists, 42% (n=76) as psychodynamic psychotherapists, and 7% (n=13) indicated other identities such as psychoanalysts, systemic psychotherapists, and addiction therapists. We used this variable to examine the differences between members with a group analytical identity and those without it (see Table 7.1). Table 7.2 presents the data in the total sample on the therapy setting, forms of contact, type of cooperation, place of work, supervision, and characteristics of the treated patients.

2.3.3 Discussion

The findings indicate that psychotherapists trained at the Institute of Group Analysis in Poland are primarily engaged in long-term individual therapy and semi-open outpatient group therapy, working predominantly in private practice and regularly participating in both individual and group supervision. Their clinical work is focused mainly on adults, most often with neurotic and personality disorders, but also with affective and psychosomatic problems, which illustrates the professional profile emerging from group analytic training.

Table 7.1 Information on age, workload and work satisfaction, certificates, and hours of supervision in the total sample (n=179) and comparisons between persons with or without primary group analyst identity.

Variable	*Total sample (n=179)*	*Group analyst identity (n=89)*	*Identity other than group analyst (n=90)*	*Test*	*p*	*Effect size*
Age	M=44.96 (SD=9.31)	M=47.65 (SD=9.57	M=42.30 (SD=8.27)	U=2754	<.001	d=.60
Experience in years	M=12.78 (SD=9.58)	M=16.47 (SD=10.27)	M=9.05 (SD=7.15)	U=2153	<.001	d=.84
Years in IGAR	M=10.97 (SD=8.44)	M=14.53 (SD=8.75)	M=7.44 (SD=6.45)	U=1813	<.001	d=.92
Workload in hours per week	M=18.98 (SD=8.61)	M=20.40 (SD=8.51)	M=17.60 (SD=8.52)	U=3205	<.05	d=.33
Work satisfaction (scale 1–10)	M=8.38 (SD=1.26)	M=8.60 (SD+1.20)	M=8.16 (SD=1.28)	U=3042	<.05	d=.36
Supervision hours per month*	M=4.91 (SD=3.05)	M=5.05 (SD=3.04)	M=4.77 (SD=3.08)	U=3685	>.05	—
Certificates						
Certificate of IAGR & other	n=31 (17%)	n=28 (32%)	n=3 (3%)	χ^2=45.37	<.001	Cramer's V=.50
Certificate of IAGR	n=47 (26%)	n=32 (36%)	n=15(17%)			
No certificate of IAGR but other	n=16 (9%)	n=3 (3%)	n=13 (14%)			
No certificate	n=85 (48%)	n=26 (29%)	n=59 (66%)			

* Values were calculated as the midpoint of the interval responses. Answer "More than 10 hours" was included in the computations as 12.

Table 7.2 Therapy setting, forms of contact, type of cooperation, place of work, supervision and characteristics of the patients treated in the total sample (n=179).

Variable	*Total sample (n=179)*	*Variable*	*Total sample (n=179)*
Setting of individual therapy		**Type of supervision**	
Short-term (up to 6 months)	n=40 (22%)	Individual supervision	n=128 (72%)
Medium-term (6–12 months)	n=64 (36%)	Group supervision	n=126 (70%)
Long-term (over a year) once a week	n=153 (86%)	Irregular peer supervision	n=51 (29%)
Long-term (over a year) with two or more sessions a week	n=87 (49%)	Regular group peer supervision	n=49 (27%)
Setting of group therapy		Regular individual peer supervision	n=31 (17%)
Short-term (up to 6 months), outpatient	n=16 (9%)	None of the above	n=4 (2%)
Medium-term (6–12 months), outpatient	n=17 (10%)	**Patient diagnosis**	
Long-term with a set end date (closed), outpatient	n=22 (12%)	Neurotic disorders	n=174 (97%)
Long-term, without a set end date (semi-open), outpatient	n=81 (45%)	Personality disorders	n=170 (95%)
Long-term, outpatient, with two or more sessions a week	n=2 (1%)	Affective disorders	n=140 (78%)
Intensive (min. 3 sessions a week – day ward or inpatient)	n=15 (8%)	Psychosomatic/somatic disorders	n=140 (78%)
Forms of cooperation		Victims/perpetrators of violence	n=87 (49%)
In a team only	n=56 (31%)	Eating disorders	n=81 (45%)
Independently only	n=51 (29%)	Schizophrenia and/or other psychotic disorders	n=48 (27%)
In both forms	n=72 (40%)	Neurodiversity	n=46 (26%)
Place of work		Sexual disorders	n=45 (25%)
Private practice or private psychotherapy center	n=156 (87%)	Addiction	n=42 (24%)
Public mental health clinic	n=45 (25%)	Disorders of organic origin	n=9 (5%)
Psychiatric hospital	n=28 (16%)	Intellectual disability	n=3 (2%)
NGO/foundation etc.	n=17 (9%)	Other disorders/problems	n=2 (1%)

Table 7.2 (Continued)

Variable	*Total sample (n=179)*	*Variable*	*Total sample (n=179)*
Place of work			
Psychological-educational counselling centre	n=14 (8%)	**Age of patients**	
School or university	n=12 (7%)	Children (0–11)	n=9 (5%)
Hospital other than psychiatric	n=6 (3%)	Youth (12–17)	n=50 (28%)
Other	n=13 (7%)	Young adults (18–27)	n=153 (85%)
Forms of supervision contact		Adults (28–74)	n=175 (98%)
In person only	n=59 (33%)	Elderly (75+)	n= 22 (12%)
On-line only	n=35 (20%)		
Both forms	n=81 (45%)		
No supervision currently	n=4 (2%)		

Around half of IGAR members declared that their primary professional identity is that of a group analyst, and nearly three-quarters reported using group analytical techniques. Therapists with this identity were typically at more advanced stages of professional development than other members: they were older, had more years of experience, and were more likely to hold an IGAR certificate. The interpretation of this finding remains open, as it may reflect a process of professional maturation (i.e., with growing experience therapists increasingly focus on long-term group analysis) or recent changes in the IGAR training program, which has incorporated short-term interventions and no longer requires certification in group analysis.

The primary limitation of the study is that the participants were likely more actively involved in IGAR than the overall membership. For instance, a larger proportion of respondents held an IGAR certificate (43%) compared to the association as a whole (29%). A second limitation concerns the study measures, which consisted of ad hoc questions with unknown reliability and validity. Nevertheless, we believe that the findings provide a reasonable approximation of the characteristics of IGAR members, including those whose primary professional identity is that of a group analyst.

Challenges and Evidence-Based Practice: Review of Existing Research and Treatment Outcomes

The first publications on group analysis in Poland emerged in the 1990s, largely through the work of Jerzy Pawlik, including his commentary "Group Analysis at Rasztów, Poland" (Pawlik, 1990), which described the country's first analytically oriented therapeutic center.

The majority of empirical research on group psychotherapy in Poland has been conducted in day hospital settings, where intensive short-term (12-week) treatment is the dominant model, and psychodynamic orientation is prevalent. Despite this, many clinicians and researchers involved in these studies (e.g., Anna Zajenkowska, Hubert Suszek, Rafał Styła, Tomasz Wyrzykowski, and Rafał Radzio) have extensive backgrounds in group analysis, which has influenced their approach to psychotherapy and research. However, most studies on evidence-based group psychotherapy in Poland do not focus specifically on group analysis.

In assessing the quantity of research on group psychotherapy in Poland, we searched databases such as PubMed and Google Scholar, as well as archives of Polish scientific journals like Psychotherapy, Psychiatry, and Archives of Psychiatry and Psychotherapy. We also searched international journals on group analysis, including *Group Analysis*. The search yielded ten empirical articles: three on psychodynamic group psychotherapy, two on eclectic group psychotherapy, three case studies of group analysis, and two articles about psychotherapists, including group therapists. For detailed results of the search, see Table 7.3.

Table 7.3 Group psychotherapy research in Poland (2011–22).

No.	*Year*	*Authors*	*Title*	*Type of treatment*	*N*
1.	2011	Prot-Klinger, K., Szwajca, K., & Biedka, Ł.	*Psychotherapy of Holocaust Survivors – Group Process Analysis*	Group analysis	–
2.	2014	Styła, R.	*Differences in Effectiveness of Intensive Treatment Programs for Neurotic and Personality Disorders: Is It Worth Monitoring the Effectiveness of a Therapeutic Team?*	6–12 weeks of approximately 5 hours of eclectic group treatment (group psychotherapy, psychodrama, psychoeducation etc.)	105
3.	2015	Styła, R.	*Shape of the Self-Concept Clarity Change During Group Psychotherapy Predicts the Outcome: An Empirical Validation of the Theoretical Model of Self-Concept Change*	Intensive eclectic group psychotherapy under routine inpatient conditions	85
4.	2015	Suszek, H., Holas, P., Wyrzykowski, T., Lorentzen, S., & Kokoszka, A.	*Short-Term Intensive Psychodynamic Group Therapy Versus Cognitive-Behavioral Group Therapy in Day Treatment of Anxiety Disorders and Comorbid Depressive or Personality Disorders: Study Protocol for a Randomized Controlled Trial*	Psychodynamic group psychotherapy vs cognitive-behavioral group psychotherapy vs wait-list control group.	199
5.	2017	Suszek, H., Grzesiuk, L., Styła, R., & Krawczyk, K.	*Who and How Conducts Psychotherapy in Poland? Part II: Results from a Nationwide Survey*	–	–
6.	2019	Prot-Klinger, K.	*Group Analytic Psychotherapy of Psychotic Patients*	Group analysis	–

Table 7.3 (Continued)

No.	*Year*	*Authors*	*Title*	*Type of treatment*	*N*
7.	2019	Rybak, W.	*Interconnected Worlds*	Group analysis	–
8.	2020	Zajenkowska, A., Barycka, J., & Chotkowska, K.	*Borderline Personality Disorder Level Predicts Change in Depressiveness After Short-Term Group Psychotherapy: A Study in a Daily Psychiatric Clinic*	Cognitive-behavioural group psychotherapy (CBT) or psychodynamic group psychotherapy (PDT)	57
9.	2021	Kalita, L. et al.	*Competences Needed to Conduct Psychoanalytic and Psychodynamic Therapies in Poland*	–	–
10.	2022	Wajda, Z., Kapinos-Gorczyca, A., Lizi⊠czyk, S., Sitnik-Warchulska, K., & Izydorczyk, B.	*Online Group Psychodynamic Psychotherapy – The Effectiveness and Role of Attachment – The Results of a Short Study*	Online group psychotherapy within psychodynamic paradigm with elements of an interpersonal approach	22

Based on the aforementioned analysis, research on group psychotherapy in Poland can be broadly categorized into three main areas:

Empirical Studies on Group Psychotherapy (Wajda et al., 2022; Zajenkowska et al., 2020; Styła, 2015; Styła, 2014; Suszek et al., 2015): these studies assess the effectiveness of various group psychotherapy approaches, including psychodynamic, cognitive-behavioral, and eclectic models, often in day hospital settings. They focus on specific clinical populations, such as individuals with borderline personality disorder, anxiety, or depression. While these studies do not primarily focus on group analysis, those groups are often conducted by group analysts and thus incorporate group analytical thinking.

Case Studies in Group Analytic Treatment (Prot-Klinger, 2019; Rybak, 2019; Prot-Klinger et al., 2011): this category includes detailed analyses of group analytic psychotherapy applied to specific patient groups, such as those with chronic psychotic states or Holocaust survivors. These studies offer both theoretical insights and practical applications of group analysis.

Research on Therapists and Training (Suszek et al., 2017; Kalita et al., 2021): this body of work examines the competencies required for conducting psychoanalytic and psychodynamic psychotherapy in Poland. It also explores the broader professional landscape of psychotherapy, including nationwide surveys on who conducts psychotherapy and how it is practiced.

These three research streams to some extent provide information on the effectiveness, development, and potential challenges of group psychotherapy in Poland. The main focus seems to be on patients participating in group psychotherapy several times a week in day wards. In many cases, this treatment is not offered in isolation but combined with other activities, such as individual therapy (usually once or twice a week) and, for example, art therapy. This makes it difficult to disentangle the specific effects of analytic group psychotherapy.

There is a clear lack of research on analytic group psychotherapy, especially randomized controlled trials (RCTs). Research specifically on group analysis remains uncommon (Chrzczonowicz-Stępień et al., 2026). Despite some conflicting ideas among group analysts about how or what research should be conducted, there is a general agreement that evidence-based practices in psychotherapy are crucial from multiple perspectives. Empirical research helps us better understand what works, how it works, and for whom – particularly in relation to specific diagnoses. It is also very important in the research field to acknowledge diagnostic changes, including the trend toward diminishing prescriptions for psychiatric problems, which is common and essential in psychoanalytic treatment. Empirical studies also provide valuable insights into patient dropout rates, prompting an exploration of why some patients struggle to fully engage in the therapeutic process. Is the difficulty primarily related to the patients themselves, or does the therapeutic method require adjustment?

All of this encourages ongoing research into the methods we use and fosters critical reflection, ensuring our practices remain both effective and adaptable. Another critical aspect is the use of outcome measures. In psychoanalytic and psychodynamic psychotherapy, one of the primary outcomes is the improvement of personality functioning. This includes both social functioning and intrapersonal dimensions, such as agency, identity, and self-complexity.

Current Project on Group Analysis in Poland

One ongoing project in group analysis that addresses aforementioned issues is a study led by Anna Zajenkowska and her team, including Katarzyna Czajkowska-Łukasiewicz and Agnieszka Chrzczonowicz-Stępień. This project aims to contribute to the development of evidence-based practices in group analysis, specifically for patients with personality disorders. Pathological personality organization can hinder the improvement in depression symptoms. A longitudinal study suggests that improvements in personality disorders (PDs) precede improvements in depression symptoms, but not the other way around (Gunderson et al., 2004). Recent research emphasizes the importance of Mentalization-Based Therapy (MBT), which has shown promising results in treating patients with PDs (Bateman & Fonagy, 2008). Developing a mentalizing stance improves the ability to process social information accurately, leading to better interpersonal functioning (Bateman & Fonagy, 2008; Karterud, 2024). Both group analysis and MBT are arguably effective approaches for improving the ability to interpret others' actions more accurately (Karterud, 2024, Lorentzen, 2014). Although MBT has been studied in randomized controlled trials, particularly in partial hospital programs (Bateman & Fonagy, 2009; Volkert et al., 2019), similar studies are limited regarding group analysis (Lorentzen, 2006; Lorentzen et al., 2013). More research is needed in intensive outpatient settings, including studies focused on group analysis. This is why the current project in Poland was initiated.

The current project investigates changes in social information processing, particularly hostile attributions, which is one of the predictors of personality functioning (Zajenkowska et al., 2024). We aim to determine whether participants become less hostile, thereby improving personality functioning, after two years of group analysis compared with MBT psychoeducation training combined with group analysis (see Figure 7.1).

Group analysis is evolving, and its current approach should not only be grounded in classical theories but also incorporate recent empirical findings on personality disorders and related theoretical frameworks. MBT consists of 12 weeks of psychoeducation, followed by approximately 1.5 years of group treatment and individual sessions if needed. The effectiveness of the initial

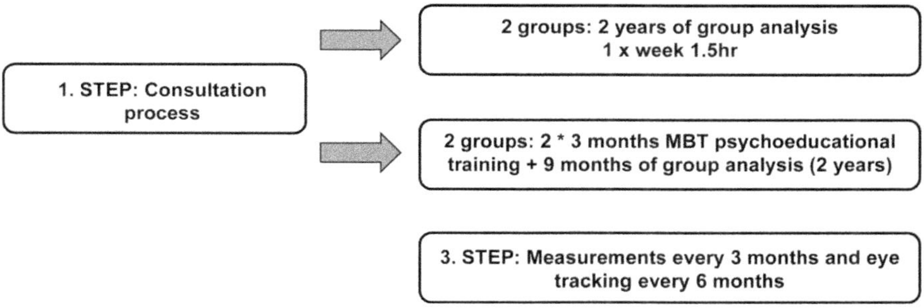

Figure 7.1 Study design.

part of the MBT treatment, specifically the six psychoeducational sessions, was recently investigated (Zajenkowska et al., 2021). After just six sessions, participants were more interested in understanding others' intentions when interpreting certain behaviors. As the training progressed, participants engaged more actively in mentalization, improving their ability to consider others' perspectives, even in situations involving disliked individuals who elicited strong negative emotions (Zajenkowska et al., 2021).

This raises the question: should we integrate methods from other therapeutic approaches, such as MBT, potentially adjusting or changing our way of working, particularly with lower-functioning patients? This would align with what Karterud (2024) describes as modern group analysis, in contrast to the classical, unmodified form of group analytic treatment. Alternatively, should we suggest a different group treatment? In our project, we aimed to check whether classical group analysis can still be helpful despite lower personality functioning. We were also curious whether adding MBT psychoeducational training before group analysis and after one year of treatment would provide superior effects for patients. Our project is built on the concept of strengthening the observing ego – not by altering the fundamental way analysis is conducted, but by incorporating a mentalization training component to clarify the concept of the observing ego. A follow-up training, in a shortened version, is introduced after one year of group psychotherapy to further reinforce the observing ego. This provides patients with an opportunity to reflect on their own experiences in the group, from both the therapist's and the patients' perspectives.

We hope that this overview illustrates how in Poland the historical dichotomy between Foulkes and Bion gradually gives way to an emerging, research-based approach – perhaps what Karterud (2024) describes as modern group analysis. Within this process, Polish group analysts continue to seek balance between the therapist's activity and passivity, individualism and collectivism, tradition and innovation, as they strive to integrate insight-oriented practice with evidence-based perspectives.

References

Bardi, A., & Schwartz, S.H. (1996). Relations among sociopolitical values in Eastern Europe: Effects of the communist experience? *Political Psychology*, 17(3), 525–549.

Bateman, A., & Fonagy, P. (2008). Comorbid antisocial and borderline personality disorders: Mentalization-based treatment. *Journal of Clinical Psychology*, 64(2), 181–194.

Bateman, A., & Fonagy, P. (2009). Randomized controlled trial of outpatient mentalization-based treatment versus structured clinical management for borderline personality disorder . *American Journal of Psychiatry*, 166(12), 1355–1364.

Bilewicz, M. (2024). *Traumaland. Polacy w cieniu przeszłości*. Kraków: Wydawnictwo WAM.

Bion, W. (1961). *Experiences in Groups and Other Papers*. New York: Tavistock Publications Limited.

Chrzczonowicz-Stępień, A., Czajkowska-Łukasiewicz, K., Adamska, Z., Kardasz, M., & Zajenkowska, A. (2026). Integrating research and therapeutic aims in long-term group-analytic treatment for personality disorders: A case study on patient selection. *Counselling and Psychotherapy Research, 26(3)*, e70190.

Foulkes, S.H. (1975). *Group-Analytic Psychotherapy: Method and Principles*. London: Gordon & Breach.

Głód, E. (2021). Kilka myśli o rozwoju psychoanalizy w Polsce w latach 1990–2020. In W.E. Kobylińska-Dehe, & K. Prot-Klinger (Eds.), *Jak Feniks z popiołów? O odradzaniu się psychoanalizy w powojennej i dzisiejszej Polsce*. Taipei: Universitas.

Gunderson, J.G., Morey, L.C., Stout, R.L., Skodol, A.E., Shea, M.T., McGlashan, T. H., Zanarini, M.C., Grilo, C.M., Sanislow, C.A., Yen, S., Daversa, M.T., & Bender, D.S. (2004). Major depressive disorder and borderline personality disorder revisited: longitudinal interactions. *Journal of Clinical Psychiatry*, 65(8), 1049.

Józefik, B. (2011). Psychoterapia jako dyskurs kulturowy. *Psychiatria Polska*, 5, 737–748.

Kalita, L., Bittner-Jakubowska, A., Buzun, E., Dworczyk, P., Giza, M., Henzel-Korzeniowska, A., Kitrasiewicz, J., Mędrzejewska, A., Szmalec, M., Witkowska, M., & Zboińska, J. (2021). Competences needed to conduct psychoanalytic and psychodynamic therapies in Poland. *Psychoterapia*, 2(197), 51–66.

Karterud, S. (2024). *Group Analysis: A Modern Synthesis*. New York: Routledge.

Klein, M. (1946). Notes on some schizoid mechanisms. *International Journal of Psychoanalysis*, 27, 99–110.

Leder, A. (2014). *Prześniona rewolucja. Ćwiczenie z logiki historycznej*. Warsaw: Wydawnictwo Krytyki Politycznej.

Lorentzen, S. (2006). Contemporary challenges for research in group analysis. *Group Analysis*, 39(3), 321–340.

Lorentzen, S., Ruud, T., Fjeldstad, A., & Høglend, P. (2013). Comparison of short- and long-term dynamic group psychotherapy: Randomised clinical trial. *British Journal of Psychiatry*, 203(3), 280–287.

Lorentzen, S. (2014). *Group Analytic Psychotherapy: Working with Affective, Anxiety and Personality Disorders*. London: Routledge.

McWilliams, N. (2004). *Psychoanalytic Psychotherapy*. New York: The Guilford Press.

Pawlik, J. (1993). *Psychoterapia analityczna. Formy grupowe*. Warsaw: PWN.

Pawlik, J. (1990). Group analysis at Rasztów, Poland. *Group Analysis*, 23(3), 328–329.

Polish Ministry of Health (2023). *Mapy potrzeb zdrowotnych*. See https://basiw.mz.gov.pl/mapy-informacje/mapa-2022-2026/.

Prot-Klinger, K., Szwajca, K., & Biedka, Ł. (2011). Psychotherapy of Holocaust survivors: Group process analysis. *Archives of Psychiatry and Psychotherapy*, 1, 21–33.

Prot-Klinger, K. (2019). Group analytic psychotherapy of psychotic patients. *Psychoterapia*, 2(189), 17–32.

Rybak, W. (2019). Interconnected worlds. *Psychoterapia*, 2(189), 33–43.

Schwartz, S.H. (2006). A theory of cultural value orientations: Explication and applications. *Comparative Sociology*, 5(2–3), 137–182.

Styła, R. (2014). Differences in effectiveness of intensive treatment programmes for neurotic and personality disorders. Is it worth monitoring effectiveness of a therapeutic team. *Psychiatria Polska*, 48(1), 157–171.

Styła, R. (2015). Shape of the self-concept clarity change during group psychotherapy predicts the outcome: An empirical validation of the theoretical model of the self-concept change. *Frontiers in Psychology*, 6, 1598.

Styła, R., Biernacki, P., Bąk, E., Kocewiak-Robalewska, K., & Olesiewicz, A. (2024). *Kim jesteśmy? Wyniki ankiety obrazującej społeczność "Rasztowa"* [Who are we? Results of the survey showing the community of "Rasztow"] Conference presentation. XX Scientific Conference of Institute of Group Analysis Rasztow. Do we play in the same orchestra? Between dissonance and harmony. Warsaw, Poland.

Suszek, H., Holas, P., Wyrzykowski, T., Lorentzen, S., & Kokoszka, A. (2015). Short-term intensive psychodynamic group therapy versus cognitive-behavioral group therapy in day treatment of anxiety disorders and comorbid depressive or personality disorders: Study protocol for a randomized controlled trial. *Trials*, 16, 1–12.

Suszek, H., Grzesiuk, L., Styła, R., & Krawczyk, K. (2017). Who and how conducts psychotherapy in Poland. Part II. Results from a nationwide survey. *Psychiatria*, 14(2), 90–100.

Volkert, J., Hauschild, S., & Taubner, S. (2019). Mentalization-based treatment for personality disorders: efficacy, effectiveness, and new developments. *Current Psychiatry Reports*, 21(4), 1–12.

Wajda, Z., Kapinos-Gorczyca, A., Lizińczyk, S., Sitnik-Warchulska, K., & Izydorczyk, B. (2022). Online group psychodynamic psychotherapy: The effectiveness and role of attachment—The results of a short study. *Frontiers in Psychiatry*, 13, 798991. doi:10.3389/fpsyt.2022.798991.

Wojciechowska, E. (2021). Cezura, pamięć, tożsamość. O przekraczaniu wyrw w transmisji psychoanalizy w Polsce. In E. Kobylińska-Dehe & K. Prot-Klinger (Eds.), *Jak Feniks z popiołów? O odradzaniu się psychoanalizy w powojennej i dzisiejszej Polsce*. Kraków: Universitas.

Wyrzykowski, T. (2021). Pierwsze grupy analityczne w Polsce. In E. Kobylińska-Dehe, & K. Prot-Klinger (Eds.), *Jak Feniks z popiołów? Odradzanie się psychoanalizy w powojennej i dzisiejszej Polsce*. Kraków: Universitas.

Zajenkowska, A., Barycka, J., & Chotkowska, K. (2020). Borderline personality disorder level predicts change in depressiveness after short-term group psychotherapy: A study in a daily psychiatric clinic. *Counselling and Psychotherapy Research*, 20(2), 380–384.

Zajenkowska, A., Nowakowska, I., Cieciuch, J., Gawęda, Ł., Rogoza, R., Pinkham, A., & Czajkowska-Łukasiewicz, K. (2025). Towards the understanding of the core of general personality disorder factor: g-PD and its relation to hostile attributions. *Development and Psychopathology*, 37(2), 696–704.

Zajenkowska, A., Prusik, M., Jasielska, D., & Szulawski, M. (2021). Hostile attribution bias among offenders and non-offenders: Making social information processing more adequate. *Journal of Community & Applied Social Psychology*, 31(2), 241–256.

Chapter 8

The Portuguese School of Groupanalysis

History, Development, and Current Challenges

Margarida França and Isaura Manso Neto

Theoretical Foundations and Cultural Links

Portuguese use the word groupanalysis – not group analysis – to refer to the psychoanalytically oriented group psychotherapy that focuses on the individual's treatment *in and through* the group. Therapeutic groupanalysis in a strict sense (Neto & França, 2021) typically involves two to three sessions per week, in slow-open heterogeneous groups of 5 to 8 individuals plus the groupanalyst, all seated in a small circle, allowing everyone to see and to be seen (Neto, 2002).

The fact that Eduardo Luís Cortesão, founder of the Portuguese Society of Groupanalysis, adopted the single word "groupanalysis" instead of the binomial group analysis, hints that this psychotherapeutic approach, as practised in Portugal, diverged from its Foulkesian foundational matrix. It incorporates a singular view about analytically oriented group psychotherapy, certainly influenced by the historical context and Portugal's culture. Groupanalysis has a strong and rich historical foundation, which dates back to 1957, when Cortesão returned to Portugal and gathered colleagues interested in Foulkes' ideas about group analysis. The groupanalytic movement holds a pivotal role in shaping the landscape of psychoanalytic psychotherapies in Portugal and the Portuguese Society of Groupanalysis and Group Analytic Psychotherapy (SPGPAG) is the only society training group analysts and group analytic psychotherapists (Neto & França, 2021).

Groupanalysis: Historical and Cultural Influences in Its Development

Portugal lived under an authoritarian regime from 1939 until 1974, known as Estado Novo, led by António Oliveira Salazar. The regime's conservative and paternalistic ideology strongly shaped mental health policies, privileging social control and institutionalization over therapeutic or community-based care. Psychiatric hospitals functioned mainly as custodial institutions, often isolating patients from society. Mental illness was approached through moral

DOI: 10.4324/9781003597674-8

and disciplinary lenses, with little integration between mental health services, primary care, or community support systems (Soares, 2008).

Censorship, restricted civil liberties, and strict regulation of academic and professional life marked this period (Almeida, 2017). This climate directly affected professionals such as Eduardo Luís Cortesão, who was prevented from pursuing a conventional hospital career due to his progressive views and interest in psychoanalysis. Through a state institute called Junta da Emigração (Emigration Bureau) he accessed international psychoanalytic training, received a British Council scholarship, and trained in London, where he met S.H. Foulkes and became a Full Member of the Group-Analytic Society in 1956 (Dinis, 2023).

The Groupanalytic Section of the Portuguese Society of Neurology and Psychiatry was founded in 1963 (Pinto & Salgado, 2001, 2002), the same year that the new Law of Bases for Mental Health attempted to decentralize services and promote the creation of mental health centres. Although unevenly implemented, these reforms coincided with the emergence of psychoanalytic movements influenced by French and Swiss traditions. In 1981, the Portuguese Society of Psychoanalysis gained IPA accreditation, and the Portuguese Society of Groupanalysis became an independent association, after years of significant influence on mental health professionals.

Cortesão's work can be understood as a form of intellectual resistance. By promoting dialogue, collective therapeutic settings, and professional networks, he challenged isolation and authoritarian control, introducing spaces for relational freedom and reflection within a repressive context (Cortesão, 2004). After the 1974 Carnation Revolution, which ended the dictatorship, these ideas gained renewed relevance. Psychiatry shifted towards more humanistic, community-based models, aligned with democratic values. Cortesão and his colleagues advocated for team-based care, day hospitals, and group psychotherapy within public services (Fragoso Mendes & Cortesão, 1957), emphasizing decentralization, interdisciplinarity, and psychosocial rehabilitation (Xavier, 2024).

During the 1980s, group work expanded in psychiatry, education, and social services as part of a broader democratization process. Group psychotherapy became a key resource to address trauma, social isolation, and the psychological effects of authoritarianism. Groupanalysis developed significantly in both clinical practice and training (Cortesão, 1989; Marques, 2016a; Neto & França, 2021). Other psychiatrists contributed to these developments, implementing intensive group models with multiple weekly sessions (Ferreira, 1965, 1989; Silva, 2003). Institutional groupanalytic interventions emerged in the 1960s and continued to evolve. An example of this is Lisbon's Santa Maria Day Hospital, where group therapeutic work is reflected in a longitudinal study assessing the impact of a groupanalytic day hospital on trainees between 1977 and 2007 (Neto, 2010). Psychotherapeutic groups were consistently rated as the most valuable activity, both for learning the therapeutic relationship and for personal development.

Portugal entry into the European Economic Community in 1986 accelerated reforms in health and social policy (Magone, 2006). However, economic priorities, persistent stigma, and a conservative social fabric influenced by Catholic values limited the broader dissemination of psychodynamic approaches (Borges Santos, 2019; Xavier et al., 2014). The expansion of psychopharmacology facilitated deinstitutionalization but also deepened divisions between biologically oriented psychiatry and psychosocial models. During the 1990s, groupanalysis remained marginal within public discourse, despite its presence in large psychiatric units and medical teaching.

The National Health Service, created in 1979, underwent slow reform, with more substantial legislative changes emerging only after 1998. Psychodynamic psychotherapy increasingly shifted to specialized settings and private practice, while public psychiatry prioritized symptom management and short-term interventions (Gameiro, 1992). In response to the heroin epidemic, community treatment centres developed in the 1990s, often integrating psychodynamic and groupanalytic approaches within multidisciplinary frameworks (Pombo & Félix da Costa, 2016; SICAD, 2019). Despite these advances, economic considerations increasingly shaped treatment choices.

In 1991 Cortesão died prematurely. Despite the already creative environment of the Portuguese Society of Groupanalysis promoted by younger members, the senior members took time to elaborate this loss, entering a period of relative destabilization. After 2000, psychodynamic group work, especially in the public sector, was also affected by economic pressures, political reforms, and institutional shifts. The 2008 global financial crisis affected Portugal significantly, resulting in greater economic stagnation, increased unemployment, and reductions in public service budgets (Correia et al., 2017). Mental health and social programmes – often reliant on public funding and multidisciplinary teams – were among the first to suffer from the austerity measures. We witnessed a shift toward individualized care models and performance-based metrics in health care that led to a decline in group-based approaches, which are harder to quantify and fund under neoliberal frameworks. The new Labor Code provisions (Lei no. 23. Portugal, 2012) introduced stricter rules for employment in public institutions. These changes reduced incentives for employers and professionals to engage in collective models. Social non-governmental institutions faced funding instability and were often forced to prioritize short-term, individual-focused interventions (Veiga et al., 2024). The rise of evidence-based medicine and standardized protocols in psychiatry and psychology favoured individual therapy over group formats. Once again, younger professionals preferred cognitive-behavioural trainings, focused on short-term results, complying with the efficacy model preconized by the current paradigm. Clinicians trained in this crisis environment often lacked exposure to groupanalytic settings, leading to a generational gap in practice. The decline of group work in Portugal after 2000 reflects a broader tension between collaborative, humanistic models and economic-technocratic pressures (Dinis, 2004).

Despite these pressures, significant groupanalytic initiatives continued to develop within public mental health services. A central example is the group-analytic framework implemented in Lisbon's main psychiatric hospital and its day hospital, under the leadership of Isaura Neto. Over several decades, this model integrated intensive group psychotherapy with other therapeutic formats, including multi-family group analytic groups, demonstrating the possibility of sustaining psychoanalytically oriented group work within institutional settings (Neto, 1993; Centeno, 1995a; Centeno, 1995b; Neto, 2009; Neto & França, 2021). Multi-family groups, as a clinical response to complex and transgenerational forms of suffering, resonate with the cultural importance of family and community in Portugal (Neto, 2017).

Still, over the past decade, psychodynamic group psychotherapy has shown signs of renewed, though modest, visibility. Groupanalytic work continues within psychiatric hospitals, private practice, and selected academic initiatives, sometimes through shorter or hybrid formats adapted to contemporary institutional realities (Marques, 2016b; OPP, 2013). Throughout this period, the SPGPAG has remained a central reference for training, supervision, and theoretical continuity, supporting the persistence and evolution of groupanalysis within Portuguese mental health care (Neto & França, 2021).

Groupanalytic Theory and Its Cultural Embeddedness

It is often stated that Portuguese divergences from Foulkesian group analysis derive from the historical and cultural context of its founders (Neto & França, 2021). Foulkes, a Jewish German immigrant in England, developed his work in the aftermath of the Second World War, following the experience of displacement and exposure to totalitarian leadership. His proximity to Norbert Elias, Gestalt and systems theory, and the second Northfield Experience contributed to the progressive distancing of group analysis from its classical psychoanalytic roots, although these were never rejected (Foulkes, 1990). At the time, group treatments were viewed as unconventional and even transgressive within traditional psychoanalytic practice.

Positioned simultaneously as a member of the British Psychoanalytic Society and as a challenger of the individual analytic model, Foulkes may have been compelled to formulate new concepts and technical pathways, such as *free-floating discussion* rather than *free association* (Foulkes, 1990). This may have contributed to his preference for presenting group analysis as a distinct treatment modality rather than as a psychoanalytic psychotherapy (Foulkes, 1990).

Cortesão's context was different. He came from a family combining traditional Portuguese academic lineages with Irish roots, introducing a more cosmopolitan dimension to his background. In Portugal, psychoanalytic and groupanalytic movements developed in parallel, reducing the likelihood of theoretical confrontation. This contrasts with Foulkes' experience in London, where he had to establish his place within a polarized psychoanalytic field marked by the Anna Freud–Melanie Klein controversies (Foulkes, 1990). These differing contexts may help explain why Cortesão attributed greater importance to the group leader's role than Foulkes did (Neto & França, 2021).

Portugal's transition to democracy after the Carnation Revolution illustrates how authoritarianism was rejected without rejecting leadership itself, provided it was grounded in democratic values. This may have facilitated Cortesão's theoretical emphasis on the role of the group leader and the formulation of the concept of *pattern* (Cortesão, 1967, 1989; Abreu-Afonso et al., 2015; Neto & França, 2021). The groupanalytic pattern includes the therapist's personality, emotional engagement, empathy, self-awareness, setting, and theoretical background, all of which, conveyed by the groupanalyst into the group matrix, will promote the development of the groupanalytic process.

The concept was discussed with Foulkes in the mid-1960s (Cortesão, 1967, 1988), who expressed reservations, perceived by Cortesão as difficulty in attributing excessive importance to the conductor's role (Cortesão, 1977). Beyond highlighting subjectivity, the pattern also stresses the analyst's responsibility toward both the group as a whole and each individual member. As treatment requests originate from individuals rather than groups, the therapist is expected to attend to individual needs within the group context (Brito, 1992; Cruz Filipe, 1992). Authors such as Billow (2003), Nitsum (2009), and Hopper and colleagues (2017) also diverge from Foulkes in their views on leadership. In Portugal the term *groupanalyst* or *psychotherapist* is preferred, reserving *conductor* for non-therapeutic or task-centred groups (Neto & França, 2021).

Influences on the Portuguese approach include Pichon-Rivière, object relations theory, interpersonal perspectives, and American psychoanalysts such as Kohut (Cortesão, 1989). Several authors emphasize the importance of transference and countertransference processes, considering therapeutic change to involve more than clarifications of present group dynamics. The groupanalyst's personal background and social engagement influence movements between the here-and-now and the there-and-then. This requires rigorous training and the capacity to engage deeply with unconscious processes. Consequently, personal groupanalysis occurs in mixed groups and lasts, on average, six years (Neto & França, 2021).

The concept of *pattern* implicitly conveys the relational turn in psychoanalysis (Ferro & França, 2021 in Neto & França, 2021). It highlights the singular relationship between analyst and each group member, as well as with the group as a whole, giving greater weight to transferential processes than in Foulkes' formulation. Through this framework, Cortesão observed the relational potential of the analytic field (Baranger, 1980) and allowed groupanalysis to address regressive phenomena alongside mirroring and ego-training-in-action.

This perspective is complemented by the concept of the *personal group matrix* or *internal relational matrix* (Leal, 1968). It refers to the internal network of relationships formed across life, originating in early family interactions and evolving through subsequent group experiences. The personal group matrix concept draws from Pichon-Rivière's idea of the internal group, highlighting the link between intrapsychic and interpersonal relations (Marques & Melo, 2020 in Neto & França, 2021; Okamoto, 2017). According to Leal (1968, 1981), transference–countertransference phenomena bring each person's internal matrix into group dynamics, with mirroring, resonance, and ego-training-in-action producing new introjections that change each member's original personal group matrix. The concept highlights the significance of relatedness in Portuguese groupanalysis as it stresses how primary relationships and interactions with various groups throughout life influence personality and present relationships deeply (França & Bivar, 2022).

Ferreira further conceptualized groupanalysis as a metatheory rather than a technique, bridging psychoanalysis and social psychiatry and emphasizing transgenerational patterns and societal structures reflected in group dynamics (Ferreira, 1992, 2004, 2015). Neto (2017) also highlighted transgenerational pathology as the unconscious transmission of unresolved relational failures, stressing the centrality of the analyst's pattern in promoting authenticity, empathy, and analytic containment. Difficult affects such as envy, guilt, jealousy, sexuality, and aggression are considered essential to address within the group setting (Neto & França, 2021).

Neto's introduction of multi-family groups into Portuguese groupanalysis, inspired by García Badaracco's multi-family psychoanalysis (2000), further illustrates this cultural embeddedness. These groups facilitate the emergence of distorted relational patterns across generations, allowing families to observe and reflect upon one another's dynamics (Centeno, 1995a, 1995b; Centeno et al., 2023; FA.M.H.E. Project Consortium, 2024). Their growing use in mental health services reflects the enduring importance of family and community in Portuguese culture.

Finally, transference and countertransference remain central in the Portuguese School of Groupanalysis (Dinis, 1994). Transferential processes are distributed across the group, creating a complex relational network in which multiple roles become available for elaboration (Dinis & Abreu-Afonso, 2021 in Neto & França, 2021). The group functions as an empathic resonance box (Dinis, 2004), The concept is a powerful metaphor for the group's ability to amplify and support individual change through collective empathy. When the groupanalyst offers a well-timed, meaningful interpretation to an individual, it does more than support that person's therapeutic journey; it sends ripples through the group, inviting others to engage, reflect, and take part in the creation of new meanings. This collective resonance transforms the group into a dynamic space where empathy is not just a quality of the analyst but a shared attribute of the entire group matrix. As the group integrates the analyst's pattern, members become agents of insight: each interpretation nurturing rational understanding and emotional commitment for all (Neto & França, 2021).

Psychodynamic, Groupanalytic, and Analytic Group Psychotherapeutic Practice in Current Times

In our view, the considerations outlined above regarding the historical and cultural context of the groupanalytic movement in Portugal are among the factors shaping the current landscape of analytic group psychotherapy and groupanalysis in the country. Other precipitating factors relate to international developments in psychoanalytic and groupanalytic theory.

From the 1990s until today, psychotherapy has been practised predominantly by psychologists rather than psychiatrists or other mental health professionals. Psychotherapeutic federations and institutional bodies responsible for regulating mental health professionals have debated several issues, such as whether psychotherapy should be considered a profession or a technique. At present, psychotherapy is not recognized as an independent profession in Portugal, but rather as a set of clinical interventions carried out by trained health professionals. However, there is no academic curriculum specifically devoted to the training of groupanalysts. Therefore, since 2008, recognition as a groupanalyst requires a degree in psychology and application to the Portuguese Psychologists' Order, which recognizes SPGPAG's training programme (Biscaia & Neto, 2023).

Following the introduction of legal provisions in 2010, questions arose concerning the official accreditation of professionals who were not psychologists but wished to practise as psychotherapists. In response, professional orders for psychiatrists and nurses established specific pathways for their members to obtain recognition and accreditation as psychotherapists. Although psychotherapy remains an unregulated profession in Portugal, it is governed by rules defined by the relevant professional bodies for psychologists, psychiatrists, and nurses, each of which provides its own accreditation procedures.

This unresolved issue is closely linked to political priorities in public mental health care. In 2017, only 917 of nearly 5,000 qualified clinical and health psychologists were employed in the National Health System (NHS) (OPP, 2018; 2020). Despite increased governmental attention, particularly following the pandemic, substantial improvements have not materialized, and only about one-fifth of registered clinical psychologists currently practise within the NHS. Most NHS psychotherapists are trained in systemic or cognitive-behavioural approaches, while fewer are trained in psychodynamic modalities (SNS, 2017).

A study on the integration of psychotherapeutic models by Vasco et al. (2011) identified two main clusters among Portuguese psychotherapists: (1) psychoanalytic and psychodynamic therapists, who show limited identification with other models; and (2) cognitive, behavioural, humanistic, and systemic therapists, who more frequently integrate across approaches. This limited integrative tendency among psychoanalytically oriented therapists may help explain their reduced presence within the NHS.

The recent increase in psychotherapists identifying as eclectic or integrative is consistent with the growing prominence of integrative models in psychotherapy (Vasco et al., 2003). This shift may also reflect the increasing emphasis on evidence-based practices in psychotherapy research, which encourages the adoption of empirically supported interventions, particularly among younger practitioners (OPP, 2013; 2020).

The Portuguese Federation for Psychotherapy (FEPPSI, n.d.) is Portugal's national representative within the European Association for Psychotherapy (EAP), bringing together 15 associations, including SPGPAG. Some major psychoanalytic associations, such as the Portuguese Society of Psychoanalysis (SPP) and PsiRelacional, have chosen not to participate, limiting psychoanalytic representation within the federation. FEPPSI is estimated to include between 700 and 800 individual psychotherapists, although exact figures are not publicly available. The federation actively advocates for legal recognition of psychotherapy as an autonomous profession, in contrast to the position of the Portuguese Psychologists' Order (OPP). The total number of Portuguese psychoanalytic psychotherapists remains unknown, as most associations do not disclose membership data.

Psychodynamic psychotherapists – including groupanalysts and group-analytic psychotherapists – work mainly in private practice or at least develop their psychotherapeutic skills there (Neto & França, 2024). Recently, there has been an increase in psychotherapeutic groups within the NHS, not always conducted by professionals with groupanalytic credentials, but often promoted by interdisciplinary teams coping with large waiting lists (OPP, 2017). Hospital administrators increasingly encourage group interventions because of their economic and organizational advantages. Nevertheless, SPGPAG remains the only scientific society dedicated to the study and development of Group Analysis and Group Analytic Psychotherapy in Portugal. The inappropriate application of analytic group techniques by professionals from diverse backgrounds without specific training poses a challenge to maintaining groupanalytic identity and may negatively influence national health policy decision making.

A small number of committed colleagues working within the NHS continue to find ways to sustain analytic group psychotherapeutic settings, including groupanalytic settings with a frequency of two sessions per week (Fialho, 2023). Groupanalytic applications with homogeneous groups continue to develop within the NHS (Neto & França, 2021), including groups for pregnant women (Madeira, 2023), individuals with infertility problems (Silva, 2024), psychotic patients in day care (Gomes, 2025), people with addictive behaviours (Farinha & Alcântara, 2024), Balint groups (Florêncio, 2017), and groupanalytic models of day hospitals inspired by the experience of Santa Maria Hospital (Neto, 2010; Graça et al., 2013).

The limited number of groupanalysts and psychoanalytically oriented therapists in the public sector restricts access to these treatments. Their long duration, perceived complexity, uneven geographical distribution, and concentration in major cities contribute to long waiting lists and limit equitable access. Moreover, there appears to be limited political commitment to changing this situation, as decision makers tend to prioritize low-cost, short-term, or pharmacological interventions, often supported by biased research, as several psychoanalytic authors have argued (Fonagy, 2003; Hoffman, 2009; McWilliams, 2019; Shedler, 2010; Wallerstein, 2015).

Working mainly in private practice or private institutions also presents advantages. Psychoanalytic and groupanalytic associations are able to maintain their independence, pursue rigorous and intensive training programmes, conduct scientific activities without external political or economic pressure, adhere to psychoanalytically grounded ethical principles, and uphold humanistic values such as dignity and patient autonomy. Recently, increased public interest in the depth offered by these approaches has led many younger patients to make significant financial sacrifices to address deep emotional and relational difficulties. In response, private insurance companies have begun to partially reimburse these treatments, and many analytically oriented associations provide reduced-cost options. SPGPAG has established a Nucleus of Applied Groupanalysis as a social response initiative to support patients with economic difficulties. Negotiated fees for patients with financial constraints are common practice among psychotherapists in Portugal.

Groupanalysis is usually conducted at a frequency of two sessions per week, while group analytic psychotherapy typically involves one weekly session. A recent survey conducted by Neto and França (2024) among SPGPAG members on perceived subjective effectiveness showed that longer duration and higher treatment frequency are considered essential for deep and lasting change, particularly when therapeutic goals are ambitious. Of the 95 associates invited, 25 valid responses were obtained. Most respondents were over 60 years old, predominantly clinical psychologists, and 72% actively conducted group therapies, mainly in private practice. No successful treatments reported lasted less than one year, and the majority (over 60%) extended beyond three years. Most groupanalysts indicated that a variable period of individual psychotherapy prior to group entry was mandatory, to establish a therapeutic alliance and ensure appropriate selection, minimizing risk to both the individual and the group (Neto, 1999). Additional factors associated with therapeutic success included patient motivation, clinical complexity, therapeutic alliance, insight, therapist empathy, technical competence, analyst maturity, and external life conditions (Neto & França, 2024).

One of the most evident challenges within the groupanalytic framework is the length of the training programme. As a member of the European Group

Analytic Training Institutions Network (EGATIN), SPGPAG ensures that international training standards are met and, in some respects, surpassed, particularly regarding personal groupanalysis. Training to become a group-analyst requires an average of six years of personal groupanalysis, which members identify as the most valued component of training (Carvalho et al., 2008). Nevertheless, this duration is not substantially different from that required by patients seeking not only symptom relief, but also a deeper understanding and transformation of psychic suffering.

SPGPAG also offers a multi-level training structure, including introductory courses, advanced training in groupanalysis, and supervision. Monthly clinical and theoretical events frequently include international speakers, and since 1989 SPGPAG has co-organized biennial Luso-Brazilian Congresses with Brazilian group psychotherapy associations. Specialized workshops, open to mental health professionals, address themes such as infertility, psychosis in institutional settings, and parenting from a groupanalytic perspective. SPGPAG also maintains an online publication with irregular periodicity.

On Research

Portuguese groupanalysts share a recognition of both the value and the challenges of research. They are in accordance with several psychoanalysts addressing the topic. Wallerstein (2015) argues that psychoanalytic research must not strictly conform to the standards of natural sciences but can be performed using diverse methodologies, valuing transparency in reporting results. Shapiro (2014) believes the complexity of clinical interactions in the psychoanalytic practice makes research challenging but not impossible. Coderch and Ávila (2021) suggest that traditional empirical methods have limitations and highlight the importance of interdisciplinary dialogue and integration. Shedler (2010) criticizes selective dissemination of research findings and public policy bias against psychodynamic approaches. Fonagy (2003) points to the lack of research tradition in psychoanalysis (and groupanalysis, we add) and expresses concern that funding and research opportunities are biased towards short-term treatments. McWilliams (2019) cautions against reducing analytic clinical work to narrow, outcome-oriented paradigms, and encourages open, collaborative inquiry with other disciplines. Some Portuguese psychoanalysts (Becker et al., 2022) highlight a critical tension: while psychodynamic psychotherapy is seen as deeply valuable, it remains underrepresented in clinical settings and research publications. We have already referred to the key factors explaining this gap, which we summarize as follows. In Portugal, psychoanalytic psychotherapies like groupanalysis are long-treatment models (Neto & França, 2021), clashing with short-term CBT models, which are easily (yet poorly, in our opinion) quantifiable as effective and thus preferred by the public health systems. Research in psychotherapy suffers from limited funding in Portugal, making it harder to conduct longitudinal studies – which is a main concern of our model but disregarded as important by other theoretical models, focusing mostly on rational behaviour and symptomatic relief. There is still, although we perceive it as improving, a disconnection between academia and clinical practice and most psychotherapists work privately, outside research networks. In the public sphere, the scarcity of psychodynamic psychotherapists and the amount of work they endure, tend to overlook research as important.

Nevertheless, many clinicians keep trying to strengthen ties between universities and clinical institutions to support data collection and training. Associations are significantly concerned about aligning with European standards on psychodynamic psychotherapies and making the few available research findings more accessible to clinicians and the public.

In general, groupanalysts contend that research into group analytic psychotherapy is essential but must employ innovative methods suited to the field's complex relationships. We advocate for transparency and methodological diversity rather than strict adherence to rigid scientific criteria, encouraging collaboration with areas such as neuroscience. Relying solely on traditional, outcome-focused models, to satisfy political or financial reasons, may overlook the subtle complexities inherent in our work. Most of us are not trained as researchers and it will be essential that we collaborate with professional researchers, remain open to learning from other disciplines, and move beyond elitist attitudes that have historically created divisions. Ultimately, research should support clinical understanding, integrate different perspectives, and maintain psychoanalytic psychotherapies, as groupanalysis, committed to freedom from constraint and preconception.

Conclusion

Portuguese culture and political history are deeply intertwined with the evolution of groupanalytic theory and practice. The adaptation of "groupanalysis" as a unique term, the introduction of core concepts like "padrão" and the "internal relational matrix", and the embrace of transgenerational and family group approaches reflect particular adaptations of Foulkesian group analysis, creating a new metatheory (Ferreira, 2004). These developments were informed by Portugal's history, which was marked by authoritarianism, revolution, and democratization and by the enduring value placed on family, community, and dialogue.

Culture and history also influence psychotherapeutic techniques, as we may conclude looking at the perception of the groupanalyst's role within the group's dynamic. The groupanalyst is not just a neutral conductor but a responsible, empathic figure whose personality, training, and engagement shape both the group's matrix and its therapeutic potential.

Regarding current practice, the landscape is complex: public mental health structures favour short-term, outcome-focused modalities, while groupanalysis thrives in private practice and in some innovative public settings. Despite challenges like limited integration into the NHS, preference for individualized treatments, and funding constraints, groupanalytic methods continue to adapt, fostered by resilient clinicians. Practices typically involve small, slow-open groups, intensive training requirements, and a strong commitment to ethical and relational values.

On research, Portuguese groupanalysts recognize the need for rigorous, transparent research but refuse to reduce complex clinical work to narrow, quantitative paradigms. We advocate for methodological diversity, interdisciplinary collaboration, and research that serves both clinical understanding and the integrity of psychoanalytic principles.

Ultimately, because we believe that the practice and theory of group-analytic psychotherapy cannot be separated from cultural, social, and historical context, we continue to thrive on demonstrating responsiveness to the field's evolution by attempting to bridge with universities, to regulate training and professional identity, and to adapt to changing models of care with groupanalytic applications in different settings.

Portugal's relatively small size and limited resources mean that Portuguese group analysts may have less influence internationally compared with colleagues in countries with larger health-care investments and more clinicians and patients, which affects the dissemination of theoretical models and research. Despite these challenges, the Portuguese School of Groupanalysis represents a major milestone in the development of group analytic psychoanalytic psychotherapy, offering a rich psychoanalytic heritage, deep theoretical understanding, and extensive practical experience shaped by Portugal's unique cultural and historical context. Preserving and promoting this legacy is crucial, as its enduring theoretical and clinical contributions continue to provide valuable insights and approaches within the broader field of psychoanalytic psychotherapy.

References

Abreu-Afonso, J., César, D., Ferreira, G., Caseiro Ferro, S.M., Motta Marques, P., Melo, J.C., Neto, I., Porto, M., Bastos Rodrigues, T., & Valente, A. (2015). Group analysis: Other sights of the conscious and the unconscious. *Journal of Psychology Research*, 5(1): 10–22. doi:10.17265/2159-5542/2015.01.002.

Almeida, A.S. (2017). A saúde no Estado Novo de Salazar (1933–1968): Políticas, sistemas e estruturas. Doctoral thesis. Universidade de Lisboa, Portugal.

Baranger, W. (1980). *Conclusiones y problemas acerca del objeto in Aportaciones al concepto de objeto en psicoanálisis.* Buenos Aires: Amorrortu.

Becker, M., Paixão, S., & Quartilho, M. (2022). Controversies on psychoanalytic Psychotherapies: Is psychodynamic psychotherapy effective for the treatment of PTSD? *Revista Portuguesa de Psicanálise*, 42(1), 58–64.

Billow, R.M. (2003). The authority of the group therapist's psychology. In R.M. Billow (Ed.), *Relational Group Psychotherapy: From Basic Assumption to Passion* (pp. 227–241). London and New York: Jessica Kingsley.

Biscaia, C., & Neto, D.D. (Eds.) (2023). *A prática profissional da psicoterapia*. Lisbon: Ordem dos Psicólogos Portugueses (OPP).

Borges Santos, P. (2019). Politics and religion under the dictatorship in Portugal (1933–1974): Rebuilding the separation between the state and the church. *Storicamente*, 14(27), 1–23.

Brito, E. (1992). O padrão grupanalítico. *Grupanálise*, 4, 7–21.

Carvalho, P., Galamba, G., & Neto, I. M. (2008). Training challenges: Portuguese experience and contribution. Survey presented at the EGATIN Study Days, 25–26 April, Oslo.

Centeno, M.J. (1995a). Analytic group psychotherapy in hospital settings: The Portuguese experience. In Proceedings of the International Symposium on Group Analysis (pp. 112–120). London: GASi.

Centeno, M.J. (1995b). Psicoterapia analítica de grupo em contexto hospitalar: a experiência do Hospital de Dia. *Análise Psicológica*, 13(2), 201–212.

Centeno, M.J., Godinho, P., & Fialho, T. (2023). The importance of multifamily groups in mental health: Presentation of the transnational project FA.M.H.E. Session presented at the Seminário Eduardo Luís Cortesão, Sociedade Portuguesa de Grupanálise e Psicoterapia Analítica de Grupo (SPGPAG), February 11, 2023.

Coderch, J., & Ávila, A. (2021). Algunas razones que explican la transformación del psicoanálisis en muchos psicoanálisis. *Revista PsiRelacional*, 1(March), 89–107.

Correia, T., Dussault, G., & Pontes, C. (2017). The effects of austerity measures on quality of healthcare services: A national survey of physicians in the public and private sectors in Portugal. *Human Resources for Health*, 15, Article 82. doi:10.1186/s12960-017-0256-6.

Cortesão, E.L. (1967). Based on the practice and theory of group-analytic psychotherapy: Some further thoughts on the concept of group matrix. *Group Analysis*, 1, 29–36.

Cortesão, E.L. (1977/2004). Uma tarde em Golders Green, *Grupanálise*, 1.

Cortesão, E.L. (1988). O Padrão Grupanalítico. *Grupanálise*, 1, 7–22.

Cortesão, E.L. (1989). *Grupanálise: Teoria e Técnica*. Lisbon: Climepsi.

Cortesão, E.L. (2004). *Um psiquiatra na revolução*. Lisbon: Editorial Notícias.

Cruz Filipe, E. (1992). Padrão grupanalítico, *Grupanálise*, 4, 23–31.

Dinis, C.V. (1994). Algumas reflexões a propósito da neurose de transferência em grupanálise. *Grupanálise*, 5, 7–18.

Dinis, C.V. (2003). O tempo e a mudança. *Revista Portuguesa de Grupanálise*, 5, 28–37.

Dinis, C.V. (2004). Grupanálise: compatibilização de protagonismos. *Revista Portuguesa de Grupanálise*, 9–16.

Dinis, C.V. (2023). *História: Contribuição do Professor Eduardo Luís Cortesão para a Grupanálise Portuguesa*. www.grupanalise.pt (accessed: 23 January 2026).

Farinha, C., & Alcântara, M.T.F. (2024). Desafios de um grupo institucional – A obrigação de estar. Paper presented at the XXIII Congresso Nacional da Sociedade Portuguesa de Grupanálise e Psicoterapia Analítica de Grupo (SPGPAG), 22–23 November, Faculdade de Psicologia da Universidade de Lisboa, Lisbon, Portugal.

FA.M.H.E. Project Consortium. (2024). *Competências e formação do condutor e do facilitador de grupo de psicanálise multifamiliar* (Erasmus+). FA.M.H.E. Erasmus+ Project Documentation. www.fa-m-he.it/wp-content/uploads/2024/06/PORT.

FEPPSI (n.d.). *Petição para a autonomia da psicoterapia como profissão*. https://peticaopublica.com (accessed: 23 January 2026).

Ferreira, A.G. (1965). *Relatório de Actividades da Secção de Grupanálise da Sociedade Portuguesa de Neurologia e Psiquiatria (1963–1965)*. Lisbon: SPNP.
Ferreira, A.G. (1989). Psicoterapias de grupo e grupanálise: suas especificidades e relações. *Análise Psicológica*, 7(3), 355–364.
Ferreira, A.G. (1992). A Matriz Grupanalítica. *Grupanálise*, 3, 45–56.
Ferreira, A.G. (2004). O problema e a procura de uma metateoria em grupanálise. *Revista Portuguesa de Grupanálise*, 17–30.
Ferreira, A.G. (2015). Group analysis and the different approaches: The Portuguese contribution – A tribute to E.L. Cortesão. *Group Analysis*, 48(4). doi:10.1177/0533316415610.
Fialho, I.C. (2023). A psicoterapia de grupo de orientação grupanalítica: Levantamento e caracterização a nível nacional em meio hospitalar e avaliação da eficácia em grupos psicoterapêuticos de diferentes dimensões. Doctoral dissertation. Nova Medical School – Faculdade de Ciências Médicas, Universidade Nova de Lisboa, Lisbon.
Florêncio, N. (2017). Balint Groups – Training and Research Groups of the Doctor–Patient Relationship. Paper presented at the 17th International Symposium of the GASi: 15–17 August, Maritim Hotel, Berlin, Germany.
Fonagy, P. (2003). Psychoanalysis today. *World Psychiatry*, 2(2), 73–80.
Foulkes, S.H. (1990). *Selected Papers on Psychoanalysis and Group Analysis*. London: Routledge.
Fragoso Mendes, J., & Cortesão, E.L. (1957). Hospitais de dia em psiquiatria. *Jornal do Médico*, 34(777), 795–798.
França, M., & Bivar, A. (2022). The Portuguese School of Group Analysis – context and concepts – Personal group matrix or internal relational matrix. *Contexts*, 97. doi:10.4324/9781003137238
Gameiro, J. (1992). *Flying over Psychiatry*. Lisbon: Editorial Notícias.
García Badaracco, J.E. (2000). *Psicoanálisis multifamiliar: los otros en nosotros y el descubrimiento del sí mismo*. Buenos Aires: Paidós.
Graça, J., Palma, M., Mendonça, C., Cargaleiro, I., & Melo, J.C. (2013). Empatia – Ferramenta pró-social explorada num grupo terapêutico. *Psilogos – Revista do Serviço de Psiquiatria do Hospital Prof. Doutor Fernando da Fonseca, EPE*, 11(2), 55–69. https://repositorio.hff.min-saude.pt/bitstreams/0a8bc90c-1c39-47f6-969d-4997f58acc23/download.
Gomes, R. (2025). Do hospital para o mundo: Possibilidades de uma psicoterapia analítica de grupo com pacientes psicóticos em contexto institucional. Paper presented at the Eduardo Luís Cortesão Seminar, January 11, SPGPAG, Lisbon.
Hopper, E., Brown, M., Friedman, R., Godby, D.C., Vincent, D., Wilson, P., & Winther, G. (2017). The Group Analytic Model. *International Journal of Group Psychotherapy*, 67(supl), S79–S90. doi:10.1080/00207284.2016.1218770.
Hoffman, I.Z. (2009). Doublethinking our way to "scientific" legitimacy: The desiccation of human experience. *Journal of the American Psychoanalytic Association*, 57, 1043–1069.
Leal, M.R.M. (1968). Transference neurosis in group-analytic treatment. *Group Analysis*, 1(2), 99–109.
Leal, M.R.M. (1981). Resistances and the group-analytic process. *Group Analysis*, 15(2), 97–110.
Madeira, L. (2023). 1+1=3 Grupos de apoio psicoterapêutico institucional na gravidez e no puerpério. Paper presented at the Eduardo Luís Cortesão Seminar, January 13. SPGPAG. Lisbon.

McWilliams, N. (2019). The future of psychoanalysis: Preserving Jeremy's Safran integrative vision. *Psychoanalytic Psychology*, 37(2), 98–107.

Magone, J. (2006). The Europeanization of Portugal (1986–2006): A critical view. *Nação e Defesa*, 115, 9–28.

Marques, P.M.B. (2016a). O modelo da escola portuguesa de grupanálise. *Análise Psicológica*, 34(2), 153–162.

Marques, P.M.B. (2016b). O modelo da escola portuguesa de grupanálise: aspetos integrativos e evolução no contexto de uma investigação conceptual-empírica sobre a matriz grupanalítica. *Vínculo – Revista do NESME Núcleo de Estudos em Saúde Mental e Psicanálise das Configurações Vinculares*, 13(12), 1–12.

Neto, I.M. (1993). O Hospital de Dia: espaço grupanalítico de intervenção psicoterapêutica. *Análise Psicológica*, 11(3), 345–356.

Neto, I.M. (1999). Selection in groupanalysis: similarities and differences: Some risks we take in group analysis. Paper presented at the 11th GAS Symposium in Group Analysis, August 1999, Budapest.

Neto, I.M. (2002). To see and be seen: an added value in Group Analysis. Paper presented at the 12th GAS European Symposium in Group Analysis, 26–31 August, Bologna, Italy.

Neto, I.M. (2009). Group analytic psychotherapy in a Portuguese day hospital: Reflections on practice and training. *Group Analysis*, 42(3), 267–280.

Neto, I.M. (2010). Moving groupwork into the day hospital setting. In J. Radcliffe, K. Hajek, J. Carson & O. Manor (Eds.), *Psychological Groupwork with Acute Psychiatric Inpatients* (pp. 325–342). London: Whiting & Birch.

Neto, I.M. (2017). Multi family group analysis – (MFGA). *Current Psychiatry Reviews*, 13(3): 165–170. doi:10.2174/1573400513666170503113353.

Neto, I.M., & França, M. (Eds.) (2021). *The Portuguese School of Group Analysis: Towards a Unified and Integrated Approach to Theory, Research and Clinical Work*. London: Routledge.

Neto, I.M., & França, M. (2024). How important is time in psychoanalytic psychotherapies? & How do we feel about time? Reflections on a survey. Presented at the EFPP Four Sections Conference: A Different World? Psychoanalytic Psychotherapy and Relatedness in Stormy Times, 27–29 September, Warsaw, Poland.

Nitsum, M. (2009). Authority and revolt: The challenges of group leadership. *Group Analysis*, 42(4): 325–348.

Okamoto, M.M. (2017). Revisitando Enrique Pichon-Rivière: grupo interno, história de origem e contexto social. Master thesis in psychology and social psychology, Pontifícia Universidade Católica de São Paulo, São Paulo.

Ordem dos Psicólogos Portugueses (2013). *Contributos da Psicologia para a(s) Crise(s): Novas Formas de Prestação de Serviços e Promoção da Saúde Mental*. Lisbon: Ordem dos Psicólogos Portugueses. See https://recursos.ordemdospsicologos.pt/files/artigos/contr_psic_crises.pdf.

Ordem dos Psicólogos Portugueses (2018, 4 January). *Despacho da Secretaria de Estado da Saúde: Organização e funcionamento da Psicologia Clínica e da Saúde no SNS*. www.ordemdospsicologos.pt/.

Ordem dos Psicólogos Portugueses (2020). *Crise Económica, Pobreza e Desigualdades – Relatório sobre Impacto Socioeconómico e Saúde Mental em Portugal*. Lisbon: OPP.

Pinto, T.S., & Salgado, F. (2001). História da Grupanálise em Portugal. *Revista Portuguesa de Grupanálise*, 3, 52–71.

Pinto, T.S., & Salgado, F. (2002). História da Grupanálise em Portugal (Part 2). *Revista Portuguesa de Grupanálise*, 7, 5–28.

Pombo, S., & Félix da Costa, N. (2016). Heroin addiction patterns of treatment-seeking patients, 1992–2013: Comparison between pre- and post-drug policy reform in Portugal. *Heroin Addiction Related Clinical Problems*, 18(6), 51–60.

Portugal (2012). *Lei no. 23/2012, de 25 de junho*. Diário da República.

Serviço de Intervenção nos Comportamentos Aditivos e nas Dependências (SICAD) (2019). *Construímos caminhos… uma história dos comportamentos aditivos e dependências em Portugal*. SICAD. www.icad.pt/DocumentList/GetFile?id=580&languageId=1.

Shapiro, Y. (2014). Psychodynamic formulation in the age of neuroscience: A dynamical systems model. *Psychoanalytic Dialogues*, 24(2), 175–192.

Shedler, J. (2010). The efficacy of psychodynamic psychotherapy. *American Psychologist*, 65(2), 98–109. doi:10.1037/a0018378.

Silva, J.A. (2003). Potencialidades da Grupanálise – quando aplicada à intervenção na e sobre a Instituição. *Grupanaliseonline.pt Ano*, 1(1), 9–12.

Silva, M. (2024). Intervenção grupanalítica breve na infertilidade: sofrimento psicológico, autoeficácia, estigma, relação matrimonial, memórias da infância e estatuto reprodutivo. Doctoral dissertation. Faculdade de Psicologia, Universidade de Lisboa. Universidade de Lisboa, Lisbon. See https://researchportal.ulisboa.pt/pt/studentTheses/interven%C3%A7%C3%A3o-grupanal%C3%ADtica-breve-na-infertilidade-sofrimento-psico/.

Serviço Nacional de Saúde (SNS) (2017). *Relatório Final do Grupo de Trabalho para análise, estudo e elaboração de propostas relativamente aos modelos de organização da prestação de cuidados na área da psicologia no Serviço Nacional de Saúde* (July 2017). RelatorioFinalModelosOrganizacaoPsicologiaSNS.pdf

Soares, M.I. (2008). A reforma dos serviços de assistência psiquiátrica. *Pensar Enfermagem – Revista Científica*, 12(2), 35–51. https://hdl.handle.net/10400.26/23995.

Vasco, A.B., Santos, O., & Silva, F. (2003). Psicoterapia sim! Eficácia, efectividade e psicoterapeutas (em Portugal). *PSICOLOGIA*, 17(2), 485–495.

Vasco, B.V., Conceição, N., Ferreira, J.F., Silva, A.N., & Vaz-Velho, C. (2011). Who are the integrative psychotherapists in Portugal and why did they become integrative? *Journal of Psychotherapy Integration*, 21(2), 123–149. doi:10.1037/a0022902.

Veiga, S., Tinoco, R., Abrantes, A., Azevedo, C.N., Figueiredo, D., Longo, G., & Lopes, H. (2024). *A psicoterapia de cariz psicodinâmico na contemporaneidade*. Porto: Instituto Politécnico do Porto. Escola Superior de Educação.

Wallerstein, R.S. (2015). Psychoanalysis as I have known it: 1049–2013. *Psychoanalytic Dialogues*, 25(5), 536–556.

Xavier, M. (Ed.) (2024). *Reforma da Saúde Mental em Portugal: Três anos de transformação*. Lisbon: Coordenação Nacional das Políticas de Saúde Mental.

Xavier, S., Klut, C., Neto, A., da Ponte, G., & Melo, J.C. (2014). Mental health stigma: Where do we stand? *Acta Médica Portuguesa*, 27(5): 646–652.

Chapter 9

Group Analytic Psychotherapy in Norway

Cultural Adaptation, Clinical Innovation, National Integration, and Research

Thor Kristian Island, Ingalill Pagliettini Johnsen and Hanne-Sofie Johnsen Dahl

Introduction

Group analytic psychotherapy in Norway represents a compelling case of how psychotherapy can be shaped by cultural values, institutional priorities, significant governmental funding, and the initiatives of dedicated individuals. This chapter explores the evolution and current status of group analytic psychotherapy in Norway, focusing on three central objectives: how it is influenced by and reflects Norwegian history and culture, how it is practiced and adapted across various settings, and how it engages with the growing emphasis on evidence-based treatment. The Norwegian example offers valuable insights into the systemic integration of group-based approaches into national health frameworks.

Historical Roots

The journey of group therapy in Norway commenced in the 1960s with the establishment of "therapeutic communities" within psychiatric institutions. These communities, significantly influenced by the pioneering work of English psychiatrists Tom Main and Maxwell Jones, laid a foundational emphasis on harnessing interpersonal relationships—both among patients and between patients and therapists—as primary material for therapeutic processing (Main, 1946, 1957). Jones championed the development of democratic therapeutic communities, advocating for a social psychiatric approach (Jones 1952, 1968, 1979). Upon its introduction in Norway, the therapeutic community model encountered initial skepticism. However, the importance of group therapy as an integral component of milieu therapy gradually gained widespread recognition within most psychiatric institutions. This apparent acceptance, however, likely represented a compromise among various orientations within psychiatry—psychoanalysts, social psychiatrists, behavioral therapists, and those with a more biological perspective creating a common

DOI: 10.4324/9781003597674-9

ground which was heavily diluted and led to an oversimplification of milieu therapeutic theory, often neglecting the irrational forces that can manifest at both organizational and group levels within psychiatric departments. Furthermore, group therapy was frequently delegated to the lower-ranking, less influential staff, such as nurses and other milieu personnel, while psychiatrists often retreated to their offices to practice individual therapy (Vaglum et al., 1982). Consequently, groups were often conducted based on a "common sense" approach, lacking a solid theoretical foundation. Sigmund Karterud's doctoral thesis in 1989 notably exposed significant uncertainty and confusion regarding these group therapies, highlighting ambiguities regarding objectives, frameworks, conduct, and, critically, in the absence of clear leadership structures—a failure in dynamic administration (Karterud, 1989). Over time, mounting concerns arose regarding the efficacy and potential harm in continuing such unstructured groups. Some psychiatrists argued that this form of therapy was confusing and potentially detrimental to patients. Another group of influential psychiatrists with psychoanalytic backgrounds maintained that group psychotherapy should remain a vital part of psychotherapeutic offerings, though proper training was required. This pressing need for formal training served as the impetus for the Norwegian Psychiatric Association to establish a committee dedicated to exploring the feasibility of establishing group psychotherapy training in Norway. Given the existing connections between the Norwegian milieu and the English therapeutic community movement, with its strong emphasis on analytical group psychotherapy, it was a natural progression to approach the Institute of Group Analysis (IGA) in London and its Overseas Training Committee to collaborate on establishing a formal training program in group analytical psychotherapy in Norway (see Island, 2022 for this history).

The Introduction of Foulkesian Group Analysis in Norway: A Contextual and Cultural Perspective

The Institute for Group Analysis and Group Psychotherapy (IGA-Norway), initially known as the Institute of Group Analysis, has played a central and transformative role in professionalizing group psychotherapy throughout the country. The beginning of the training program for Foulkesian group analytic theory and practice in Norway was met with considerable enthusiasm, rapidly gaining prominence and leading to a substantial demand for training. There was also the widespread establishment of group therapies across psychiatric institutions nationwide. However, this initial enthusiasm was occasionally tempered by a degree of skepticism, with concerns articulated about potential "colonization" by English therapeutic models. A similar concern appeared among other training institutes in Europe as well, which finally led to the founding of the European Group Analytic Training Institutions Network (EGATIN) as a network intended to counteract excessive dominance by the IGA in London (Voyatzaki, 2006).

Cultural Resonance

Concerns about colonization reflected perhaps a deeper unconscious, apprehension rooted in the Norwegian national psyche (Island, 2020) and the collective social unconscious (Hopper, 2003; Hopper & Weinberg, 2011; Weinberg 2007). This apprehension underscored a historical aversion to external dominance. Norway's historical trajectory, marked by periods of both independence and protracted subjugation, significantly influenced the reception of group analysis. After a period of prominence during the Viking Age, Norway was subsumed into a union with Denmark, assuming a subordinate role for 400 years until 1814, a period that suppressed Norwegian cultural and national identity (Glenthøj, 2008). The subsequent cession of Norway to Sweden following the Napoleonic Wars, despite offering a degree of autonomy, did not fully realize Norwegian aspirations for complete independence, which were only achieved in 1905 with the dissolution of the union. Consequently, a deep-seated skepticism towards unions necessitating submission to external ideologies and supranational powers seem to characterize Norwegian national consciousness. These historical roots offer possible insight into Norway's national apprehension toward ceding of self-determination and the continued non-membership in the European Union, as evidenced by two referendum rejections in 1972 and 1994, and a persistent reluctance to fully integrate with broader European frameworks. However, this opposition is currently challenged by the imperative of supranational cooperation to address contemporary regional and global challenges pertaining to climate change, pandemics, and the escalating fear of war in Europe.

Nevertheless, the early groundwork proved to be a fertile environment for the subsequent introduction and widespread acceptance of Foulkesian group analysis (Foulkes & Anthony, 1957; Foulkes, 1964; Pines, 1983), an approach that found deep resonance with core Norwegian cultural values (Schwartz, 2006; Gullestad, 1992). According to Schwartz, culture consists of enduring patterns of shared values and beliefs transmitted across generations. These cultural patterns deeply influence societal organizations, communications, and therapeutic practice (Schwartz 2006)

Today, Norway consistently ranks high in universal cultural values such as egalitarianism, autonomy, and harmony, while simultaneously exhibiting a low power distance index (Schwartz 2006). These deeply ingrained societal characteristics resonate with the fundamental principles of Foulkesian group analysis (Foulkes, 1964; Pines, 1983), which champion reciprocity, active participation, and democratic engagement. In group analysis, the therapist assumes a facilitative role, acting as a "conductor" rather than an authoritarian leader, guiding group dialogue and fostering shared reflection. This non-hierarchical stance is particularly compatible with Norwegian cultural norms that favor low power distance and a consensual, collective approach to decision making. This inherent cultural fit has, arguably, created exceptionally favorable conditions for the growth of group analysis throughout Norway. The ethos of the Norwegian welfare state, with its strong emphasis on collective solutions and robust social support networks, further reinforces the group analytic notion of the group itself serving as a vital holding structure for individual development and collective healing.

Contextual Perspective

Against this backdrop, the Norwegian group analytic community approached the adoption of Foulkesian group analysis with a nuanced perspective, driven by the imperative to adapt this therapeutic modality to distinct Norwegian contexts, fostering what might be termed "applied group analysis," while simultaneously contributing to its theoretical and practical evolution (Island in press, Karterud 2024). This approach rejected a rigid adherence to Foulkesian principles, viewing group analysis not as a dogma or static practice, but as a dynamic framework open to integration with other theoretical perspectives, such as self-psychology and mentalization-based theory. This integrative approach was exemplified by the 1999 EGATIN study days in Oslo, themed "*One Group Analysis or Many? The impact of theory on group analytic practice*," which facilitated a plurality of theoretical and practical perspectives.

While Foulkes' conceptualization of humans as social beings and his group analytic framework remain influential in Norway, there has been a consistent emphasis on adapting and modifying these principles for application within the Norwegian public mental health, without compromising core tenets.

The IGA's training model is distinguished by several key features:

- **Interdisciplinary Inclusion:** From its very inception, the training program was conceived to be interdisciplinary, ensuring that health care professionals directly involved in conducting group therapy received comprehensive and formalized education. This commitment to interdisciplinary training reflects a pragmatic recognition of the diverse clinical workforce engaged in group therapy as well as reflecting cultural values that de-emphasize hierarchical structure in Norway.
- **Block-Based Structure:** To effectively accommodate professionals hailing from all corners of the country, the IGA pioneered a block-based training format. Candidates convene five times annually for intensive extended weekend sessions, typically lasting three to four days. These immersive sessions encompass a blend of traditional training components, including self-experiential small groups, supervision, theoretical and literature review, and daily large groups. This structure minimizes travel burden and allows for concentrated learning experiences.
- **Modular and Adaptive Curriculum:** While the original vision was to train fully certified group analysts through a comprehensive five-year program, it became evident that the demands of public mental health services made

> it challenging for many candidates to fulfill such a lengthy commitment. In response, the IGA demonstrated adaptability by developing a modified, more flexible training pathway: a three-year applied group analytic psychotherapy track. However, from 2010 there was a significant decline in candidates seeking to become group analysts. And in 2014 IGA established an expert committee to consider health policy guidelines and needs in public mental health care, evaluate the prevalent training program, and suggest different models of adjustment to meet the needs of managers, training candidates, and above all, the needs of patient population (see Karterud et al., 2025 for a thorough description of these changes). Through many scrupulous, careful, and at times heated discussions, the committee came up with a new model. Since 2017, the training has been consolidated into a tiered certification structure to meet the diverse needs of individual candidates and their workplaces. For novices in the field, the training commences with a one-year introductory level, providing basic skills and theoretical grounding. Upon completion, candidates can advance to a two-year Level A, which qualifies them to work as group psychotherapists in various psychiatric institutional settings. An additional two years (Level B) and a diploma thesis (Island & Karterud, 2013) are both required for full qualification as a group analyst. In the new training program the candidates choose between two paths on Level B: the traditional path where they start their own slow-open analytic group with no definite ending, or they may choose to run an analytic long-term group together with a colleague and, in addition, conduct their own short-term analytic group. Both paths imply long-term analytic processes as well as starting one's own group. This implementation of the two paths has been a real achievement, and again there are many candidates who continue to Level B (Karterud et al., 2025).

As of today (2025) 265 group analysts have completed the 4–5 years training and written their diploma paper. These group analysts may undertake a one-year supervision training course, qualifying them to teach and supervise within the IGA. This tiered system ensures both accessibility and depth of training. Additionally, the institute provides specialized modules in Mentalization-Based Treatment (MBT), group therapy for drug and alcohol addiction, and focused short-term group therapy, showcasing its responsiveness to evolving clinical needs and contemporary therapeutic advancements.

Beyond its core training, the IGA also offers regional one-year programs with lectures and supervision for health personnel across the country, significantly broadening access to knowledge about group therapy in various contexts, including municipal health services. This program has been immensely popular and has run yearly in a different part of Norway since 1998. However, times are changing and sadly there have been too few applicants to run the program in 2025 and 2026. Less group psychotherapy and more psychoeducational courses are run in the public sector. IGA are again seeking to develop and adapt without losing our focus on helping groups to be helpful for individuals in need. In Norway, all doctors specializing in psychiatry (residents) must fulfill three years (105 hours) of psychotherapy supervision. The one-year introductory course at IGA is equal to one year of psychotherapy supervision. In addition, all psychiatric residents must complete a two-day introduction to group psychotherapy. These introductory courses receive highly positive evaluations and may be one reason why there are quite a few psychiatrists becoming group analysts (125 out of a total of 337 group analysts). The national focus and all the specialized offerings highlight IGA's commitment to broad dissemination and clinical relevance.

- **National Reach and Specialized Offerings:** The deliberate decision to name the institute "IGA Norway" rather than "IGA Oslo" reflects a significant post-war political ambition to foster national unity by bridging urban and rural regions and ensuring equitable access to professional training nationwide. This was especially important in making group therapy accessible for patients around the country, not only for those living in the main cities, and thus gaining a solid stand and reputation within the public health system and in line with political guidelines. By establishing a national institute, we were able to gather expertise and resources instead of having several local institutes competing with each other.

Current Practice and Clinical Innovation

Group analytic psychotherapy is widely and robustly practiced across both public and private sectors in Norway. In public outpatient clinics, therapists frequently conduct long-term groups, often specifically tailored for patients with personality disorders. Conversely, private practitioners may offer "slow-open" groups characterized by heterogeneous memberships. Group sessions typically occur on a weekly basis for 90 minutes, and can be either open-ended or time-limited, commonly spanning one-and-a-half to three years.

Psychiatric day hospitals have historically been central to the provision of long-term group therapy, particularly for patients diagnosed with personality disorders. The Norwegian Day Hospital Network, established in 1992, further exemplifies clinical innovation and collaboration in group therapy (Karterud et al., 2025). Comprised of highly specialized clinicians, including group analysts, this network was founded on the recognition of a critical need for collaboration in quality assurance, knowledge exchange, research, and development. Over time, these day units evolved into dedicated group treatment units, characterized by close collaboration in clinical practice and, notably, a robust commitment to research. This collaborative effort led to the creation of a substantial database on treatment outcomes, serving as a cornerstone for ongoing empirical research in the field. A significant proportion of patients treated within these group units presented with personality disorders. The preferred mode of group treatment in the different units of the network developed gradually towards MBT, often combined with individual psychotherapy. In addition, these units provided a range of group modalities for different clinical conditions (short-term, long-term, psychoeducational, trauma-focused, for ADHD, etc.). Research conducted within this network demonstrated that patients with borderline personality disorder had significantly better outcome in MBT programs that combined psychoeducation with group and individual treatment, compared to psychodynamic groups alone (Kvarstein et al., 2015). Reflecting this evolving clinical focus, the network formally changed its name to the "Network for Personality Disorders" in 2018.

Successful implementation in these settings, however, largely depends on the leadership possessing adequate group analytic training and insight, particularly given the complex relational dynamics inherent in treating patients with severe personality disorders.

Beyond long-term groups, short-term closed groups are also prevalent, targeting specific diagnostic categories such as ADHD, anxiety disorders, and trauma. These shorter interventions are more commonly found in outpatient and community mental health centers (CMHCs), reflecting a growing emphasis on focused and time-efficient treatments. Group therapy is also offered as part of on-going treatment programs to other patient groups, including drug and alcohol abuse, eating disorders, and in more acute settings in hospital wards. The setting varies greatly across the country and from clinic to clinic, but a common factor is that the treatment is getting shorter within the public sector, even for personality disorders.

A significant indicator of the widespread recognition and success of group therapy in Norway is a comprehensive 2022 government review of mental health services. This review, which solicited feedback from regional health authorities and district psychiatric centers, revealed that group-based treatment programs received the highest satisfaction ratings among 58 identified programs, underscoring its high level of recognition and appreciation within the Norwegian mental health care system (Regjeringen.no, 2023; Karterud et al., 2025).

The Institute for Group Analysis and Group Psychotherapy (IGA) in Norway currently benefits significantly from public funding provided by the Directorate of Health. This crucial financial support enables broad access to training and has been pivotal to the institute's institutional sustainability. This blessing also carries certain implicit conditions and potential constraints. Funding is often contingent upon alignment with national guidelines, which increasingly prioritize shorter, symptom-focused interventions. Awareness regarding this needs to be kept in mind in the continuing development of the institute. The IGA is committed to providing training that aligns with the needs of the health care system while still seeking to maintain fidelity to its analytic ideals and potentially risk funding cuts, rather than adapt its curriculum and potentially dilute its theoretical foundation.

Challenges and Evidence-based Practice

Despite the widespread acceptance and documented effectiveness of group analytic psychotherapy in Norway, it faces considerable challenges. These include increasing bureaucratic pressure to prioritize short-term, measurable treatments, a lack of trained colleagues in rural areas, courses rather than psychotherapy, and administrative overload for therapists. The shift toward more standardized, quantifiable outcomes in mental health services poses a threat to the nuanced and relationally anchored work that group analysis represents.

The evidence-based practice (EBP) movement, though conceptually supportive of integrated knowledge, has increasingly equated evidence with randomized controlled trials (RCTs) and short-term treatments. Sackett et al. (1997) originally defined EBP as the integration of clinical expertise with the best available evidence, emphasizing relevance and context. However, the current application of EBP often favors symptom-focused shorter interventions due to their compatibility with RCTs and structured outcome measures, rather than treatment intended to enhance personality development.

Despite these prevailing treatment guidelines and the pressures favoring shorter, manualized approaches, extensive group psychotherapeutic activity persists and thrives within Norwegian public mental health services. This is evidenced by the robust network of group therapeutic units, which continue to operate effectively. Practicing group analysts in Norway reveal a strong and unwavering commitment to group analysis, even in the face of institutional pressures.

A recent survey of 35 certified group analysts out of a total of 151 members in IGA indicated that the majority are actively involved in public mental health institutions, particularly in outpatient clinics and semi-private specialist services. Only a small minority of respondents worked exclusively in private financed practice, strongly underscoring the deep public-sector anchoring of the field in Norway. Group analysts in private practice typically work independently, conducting slow-open analytic groups that are heterogenic in nature regarding diagnoses, gender, and age. In contrast, group analysts in outpatient clinics reported that they often collaborate with colleagues in co-therapy, conducting time-limited slow-open groups, lasting one-and-a-half to three years. These groups mainly focus on personality disorders, particularly borderline and avoidant personality disorders. Treatment for personality disorders may include some form of psychoeducation before they start in modified psychodynamic groups, integrative treatment groups, or models developed specifically for these disorders like MBT. The survey indicates that some group analysts in private and outpatient settings also facilitate 22 sessions of Focused Group Analytic Psychotherapy as described by Lorentzen (2022).

The analysts in the survey frequently highlighted several systemic challenges, including insufficient support from management, difficulties in recruiting appropriate patients (especially men), and the pervasive marginalization of long-term therapies due to increasing efficiency demands. Many patients have received short-term interventions and seek longer treatments for relational and emotional difficulties. Therapists also express concern about a general lack of understanding among health administrators regarding the intricate mechanisms and benefits of group therapy. Some report working in professional isolation, with minimal collegial infrastructure for support and collaboration. Nevertheless, the responses in the survey reflect a strong professional identity and a profound commitment to the group analytic modality. Many therapists emphasize the personal and clinical value derived from participating in conferences, supervision groups, and engaging in academic reading. There is also a widely expressed need for more robust research evidence to secure legitimacy and effectively advocate for necessary resources. Particular interest lies in research exploring patient change processes, long-term outcomes, and comparative effectiveness studies of analytic versus manualized therapies. Overall, the responses reflect a mixture of pride, challenges, and aspirations regarding group psychotherapy practice, alongside a shared desire to enhance awareness and support for the effectiveness of group therapy within the mental health community.

Despite the methodological challenges inherent in conducting research on group analytic psychotherapy—given its distinct treatment focus and less direct emphasis on immediate symptom reduction—Norway has produced a notable body of research in this domain. Pioneering work, particularly by Steinar Lorentzen and his colleagues, has contributed extensively to the field. Lorentzen has published widely on both long-term and time-limited group analytic psychotherapy, focusing on critical aspects such as treatment effectiveness, dropout risk, and patient characteristics (Lorentzen, 2014, 2022). However, much of this valuable research remains largely unrecognized by health bureaucrats and guideline developers, further highlighting the ongoing struggle for recognition within the EBP paradigm.

Future Directions and Reflections

As the field of group analytic psychotherapy in Norway continues to evolve, several critical questions emerge that will shape its development in the years to come. The increasing integration of digital technologies into health care, including the advent of online group therapy, poses both opportunities and challenges for group analytic practice (Weinberg, 2025). While some therapists have begun experimenting with online formats, many express concern that the depth and immediacy of analytic processes may be compromised when group members are not physically present. During the COVID-19 pandemic from 2020 to 2022, IGA did not stop our training, and six of ten block sessions were run on digital platforms. This was a challenge, but most candidates expressed gratitude for the continued training through the demanding and grim period. Future research and practice development will need to explore how the core tenets of group analysis—such as resonance, containment, and transference—are maintained or altered in digital contexts.

Additionally, the demographic shifts in Norwegian society call for renewed attention to cultural competence in group analytic training and practice. As Norway becomes increasingly diverse, group therapists must be equipped to work across differences in ethnicity, religion, language, and social class. This also requires theoretical innovation, ensuring that group analytic frameworks are sufficiently inclusive and adaptable to pluralistic realities. Questions arise about how to address intergenerational trauma in immigrant communities, how to facilitate group cohesion in culturally heterogeneous settings, and how societal dynamics such as racism and marginalization may be mirrored and worked through in the group space. The Norwegian training program is still challenged to recruit a broader group of clinicians in terms of multicultural background.

Another pressing area is the integration of group analysis within interdisciplinary teams. As mental health services increasingly adopt collaborative models, group analysts must define their unique contributions while also finding common ground with professionals from other paradigms. This includes psychiatrists, clinical psychologists, social workers, nurses, and peer support workers. Clarifying the role of group analysis within these contexts can help solidify its standing and ensure that it complements rather than competes with other modalities.

Furthermore, the sustainability of public funding for long-term training programs remains uncertain. While the current support from the Department of Health and Human Services has enabled widespread access and institutional growth, economic pressures and shifting political priorities may threaten these resources. If public funding were to diminish, the field could risk a re-privatization of advanced training, making it accessible only to those who can afford it. This would run counter to the egalitarian spirit of group analysis as it has been developed in Norway. Consequently, the community must continue advocating for the value of long-term, relational therapies within public health discourse, emphasizing their preventative and transformative potential.

The generational transfer of knowledge and leadership within IGA Norway also represents an important issue. As many of the institute's founders and early contributors approach retirement, efforts must be made for the continual support of the next generation of analysts, educators, and researchers. This includes mentorship programs, scholarly collaboration, and support for early-career professionals to engage in academic publishing, supervision, and training roles. That is illustrated by the collaboration between the first, the third, and current directors in writing this paper.

Finally, the articulation of group analytic values in response to societal crises—including political polarization, ecological anxiety, and increasing mental health problems among youth—demands renewed reflection. Group analysis is uniquely positioned to address collective processes such as alienation, distrust, and fragmentation. It offers a language and a practice for rebuilding relational networks and fostering psychological resilience at both individual and systemic levels. As such, it may prove to be not only a clinical tool but a civic resource.

Conclusion

Norway's robust group therapy infrastructure exemplifies a well-integrated model that effectively bridges training, clinical practice, and research. Its success can be attributed, in large part, to several interwoven factors: the development of flexible and modular training programs meticulously aligned with pressing clinical demands, the cultivation of a research-informed clinical network, particularly effective in treating complex personality disorders, and the governmental recognition of group therapy's inherent values and thus the continuous economic funding from the Department of Health. In the future, these fundings will be increasingly connected to research findings. Economic support from mental health institutions will also depend on documented effect.

Nonetheless, the establishment and growth of the field have also depended on institutional entrepreneurship. Key psychiatrists such as Sigmund Karterud, Steinar Lorentzen, and the institute's long-serving general secretary Thor Kristian Island played pivotal roles. Through persistent professional engagement, promoting, academic publication, and curriculum development, these individuals secured funding, institutional legitimacy, and the integration of group analysis into national health policy.

The field of group analytic psychotherapy in Norway stands at a critical juncture. With its strong theoretical foundation, cultural compatibility, and institutional infrastructure, it is well positioned to meet emerging clinical and societal needs. However, this will require adaptive leadership, sustained advocacy, and a commitment to both innovation and tradition. The interplay between public health systems, academic research, and therapeutic communities will continue to shape the contours of group analysis in Norway—and possibly serve as a model for other countries seeking to embed relational, democratic, and depth-oriented therapies into their own mental health landscapes.

While analytic group psychotherapy remains often underutilized globally, Norway's experience demonstrates its potential as an important component of public mental health treatment. The Norwegian system has managed to institutionalize group therapy in a way that is both highly effective and sustainable, benefiting from a high level of public investment in mental health. How can the depth and relational richness of group analysis be preserved in an era increasingly driven by demands for efficiency? What compromises, if any, are acceptable in the name of evidence-based practice and short-term outcomes? And, crucially, can group analysis, in its fullest and most authentic sense, remain both broadly accessible and true to its core theoretical foundations amidst evolving health policy landscapes? Continued research is essential to further refine group therapy models, particularly in the context of emerging digital and hybrid care systems.

References

Foulkes, S.H. (1964). *Therapeutic Group Analysis.* London: George Allen & Unwin.

Foulkes, S.H., & Anthony, E.J. (1957). *Group Psychotherapy: The Psychoanalytic Approach.* London: Penguin.

Glenthøj, R. (2008). *En moderne nations fødsel: Norsk national identifikation hos embedsmænd og borgere 1807–1815* [*The Inception of a Modern Nation: Norwegian National Identification of Assets and Citizen 1807–1815*]. Odense: Syddansk Universitetsforlag.

Gullestad, M. (1992). *The Art of Social Relations: Essays on Culture, Social Action and Everyday Life in Modern Norway.* Oslo: Scandinavian University Press.

Hopper, E. (2003). *The Social Unconscious: Selected Papers.* London: Jessica Kingsley.

Hopper, E., & Weinberg, H. (Eds.) (2011). *The Social Unconscious in Persons, Groups and Societies, Vol 1: Mainly Theory.* London: Karnac.

Island, T.K. (2022). *IGA 1992–2022. 30 års suksesshistorie* [30 years success story]. http://fliphtml5.com/bxvnu/rasg/basic.

Island, T.K., & Karterud, S. (2013). From group analytic practice to group analytic text: On writing a group analytic diploma paper. *Group Analysis*, 46, 439–451.

Island, T.K. (2020). Norway: Between grandiosity and inferiority. In A. Zajenkowska & U. Levin (Eds.), *A Psychoanalytic and Socio-Cultural Exploration of a Continent: Europe on the Couch.* London: Routledge.

Island, T.K. (in press). Norway: National reach, international roots, and the Norwegian model of group analytic training. In V. Harte (Ed.), *Group Analysis Across Borders: Dialogues on Culture, History, and Transformation.* London: Karnac.

Jones, M. (1952). *Social Psychiatry: A study of Therapeutic Communities.* London: Tavistock.

Jones, M. (1968). *Beyond the Therapeutic Community.* New Haven: Yale University Press.

Jones, M. (1979). The therapeutic community, social learning and social change. In R.D. Hinshelwood & N. Manning (Eds.), *Therapeutic Communities.* London: Routledge.

Karterud S. (1989). Group processes in therapeutic communities. Doctoral dissertation, University of Oslo.

Karterud, S. (2024). *Group Analysis: A Modern Synthesis.* London: Routledge.

Karterud, S., Ness Bjerke, S., Normann-Eide, T., & Ulland, A. (2025). Group treatment is favoured by Norwegian mental health leaders. *Group Analysis.* doi:10.1177/05333164241300693

Kvarstein, E., Pedersen, G., Urnes, Ø., Hummelen, B., Wilberg, T., & Karterud, S. (2015). Changing from a traditional psychodynamic treatment programme to mentalization-based treatment for patients with borderline personality disorder. Does it make a difference? *Psychology and Psychotherapy: Theory, Research and Practice*, 88(1), 71–86.

Lorentzen, S. (2014). *Group Analytic Psychotherapy.* London: Routledge.

Lorentzen, S. (2022). *Focused Group Analytic Psychotherapy: An Integration of Clinical Experience and Research.* London and New York: Routledge.

Main, T. (1946). The hospital as a therapeutic institution. *Bulletin of the Menninger Clinic*, 10, 66–70.

Main, T. (1957). The ailment. *British Journal of Medical Psychology*, 30, 127–145.

Pines, M. (1983). *Reflections on Group Analysis*. London: Routledge.

Regjeringen.no. (2023). Rapport om tematisk organisering av psykisk helsehjelp. Seewww.regjeringen.no/no/dokumenter/fornkle-og-forbedre-rapport-om-tematisk-organisering-av-psykisk-helsevern/id2993928/?ch=1.

Sackett, D.L., Richardson, W.S., Rosenberg, W., Haynes, B.R. et al. (1997). *Evidence-Based Medicine: How to Practice and Teach EBM*. London: Churchill Livingstone.

Schwartz, S.H. (2006). A theory of cultural value orientations: Explication and applications. *Comparative Sociology*, 5(2), 137–182.

Vaglum, P., Friis, S., Jorstad, J., Karterud, S., & Lorentzen, S. (1982). From a panacea to a special treatment method. *The International Journal of Therapeutic Communities*, 1, 24–32.

Voyatzaki, Z. (2006). On the history of EGATIN. *Group Analysis*, 39, 108–120.

Weinberg, H. (2007). So, what is this Social Unconscious Anyway? *Group Analysis*, 40(3), 307–322.

Weinberg, H. (2025). Resistance to online group analysis – is there anything new under the sun? *Group Analysis*, 58(1): 49–69.

Chapter 10

Group Analysis in Lithuania

Historical Roots and Contemporary Practice

Ilona Laurinaitytė, Eugenijus Laurinaitis and Rūta Klimašauskienė

Introduction

Group psychotherapy is an important form of therapy that significantly contributes to the accessibility of mental health services, particularly by offering effective support to diverse population groups (Whittingham et al., 2021). According to a report by the American Psychological Association, group therapy is as effective as individual therapy in treating various issues and, in some cases, may even be more effective than individual psychotherapy (Pappas, 2023). Currently, there is a wide range of group therapy approaches, which vary not only in their theoretical frameworks but also in practical application models and professional training standards. However, the cognitive-behavioural therapy (CBT) paradigm has received the most attention in scientific literature, often being associated with particularly high therapeutic effectiveness. However, research findings also indicate that other therapeutic approaches, such as psychodynamic group therapy, can be equally effective (Glicken & Robinson, 2013). Moreover, the lack of scientific studies evaluating the efficacy of group analysis and analytic/dynamic group psychotherapy highlights the need for further research using both qualitative and quantitative methods (Blackmore et al., 2009). Accordingly, this chapter aims to provide an overview of the emergence of group analysis in Lithuania, the specific features and challenges of specialist training, with a particular focus on the characteristics of applied psychoanalysis training programmes. The chapter also discusses the specific nature of the work conducted by psychodynamic group psychotherapists and group analysts, as well as their perspectives on the future of group therapy.

Historical and Cultural Contexts of Group Analysis Development in Lithuania

Group analysis is a form of psychoanalytic psychotherapy that examines the relationships between individuals and their social networks. In Lithuania, its foundations are largely based on the ideas of S.H. Foulkes and his followers.

DOI: 10.4324/9781003597674-10

The history of group analysis in the country begins with the first contacts with the founders of the European Group Analytic Training Network (EGATIN) in 1989 in Amsterdam. This connection was established (by one of the authors of this chapter, E.L.) during the 11th International Congress of Group Psychotherapy.

After the initial contact, efforts began to find group analysts who could come to Lithuania to introduce local professionals to this branch of psychotherapy. The first to respond to the invitation was Raymond Blake from London, a passionate enthusiast for expanding group analysis to Eastern Europe. In the summer of 1991, he conducted the first multi-day seminar on group analysis in Vilnius, focusing on theoretical concepts and practical applications. A year later, he was joined by Rita Lynn, a Lithuanian-born and fluent Lithuanian-speaking group analyst. These seminars prompted the establishment of a group analysis section within the Lithuanian Group Psychotherapy Association (LGPA), which studied theoretical literature and conducted group intervisions[1] for several years. This section consistently involved around a dozen professionals, and this enduring interest led EGATIN to organise one of its "Study Days" in Vilnius in June 1992. Notable representatives of this approach participated in the event: Malcolm Pines and Sylvia Hutchinson from London, Werner Knauss from Heidelberg, Rudi Olivieri Larsson from Zurich, Jerzy Pawlik from Warsaw, Tore Kristian Island, and Steinar Lorentzen from Oslo.

For several years, a training project was coordinated with the Institute of Group Analysis in Norway (IGA-Norway), whose representatives expressed a commitment to start training. Steinar Lorentzen contributed especially to this project's success, securing funding from the Norwegian Psychiatry Development Fund for the first training year in Vilnius. S. Lorentzen, authorised by the IGA-Norway, began supervising this programme for professionals from all the Baltic countries. A local organisational committee was formed in Lithuania to handle the main organisational and coordination tasks in the Baltic countries. In the fall of 1995, a group of 30 candidates from Lithuania, Latvia, and Estonia began introductory training in group analysis in Vilnius. In 1997, further funding was secured from the Nordic Council, and the training continued into an advanced (second) level.

Additionally, from 1998, the IGA-Norway invited the first Lithuanian group analysts to teach in the course, which subsequently took place under the postgraduate training framework of Vilnius University. Since 2002, the entire course has been conducted in Lithuanian by Lithuanian professionals.

It should be noted that, at that time, group therapy was quite a rare phenomenon in the Baltic states, partly due to cultural norms of privacy and emotional restraint. Many people felt uncomfortable discussing personal issues in front of others, while the distrust that had taken root during the years of Soviet occupation under conditions of enforced collectivism, where openness could once pose social or political risks, made self-disclosure difficult. On the one hand, the newly emerging psychoanalysis-based group therapy gradually became a space in which collective trauma could be identified and processed. On the other hand, this form of psychotherapy fostered an atmosphere of trust and cooperation. All trainers of the first stage (strictly Scandinavian) of group analysis training in Lithuania were the graduates from the courses conducted by group analysts from London – the first original training community in Europe. The importance of this fact was expressed in the strategic goals of this Baltic training programme, among others, to implement the democratic way of thinking and behaving both in therapy groups and in society at large. Considering the clusters of cultures described by Schwartz (2006), all three Baltic states should be included in the formerly Soviet-occupied states'[2] value system, but reality appeared to be more complicated, and all three nations differed a little in their values, especially concerning the learning and implementation of group analysis (GA) in practice. For example, Lithuania has always been the most homogeneous country in terms of ethnicity (even today, ethnic Lithuanians make up 85% of the country's population, while Estonians make up 69% in Estonia and 62% Latvians in Latvia). In addition, historically, Roman Catholicism predominated in Lithuania, whereas Lutheranism/Protestantism was more characteristic of Estonia and Latvia. These religious differences, in turn, have a significant influence on prevailing values, particularly with regard to tendencies toward individualism or collectivism, concepts of autonomy, and the importance of social context. On the other hand, the values and behaviour of the Scandinavian teachers were not exactly typically Nordic but carried some important part of the English value system. In conclusion, at the beginning of group analysis training and practice in the Baltics, a complex mixture of values and professional standards existed.

On the other hand, since the very beginning of training in group analysis, the theory and literature were based on Foulkes' texts and ideas. Until now, the primary source of literature has been English-language texts, with some minor additions of presentations from EGATIN Study Groups, Lithuanian Group Analysis Society conferences, and articles from the *Journal of Group Analysis.* This specificity demonstrates itself when compared to e.g. Austrian, German, Italian, or American approaches while reading literature and/or discussing in person.

Currently, theoretical and practical group analysis training in Lithuania is conducted at two levels: initial qualification level and advanced qualification level. Considering all organisational and financial challenges, this training project is a successful attempt to implement group analysis among the Baltic countries.

In 1999, an independent Lithuanian Group Analytic Society (LGAS) was established, taking on active organisational and promotional roles to popularise group analysis and unite practising professionals. LGAS organises several activities, including annual summer schools focused on group analysis. These summer schools are held biannually in Lithuanian and biannually in English.

Group Psychotherapy Training Programmes Implemented by LGAS

Currently, the LGAS, in collaboration with Vilnius University, offers several training programmes for professionals working with groups: the Psychodynamic Group Psychotherapy Programme, the Group Analysis Programme, and the Programme for Working with Adult Groups in Organisations.

These training programmes are organised in blocks, five blocks per academic year. The length of each block is three days, usually from Thursday to Saturday. All mentioned training programmes are delivered in the Lithuanian language. In addition to block training sessions, participants of all training programmes are required to complete a specified number of intervision hours. Intervisions are peer groups in which work cases from psychotherapeutic or organisational practice (depending on the study programme) are discussed among peers, without a supervisor. Intervision groups bring together students from different courses; the intervision groups for Group Analysis and Group Psychotherapy participants are shared, while those enrolled in the Working with Adult Groups in Organisations programme usually form separate intervision groups.

All programmes' activities take place during the same block. Participants attend supervision sessions and theoretical lectures according to their respective programmes. Students from different programmes share the same small groups, while all participants join together in a common large group. For participants in the Working with Adult Groups in Organisations programme, this is an excellent opportunity to understand how psychotherapist programme participants view the same processes and behave in various group situations, and to learn from their experience. Participants of the Working with Adult Groups in Organisations programme learn to recognise and understand subconscious processes and psychodynamic phenomena and factors when working with groups. Group Analysis and Group Psychotherapy training programmes are also enriched by the opportunity to learn with a more diverse range of participants, coming not only from a clinical background, but from a much broader context. This brings more diversity to the training programmes and enriches them with different perspectives and a variety of experiences.

The Psychodynamic Group Psychotherapy Programme (a four-year course of study) is intended for medical specialists and residents, psychologists with a master's degree, as well as professionals with master's degrees in social work or nursing who are interested in working with groups and understanding group processes. The programme aims to provide both theoretical and practical training to prepare psychodynamic group psychotherapists for independent professional practice within health care institutions.

The Group Analysis Training Programme (two years of study) aims to provide both theoretical and practical preparation for specialists in group analysis. It prepares them to work independently in psychotherapeutic analytic groups within psychiatric or medical institutions, applying the theory and methods of group analysis. Admission to this programme is open to individuals who have successfully completed the Psychodynamic Group Psychotherapy Programme.

The Programme for Working with Adult Groups in Organisational Settings (three years of study) aims to equip participants with the skills required to work with employee groups in non-clinical organisations, drawing on both analytic and systemic approaches.

The Programme for Working with Adult Groups in Organisational Settings did not emerge immediately. When the training programme for group psychotherapists was being developed and implemented in Lithuania, it included an introductory course as part of its structure. This one-year introductory study programme was intended for individuals interested in the field of psychodynamic group psychotherapy but lacking the necessary professional qualifications. This study format proved popular among participants, and the training programme was able to meet their needs. This programme offers a wide range of opportunities for specialists and managers in various fields, from training lecturers working individually with adult groups, organisational consultants, internal training specialists, and human resources specialists to managers of organisations or their divisions.

It was observed that, after completing these foundational courses, participants often felt inspired to deepen their expertise in the field, with some pursuing studies in psychology or social work. Moreover, within the Psychodynamic Group Psychotherapy Programme, there were some participants who were employed in organisational rather than clinical settings, and the requirement to lead clinical groups presented challenges for them. Thus, the idea for the organisational programme emerged as a response to two key needs: to support these professionals in further developing their qualifications for working with groups, and to offer them the opportunity – through personal experience in small groups – to gain a deeper understanding of themselves, of others, and of how groups function.

The first Programme for Working with Adult Groups in Organisational Settings cohort was launched in 2014. The model for this programme was drawn from the Nordic countries (such as Denmark and Norway). Its initial structure closely resembled the psychotherapist and analyst training programmes: theoretical lectures, supervision, small therapeutic groups, a large group, and intervision.

Over time, the structure of the programme for Working with Adult Groups in Organisations evolved naturally. The teaching team expanded, and new formats were introduced, including seminars, organisational observation, and an increasing amount of literature focused on organisational contexts. The training content progressively aligned more closely with the needs of professionals working with groups in organisational settings: strengthening self-awareness and awareness of others through experiential learning, gaining deeper insight into group processes and systemic approaches, and making sense of one's role as a leader or group facilitator. These developments reflected the programme's capacity for reflection and transformation, continuously identifying effective and ineffective practices and adapting them accordingly.

Development of the Training Programme on Working with Adult Groups in Organisations

During the preparation of this article, five expert interviews were conducted with individuals closely involved in the Programme for Working with Adult Groups in Organisational Settings. Three of the experts were current or former teachers and/or members of the programme's training committee, while the remaining two were graduates of the organisational programme.

Interviews with the programme's teachers revealed that the initial stages of the organisational programme were challenging and marked by uncertainty and anxiety within the teaching team. A key concern was what meaningful contributions psychotherapists could offer to professionals working with groups in organisational settings. A narcissistic phenomenon was also experienced – anxiety about the potential failure of the programme and the difficulty of attracting participants. This manifested as resistance to the programme among some teachers. However, over time, the programme grew, became successful, and attracted a steady interest from participants. The teaching team's confidence strengthened, and the outcomes of the programme demonstrated that psychoanalytic knowledge about group work could be extremely valuable, extending far beyond the boundaries of clinical practice.

The first graduates of the Programme for Working with Adult Groups in Organisational Settings completed their studies in 2016. Between that time and 2025, a total of 30 participants have completed the programme. As of 2025, the current ratio of applicants to the organisational programme compared to psychotherapy programmes is approximately 4:1, i.e., four candidates apply to the organisational programme for every one candidate applying to the psychotherapeutic and/or psychoanalytic programmes. This growing interest is also reflected in the current participant ratio across first-year cohorts, which stands at around 3:1 in favour of the organisational programme. At the time of this analysis in 2025, 28 trainees are enrolled in the organisational programme, 18 in the group psychotherapy programme, and five in the group analysis programme. From 2013 to 2025, the following number of participants have completed the psychotherapy and group analysis programmes: 56 graduates from the group psychotherapy programme and 23 graduates from the group analysis programme.

The successful implementation of the organisational programme demonstrates that it not only meets a need for knowledge but also creates value and provides practical benefits. Interviews with programme graduates revealed a clear consensus regarding the usefulness of the studies for self-awareness and personal growth. Participants reported a deeper understanding and internalisation of their roles within groups, alongside a greater capacity to recognise and comprehend group processes. Moreover, the studies are experiential and closely linked to practice and personal experience, rather than being limited to the analysis of theoretical knowledge. As a result, participants learn to view group processes from multiple perspectives: through lived experience, interpersonal connections, and the dynamics between group members and groups themselves. This fosters curiosity and a desire to explore what is happening within groups more deeply.

The interviewed experts emphasised that, during the course of these studies, participants develop and experience deep, supportive relationships. This is considered one of the programme's added values, as it helps participants find greater meaning in their professional activities. Another key strength of the programme is its openness to professionals from diverse fields, creating broad opportunities for sharing different experiences. However, this diversity also presents challenges, particularly in managing and balancing the varied expectations, needs, and capacities of participants from such a wide range of professional backgrounds.

An important aspect of programme implementation is that some curriculum components are shared among participants from all specialisations, such as small group sessions, large group sessions, and theoretical lectures. For students of the organisational programme, this provides an excellent opportunity to gain insight into how those enrolled in psychotherapy programmes perceive the same processes, and to learn from their experience. Participants in the organisational programme are trained to recognise and understand unconscious processes and psychodynamic phenomena in group work. The fact that they gain knowledge of subjects typically studied by psychotherapists, such as human development, defence mechanisms, personal and group psychodynamics, and more, is highly valuable. The unique feature, appeal, and benefit of the organisational programme lies in offering precisely this type of knowledge, rather than more conventional managerial content (e.g., marketing, strategy). The psychotherapy and psychoanalytic training programmes are enriched by the opportunity to learn alongside a diverse group of participants from both clinical and broader professional contexts. This brings greater diversity into the learning process and enhances the programmes through varied perspectives and shared experiences. In recent years, discussions have emerged regarding the future of these study programmes, particularly around attracting a wider audience. However, while expanding access is desirable, there is a risk of over-commercialising the programmes, which could diminish their distinctiveness and value, particularly the deeply personal experiential component that is central to their impact. Furthermore, the current organisational, psychodynamic group psychotherapy, and group analysis programmes are supported by a large teaching team (currently comprising 22 instructors). Expanding the programmes would therefore also require expanding the teaching staff, which presents challenges in terms of finding and recruiting suitably qualified professionals.

The aspect of adapting the programme for a broader circle of potential participants raises several related questions. Despite the programme's evident value, experts note that there is still a considerable degree of caution and even certain apprehensions among managers about enrolling in it. In the experts' view, a manager must be highly mature to join this programme, as it tends to expose and reveal deeper layers of one's personality. Managers come seeking knowledge but receive much more in practice – self-awareness, the experience of forming and maintaining deep interpersonal connections. Nevertheless, this process of self-discovery is often challenging and not without pain.

A broader context influencing this caution involves the country's and society's cultural and value dimensions. According to Schwartz (2006), the values emphasised by a society are a crucial factor in understanding its culture, while culture itself forms the core that shapes a society's beliefs, perceptions, practices, norms, and institutions. Research based on Hofstede's cultural dimensions indicates that Lithuanian society tends to be individualistic (Dülmer et al., 2023; Mockaitis, 2002). According to Schwartz's (2006) value scale, *affective autonomy* is a value orientation associated with this dimension, indicating that greater emphasis is placed on individual perspectives and opinions rather than on the group. Another dimension that complements this aspect of individualism is the tendency toward *egalitarianism* – concern for others and their well-being. Lithuania's score on this dimension is somewhat lower compared to other countries (35th out of 50) (Mockaitis, 2018). These broader contextual factors and the prevailing tendency toward individualism may also serve as unconscious barriers to engaging more deeply with the topic of group psychodynamics.

Institutional governance of the programmes presents yet another future challenge. At present, various psychotherapy training programmes representing different approaches are being implemented in Lithuania, either by various institutions or by different departments within the same institutions. A significant number of teachers work across multiple psychotherapy training programmes, e.g., in both group psychotherapy and individual psychotherapy training. From an institutional governance perspective, there is potential for greater integration of these programmes, which could involve unifying teaching teams and pooling administrative resources. Such consolidation would also contribute to a more systematic and coherent implementation of psychotherapy training programmes on a national scale.

In summary, the training programmes implemented by the LGAS contribute significantly to promoting the idea and value of group psychotherapy not only among professionals but also in the broader society. These programmes help foster a more positive general attitude towards psychotherapeutic groups and reduce prevailing stereotypes that view group work as difficult, complex, or incomprehensible.

Overview of the Practice of Psychodynamic Group Therapists and Analysts

In order to explore the specific characteristics of psychodynamic group therapy and group analysis practice in Lithuania, an online survey was conducted among professionals leading such groups. The survey included 19 psychotherapists (representing 25.7% of LGAS members), of whom nearly three-quarters (74%) were women. The majority of participants (79%) were between the ages of 36 and 65, while the remaining respondents were evenly split between younger and older age groups. The surveyed specialists obtained their group psychotherapist qualifications between 1994 and 2024, with an average of 15.7 years of experience in psychotherapeutic group work. It is worth noting that nearly half of the respondents (47%) qualified for group analysis.

Regarding the characteristics of the groups, it was observed that all survey participants conducted sessions lasting 90 minutes. For the majority (94%) of the groups, sessions are held once a week. Notably, nearly one-third of the specialists (31.6%) lead more than one group. In most groups (68%), the number of clients ranges from 6 to 8, while in other cases it varies from 5 to 12. The duration of the groups also varies greatly, from 6 months to 25 years. Most groups (89%) take place in private practice settings, where clients pay for therapy using personal funds. Payment practices for group therapy sessions are diverse; however, the most common arrangements include payment at the end of each month for that month's sessions (63%) or payment in advance for the upcoming month (21%).

Among the most commonly reported issues presented by group participants, specialists identified neurotic, affective, and personality disorders, as well as relational difficulties, loneliness, and psychosomatic problems. The vast majority of psychotherapists did not combine group psychotherapy with other individual treatment methods (e.g., MBT – Mentalisation-Based Therapy, DBT – Dialectical Behaviour Therapy, CBT – Cognitive Behaviour Therapy, etc.). However, some clients were taking medication prescribed by another specialist. A few respondents noted that they had recommended EMDR (Eye Movement Desensitisation and Reprocessing) therapy or applied the CAMS approach (Collaborative Assessment and Management of Suicidality) in cases involving suicide risk.

It should be noted that all psychotherapists are confronted with the collective trauma caused by the Soviet occupation, which continues to influence societal values, particularly in the context of Russia's aggression against Ukraine. The invasion has revived old fears of losing freedom but has also strengthened national resilience, solidarity, and commitment to democratic values. Psychotherapists in our country are increasingly addressing these inherited wounds, linking personal healing with collective memory and the restoration of an authentic cultural identity.

When asked about the advantages of this form of psychotherapy, group therapists emphasised its effectiveness and therapeutic value for the majority of clients. Particularly encouraging are the long-lasting changes observed in clients who have completed therapy. The primary reason individuals seek group therapy is a disrupted relationship with themselves and with others. Within the group setting, a wide range of intense emotions and behavioural patterns emerges, allowing individuals to explore and better understand their difficulties and strengths in the "here and now" through interaction with others. This process facilitates the working through and reorganisation of traumatic experiences. Specialists highlighted the power of the group as a whole, the potential for universal experiences, a sense of belonging, and the diverse manifestations of projection and transference. Once a positive bond has formed, the relational experience within the group can be stronger than in individual therapy, and group members particularly value the support they receive from one another. Clients are able to reflect collectively and inspiringly on their contribution to group dynamics and receive broader feedback. Feedback from peers within the group often resonates differently and is easier for clients to accept. A significant advantage of group therapy is its cost-effectiveness, for it is generally less expensive than individual therapy, which not everyone can afford. Furthermore, it allows for support to be provided to a larger number of individuals at the same time.

Fewer disadvantages of group therapy were identified, with most of them relating to challenges in participant selection. On the one hand, group therapy is not suitable for all clients, for instance, those with pronounced personality disorders or individuals currently in crisis. On the other hand, it can be difficult to foster participants' motivation to commit to long-term attendance, as therapeutic change tends to occur gradually. Moreover, explaining the value of exploring unconscious processes is often challenging, particularly as the significance of such work may not be immediately evident to those without a professional background. Nonetheless, these issues can be significantly reduced by emphasising the careful selection of future group participants, providing education about the process, and actively supporting and encouraging participant motivation.

Specialists also identified several challenges encountered in the course of leading group therapy sessions. One of the most significant issues was the difficulty in attracting new group participants, particularly due to problems in disseminating information about group therapy. The challenge was ensuring visibility within today's overwhelming flow of information. It was also noted that psychodynamic group therapy, in general, struggles to compete with approaches such as CBT or other methods that promise rapid and tangible results. In addition, some specialists reported challenges related to their own competencies, for instance, the sudden shift to online therapy during the COVID-19 pandemic, a completely new mode of working for which they were unprepared; a lack of experience with specific patient groups; issues related to maintaining confidentiality in small towns; the limited availability of professional literature in Lithuanian; and the absence of a publicly accessible list of qualified supervisors.

The role of the LGAS is regarded as significant both in training psychodynamic group therapists and analysts, and in representing the interests of its members within various professional organisations. LGAS also plays a key role in organising national and international conferences and events in the field of group analysis. In doing so, it contributes to ensuring the quality of training programmes, supports continuing professional development, and helps sustain the professional identity of its members. At the same time, particular emphasis is placed on the informal dimension of LGAS membership, which fosters a sense of community, provides peer support, and encourages the sharing of professional experience.

In summary, the specialists noted that a great deal of meaningful work has been accomplished over the past three decades, resulting in the development and ongoing implementation of an excellent training programme for group therapists. This programme integrates not only psychotherapists working in clinical practice but also professionals employed in organisational settings. In doing so, it helps to promote a culture of tolerant, dynamic thinking across various social groups. Nonetheless, concerns were expressed regarding the persistent difficulty in attracting new candidates. Among the many psychotherapy programmes available in Lithuania, this one is rarely the first choice, and group therapy continues to be valued less than individual therapy. Despite this, the specialists who participated in the survey expressed faith and hope that the programme for training group therapists in this approach will continue to thrive and gain wider recognition among professionals. It is also encouraging that analytic group psychotherapy is becoming increasingly accessible to a broader population in Lithuania, and that patients can now receive group therapy funded by the national health insurance system.

Notes

1 Intervision is the discussion of cases in a group of peers, while maintaining confidentiality and professional ethics. Usually, the intervision group is 5–8 participants. During intervisions, they share their cases, link theoretical and practical aspects of their work, and try to find ways to address the professional difficulties they've faced in the shared case. Each group member can share their opinion, thoughts, and feelings related to the case discussed.

2 Although Schwartz (2006) originally used the term "*post-Soviet*" to describe the value system, this designation may be misleading in reference to Lithuania and the other Baltic countries, as it does not accurately reflect their historical experience (Sagatienė, 2023). These states did not voluntarily join the Soviet Union but were incorporated as a result of occupation, accompanied by widespread repression and genocide.

References

Blackmore, C., Beecroft, C., Parry, G., Booth, A., Tantum, D., Chambers, E., Simpson, E., Roberts, S., & Saxon, D. (2009). *A Systematic Review of the Efficacy and Clinical Effectiveness of Group Analysis and Analytic/Dynamic Group Psychotherapy.* Sheffield: University of Sheffield, Centre for Psychological Services Research, School of Health and Related Research.

Dülmer, H., Schwartz, S. H., Cieciuch, J., Davidov, E., & Schmidt, P. (2023). Testing Schwartz's model of cultural value orientations in Europe with the European social survey. *Survey Research Methods*, 17 (4), 447–417. doi:10.18148/srm/2023.v17i4.8031.

Glicken, M.D., & Robinson, B.C. (2013). Treating work-related problems. In M.D. Glicken, & B.C. Robinson (Eds.), *Treating Worker Dissatisfaction During Economic Change* (pp. 201–218). Cambridge, MA: Academic Press. doi:10.1016/b978-0-12-397006-0.00011-7.

Mockaitis, A.I. (2002). The national cultural dimensions of Lithuania. *Ekonomika*, 59, 67–77. doi:10.15388/Ekon.2002.17007.

Mockaitis, A.I. (2018). A portrait of Lithuanian societal values. https://mockaitis.com/2018/08/16/a-portrait-of-lithuanian-societal-values/.

Pappas, S. (2023). Group therapy is as effective as individual therapy and more efficient. Here's how to do it successfully. *Monitor on Psychology*, 54(2). www.apa.org/monitor/2023/03/continuing-education-group-therapy.

Sagatienė, D. (2023). Challenging the 'post-Soviet' label and colonial mindsets: NATO summit in Vilnius. *Verfassungsblog: On Matters Constitutional*, July 11, 2023. doi:10.17176/20230711-231150-0.

Schwartz, S.H. (2006). A theory of cultural value orientations: Explication and applications. *Comparative Sociology*, 5(2–3), 137–182. doi:10.1163/156913306778667357.

Whittingham, M., Lefforge, N.L., & Marmarosh, C. (2021). Group psychotherapy as a speciality: An inconvenient truth. *American Journal of Psychotherapy*, 74(2), 60–66. doi:10.1176/appi.psychotherapy.20200037.

Chapter 11

The State of Group Analysis in Greece Today

Apostolis Angelopoulos, Eirini Ioannovich and Margarita Kritikou

Greek Society

Greek society has been undergoing rapid changes over the past few decades. In less than three generations, Greece shifted from a traditional agrarian economy – where small family holdings and strong kinship bonds formed the core of social life – to a society dominated by urbanization and the service sector. In the 1960s, nearly half of all Greeks worked in agriculture; today agricultural production accounts for less than 4%, while the service sector – led by tourism, transport, and financial services – constitutes 80% of economic activity.

Urbanization proceeded at a rapid pace: hundreds of thousands left the countryside for major urban centres – especially Athens (now home to more than 35% of the Greek population) and Thessaloniki – or emigrated abroad.

This transition was not only economic but also profoundly social, reshaping lifestyles, family structures, and collective identities.

The family, once a productive and collective unit, gradually evolved into a more nuclear, consumer-oriented one. Women increasingly entered education and the labour market, playing an increasingly active role in social life and transforming social roles that had seemed immutable for centuries.

The development of the welfare state from the 1980s expanded access to education, health care, and social benefits. At the same time, increased access to higher education gave rise to new expectations of upward mobility.

Greek society also shifted toward more consumerist and individualistic ways of life: housing, cars, leisure services, and, later, technology became markers of social status. However, the severe financial crisis of the 2010s starkly revealed the instability of this model, with soaring unemployment (especially among young people), a dramatic decline in incomes, and an intensified "brain drain" toward other countries. The crisis shook people's trust in political institutions, rekindled old social traumas associated with the post-Civil War divisions (1946–49), heightened social insecurity, and further strained family bonds and social identities.

DOI: 10.4324/9781003597674-11

Although economic indicators have gradually improved, Greek society – deeply scarred by the crisis and the subsequent COVID-19 pandemic – continues to struggle toward recovery. It is a society in transition, a society in search of meaning.

Greek Mental Health Policy and Practice

The mental health system in Greece has also undergone gradual transformation since the 1980s. Forty years ago, the national network of services was rudimentary and inadequate, operating under poor conditions. The Hellenic Psychiatric Reform was launched as a national programme to establish community psychiatry, close large psychiatric hospitals, and deinstitutionalize long-term patients. While this reform modernized infrastructure and created new services, the main emphasis was placed on discharging patients rather than a robust network of community services (Anargyros et al., 2021).

The decade of economic recession and financial crisis (2009–19) further undermined progress. Between 2010 and 2019, per capita health care expenditure in Greece fell by nearly 30%. In 2010, Greek per capita health spending was about 70% of the European average, but by 2019 it had dropped to less than 50%. According to the OECD (2021), Greece also allocates a smaller share of its health budget to mental health compared to other European countries (3.9% vs. 6.7%).

Workforce capacity shows a strong reliance on psychiatrists, with higher availability than the EU average (0.26 vs. 0.18 per 1,000 population). However, the numbers for mental health nurses (0.13 vs. 0.52) and psychologists (0.09 vs. 0.53) are far lower. This imbalance reflects the continued dominance of the biomedical model in the public mental health system.

A recent study confirms that Greece performs poorly on essential service indicators such as integration of mental health into primary care, implementation of policies, prevention strategies, and data collection (Kotsis et al., 2024). Before the COVID-19 pandemic, approximately 19% of the population experienced a mental health condition – the third-highest rate in the European Union (OECD, 2023).

Patterns of service use further highlight systemic gaps. Outpatient prescriptions for psychotropic drugs doubled between 2015 and 2021, with prescriptions for antidepressants nearly tripling. At the same time, unmet needs are slightly above the European average (70% vs. 67.2%), largely due to financial barriers, long waiting times, and transportation difficulties. Access to services remains limited: only 4.1 per 1,000 people use public mental health services compared to an EU average of 31.5 per 1,000. This discrepancy is due to the undermining of public mental health services and the fact that the overwhelming majority of mental health needs are ultimately addressed in the private sector, which remains difficult to monitor.

The burden of poor mental health is particularly evident among younger generations. Surveys show that 38.9% of people aged 17–24 and 25% of those aged 25–39 identify mental health as their most pressing concern (Kolostasis, 2022).

It is evident that the public mental health system in Greece primarily deals with severe mental pathologies while failing to meet the broader and growing mental health needs of the population. Public services remain underfunded, fragmented, and overly reliant on the biomedical model.

Psychoanalysis is not recognized as a principal therapeutic model or part of the official mental health network in Greece. Naturally, this applies to Group Analysis as well. Recent research shows that the presence of psychoanalytic psychotherapy in Greek institutions, despite its introduction in the 1950s, is often situational and highly dependent on the dedication and efforts of individual professionals and/or specialist teams (Panagiotopoulou, 2021). Similarly, the influence of psychoanalysis in education – especially in national universities – remains limited. This is also one of the reasons why psychotherapy research in Greece is relatively underdeveloped.

It is already clear that the majority of psychotherapeutic practice and training in Greece occurs in the private sector. This is also consistent with the broader structure of the Greek economy and the corresponding mentality: the percentage of Greeks who are self-employed is more than double the EU average (according to the European Union's statistical agency, 31.9% of Greeks are self-employed compared to the EU average of 15%).

Institutes offering group analytic training are either professional associations or non-profit private organizations. Analytic Group Psychotherapy is provided mainly by self-employed specialists and, occasionally, by private firms.

Psychotherapy session fees are entirely private; neither state subsidies nor insurance companies cover them. The same applies to psychoanalytic and group analytic training.

The average cost in the private sector of an individual psychotherapy session ranges from 40 to 50 euros, while the minimum daily wage stands at 29.04 euros. Nevertheless, more and more people seek psychotherapy services, and hundreds of new specialists have entered the profession since 2010. In fact, three new public Psychology faculties have been established in different cities over the past five years. In addition, at least ten private colleges, in collaboration with foreign universities, offer Psychology programmes and related degrees.

Greek law grants licences to practice psychotherapy to any graduate of Psychology or Psychiatry, without requiring supervision or specialized psychotherapy training. Moreover, certifications for training in psychotherapy, psychoanalysis, and group analysis are recognized only by international organizations such as the IPA or EGATIN and not officially recognized by the Greek state.

Group Analysis in Greece

Although psychoanalysis had already had a long history (dating back to the 1930s) in Greece, its institutional representation followed the return to Greece of many psychoanalysts from mainly Britain, France, Germany, Italy, and

Switzerland after the fall of the dictatorship (1967–74). Their homecoming marked a restart of psychoanalysis in the country, exemplified by the founding of the Hellenic Society for Psychoanalytic Psychotherapy (HSPP) in 1977, and the Hellenic Psychoanalytic Society (HPS) in 1984, which became a provisional member of the International Psychoanalytic Association (IPA).

Around the same period – in the late 1970s and early 1980s – psychiatrists I.K. Tsegos and M. Josafat, both trained in Group Analysis in London, founded in Athens:

- The "Open Psychotherapeutic Centre" (OPC, 1980) and the "Institute of Group Analysis Athens" (IGAA, 1982) (Tsegos).
- The "Hellenic Institute for Group Analytic and Family Psychotherapy" (HIGA&FP, 1983) (Josafat).

The following decades witnessed a series of splits within the aforementioned institutes and societies. These divisions stemmed from differences in theoretical beliefs, interpersonal conflicts, competitive dynamics, and authoritarian behaviours. Such phenomena led to the creation of subgroups and internal divisions:

- The IGAA, through a series of splits, gave rise to at least four new institutes still in operation today. Two of these belong to the EFPP Greek National Network: the "Hellenic Organization for Education & Psychotherapy in Group Analysis – HOPE in GA" (2005) and the "Institute of Group Analysis 'S.H. Foulkes'" (2016).
- Similarly, the HSGA&FP engendered at least three new institutes through splits, among them the "Hellenic Society for Psychoanalytic Group Psychotherapy – HSPGP" (2014) and the "Hellenic Training Institute for Group & Family Analytic Psychotherapy – EL.EK.IN" (2023), which, alongside HSGA&FP, are also members of the EFPP Greek National Network.

Today, out of the eight group analytic institutes operating in Greece, five are active members of the EFPP. Two of them include the term "Group Analysis" in their official names, while three use the terms "Analytic" or "Psychoanalytic Group Psychotherapy". (The three institutes not currently active within the EFPP Network also use the term "Group Analysis" in their names.)

In two of the five EFPP-member institutes, there are direct references not only to S.H. Foulkes' tradition of *Group Analysis* but also to the French school of *Psychoanalytic Group Psychotherapy*, particularly the contributions of D. Anzieu, R. Kaës, and E. Pichon-Rivière.

The recent dialogue initiated among the institutes through the EFPP National Network has highlighted many similarities in their functioning, along with some differences – mainly related to institutional issues, leadership models, and the specific implementation of EGATIN's general guidelines for training programmes.

It is evident that the causes shaping this mosaic of group analytic institutes in Greece are multiple and multilayered; however, the very process of schisms was experienced traumatically by the participants. Phenomena such as authoritarian leadership, scapegoating, fraternal hordes, rivalries, and unresolved conflicts seem to have lacked frameworks within which they could be contained and processed in the original institutes. As Mylona & Moraitou (2022) note, the new institutes emerged from the desire to belong to a professional group, to counterbalance loss and rage, and find new ways of thinking and coexisting, while simultaneously serving as endeavours "to metabolize" the cumulative traumas. The lack of processing and elaboration of these historical splits has resulted in the formation of un-metabolized affects lying at the foundation of the institutes that arose.

Efforts to restrain and mitigate defensive movements, such as repetition compulsion or identification with the aggressor, have not been successful, largely because inter-network dialogue remains absent. In this context, the establishment of the EFPP Greek National Network (2022) becomes crucial: it offers a space where the "origin trauma" can be acknowledged, given meaning, and transformed into a shared narrative object. Only then can a dialogue develop that supports and is supported by communication, collaboration, and creativity – converging on commonalities while accepting differences.

The Models of the Institutes

Although group analysis in Greece presents a seemingly traumatic and fragmented picture in relation to the institutes representing it, its development aligns closely with the patterns of recent Greek economic and social history. This, in turn, points to a dynamic interplay of economic, social, and cultural forces that have shaped its evolution. Let us examine their models from this perspective.

The first group analytic structure in the early 1980s followed a model of a therapeutic centre offering outpatient analytic groups, a non-residential therapeutic community, and group analytic training. *This model served as an alternative to the outdated and inhumane psychiatric institutions of the time.* Its impact was significant, both in the therapeutic culture among mental health professionals and in the lives of those engaged in Analytic Group Psychotherapy and therapeutic communities. It also inspired pioneering group analytic projects with psychotic patients in public mental health units during the 1980s.

Today, this model remains active in more than one group analytic institute. Although its effectiveness is evident, its development has largely been confined to a singular centre with strong leadership, limited expansion into broader communities and, overall, it was not espoused by mental health and community services.

At the same time, the second institute established in the early 1980s was based exclusively on providing training in group analytic and psychoanalytic family therapy. Group therapy was conducted within the institute itself and primarily addressed professionals participating in the training programmes. This was also a leader-centred model, functioning in a complementary way to other psychoanalytic institutions. Its contribution to "sensitizing" psychiatrists and other mental health professionals to psychoanalytic psychotherapy and group analysis was notable.

Over the following decades, several new institutes emerged, primarily as a result of splits from both original institutes. Some of these new institutes tend to replicate the same models, although there is a growing tendency toward more collective and less leader-centred organizational forms.

Nevertheless, most institutes appear to be oriented primarily toward training rather than the organization of clinical structures. We could characterize this model as "*network-based*": Members' private practices serve as focal points for group analytic networks. Trainees participate in group analytic groups alongside other patients within the trainer-analysts' *private practices* in most institutes. Trainees are encouraged to establish analytic groups, experiential groups, and other group activities in *local community mental health or social welfare services* whenever possible. They are also encouraged to start their own *private practices*, which represent the main field for psychotherapy and group analysis in Greece.

This method encourages trainees and graduates to become more active in community-based group initiatives, which in turn "disseminates" group analysis into various areas of professional activity.

However, out of the five EFPP member institutes, only two offer training programmes in object-mediated group work (e.g., painting, music, rhythm-movement, photo-language, myth and storytelling, creative writing, psychodrama), which have proven highly effective in community settings with diverse populations.

Additionally, only one institute places emphasis on working with medium-sized and large groups, incorporating them actively into their training programmes (Loutsos, 2016).

It appears that the newer network-based models are better suited to the ever-increasing mental health needs of the general population that remain unmet by state planning, while simultaneously motivating an increasing number of individuals not diagnosed with psychiatric conditions to seek psychotherapy. This search occurs locally and is guided more by incidental indicators of "quality", such as those found on the internet or drawn from the experiences shared through the personal networks of relatives and friends.

Group Analysis in the Public Sector

The network-oriented model is also, mainly, the reason why none of the five EFPP-member institutes currently operates a therapeutic community, whereas at least two of the other institutes maintain non-residential therapeutic communities. Although the literature supports the notion that a group analytic unit with a therapeutic community can be financially viable (Karapostoli et al., 2012), other attempts to establish private therapeutic communities over the past 20 years have not borne fruit, mainly due to financial reasons.

Therapeutic communities within public institutions seem to follow the typical trajectory of many psychoanalytic initiatives: they are created and flourish for a time thanks to the enthusiasm and tireless work of their founders, but often lack institutional entrenchment, leading to their gradual decline or administrative dissolution once their founders retire or move on.

In general, group analysis in the public sector in Greece has contributed a rich array of applications within community services and mental health structures. Analytic and experiential groups have been conducted in mental health units and across a wide range of professional fields and special populations, including migrants and refugees, the elderly, children and adolescents, pregnant women, patients with rheumatic diseases, neurological patients and their caregivers, cancer patients, individuals struggling with substance addiction, etc.

Numerous object-mediated groups (involving art, music, group analytic psychodrama, etc.) have been organized across different types of community services. Supervision and professional support groups have been implemented within psychiatric units, drug addiction and prevention centres, general and military hospitals, educational institutions, welfare services, and other settings.

All these activities have had a positive impact on the lives of participants. However, they have rarely managed to operate in the long term or to achieve institutional sustainability.

Notable exceptions include:

- *Athens University Clinic of Psychiatry*: Since the early 1980s, the clinic has introduced group psychotherapy for hospitalized patients. Following the movement of deinstitutionalization, it established a Day Hospital and the first Community Mental Health Center in Greece (based on the catchment area model). These units primarily served chronic psychotic outpatients, offering an integrated therapeutic programme that included medication, group and family psychotherapy, occupational therapy, and vocational rehabilitation programmes.
- *Athens University Clinic of Psychiatry*: The "Athens Project", a pioneering initiative for the treatment of severe personality disorders, later developed into a full department. It provided comprehensive therapeutic services for these challenging patients, combining medication, individual and group psychotherapy, and art therapy. For more than 30 years, it also functioned as a major educational and training hub for mental health professionals. More recently, by expanding its scope, it established a specialized unit for adolescents.

- *Naval Hospital of Salamis*: For nearly 20 years, it sustained a group analytic inpatient therapeutic community programme, offering an innovative model of psychiatric care within the military health system.
- *251 General Air Force Hospital*: For the past decade, its psychiatric ward has maintained group analytic inpatient and outpatient programmes, demonstrating a commitment to the integration of psychodynamic group approaches into institutional psychiatric care.

Group Analysis as Private Practice

However, the greatest volume of group analytic work in Greece takes place in the private practices of institute members, as psychotherapy in Greece, in general, has developed mainly within the private sector – reflecting the overall structure of the Greek economy.

From a survey among institutes, it appears that most analytic groups operate on a weekly basis, except for one institute that also employs the model of two sessions per week. Group sizes typically consist of 7±2 members (including the conductor), with larger groups being relatively rare. These groups include individuals from diverse social backgrounds, of different ages and origins, and presenting with various treatment needs and diagnoses.

Group analysis in Greece is generally a long-term psychotherapy. According to the institutes' responses, it typically lasts between 5 and 7 years, and in some cases even longer.

Individual psychotherapy usually precedes group psychotherapy, culminating in the integration of the client into the group. However, in some clinical practices, there may be an initial transitional period where both individual and group therapies run in parallel. The duration of individual psychotherapy can vary significantly, depending on the client's needs and the analyst's clinical approach. Generally, parallel individual psychotherapy is rarely recommended for members of analytic groups but may occur and is dependent on each individual case.

Regarding group conductors, it appears that it is rare to have a co-conductor in private practice, although it is not entirely excluded. The co-conductor model is more commonly used in public sector settings or for training purposes within the institutes.

In private practice, a typical process involves a client starting with individual sessions with a therapist, then negotiating participation in an analytic group conducted by the same therapist in the same private office.

Among the institutes, there are differences concerning the emphasis placed on individual analysis. In some institutes, individual psychoanalytic psychotherapy is considered an essential and autonomous therapeutic process that complements group analysis. In others, the model follows what Nitsun (2001) describes as "group analytic individual psychotherapy", which begins with individual sessions and culminates in group participation. These differences are reflected in the requirements imposed on trainees: in some institutes, undergoing individual psychoanalytic psychotherapy is mandatory; in others, it is not.

Virtual Groups

From the dialogue among the institutes, it appears that in recent years – especially following the COVID-19 pandemic – online analytic groups have been established. These groups mainly serve:

- Greeks living in rural areas, where psychotherapeutic services are scarce.
- Greek emigrants, whose population almost tripled during the economic crisis (over 500,000 Greek citizens have left the country since 2010), and who often face cultural and linguistic barriers that hinder access to psychotherapy services abroad.

Among group analysts in Greece, there is no unified position regarding online therapy, and significant reservations exist concerning the difficulties and quality of such practice.

Critics emphasize:

- The lack of physical presence and bodily experience.
- The absence of the "circle" formation.
- The diminished eye contact.
- The communication difficulties inherent in the medium.

On the other hand, group analysts who conduct online groups focus on the possibilities for relatedness – embracing all the advantages and disadvantages of the medium – and approach these phenomena as new forms of resistance emerging within the group analytic framework.

Regardless, online analytic groups represent a new development that responds to real needs, attracts the younger generations of both analysands and analysts, and, although it has already appeared internationally in clinical practice, it still requires systematic communication and further study (Weinberg et al., 2024).

Research

As already noted, analysands in Greece usually reach analysts' private practices through a "random" process rather than via an organized referral system. Even when someone has previously contacted a public mental health service and has been recommended psychotherapy, they will typically seek a private therapist, relying either on family and social networks or – for younger generations – on internet searches.

This randomness in referrals, along with the dispersed nature of clinical practice, does not favour the systematic conduct of research on the effectiveness of group analysis.

However, the main reason why research in Greece on group analysis remains at a rudimentary stage is that psychotherapy research in general is still in its early steps.

Group analytic institutes, as we have seen, are private organizations or collectives. They lack the resources and personnel required to conduct valid research or even to adapt existing research "tools" from abroad to the Greek reality. University institutions connected to mental health, which might fund such research, are mostly oriented toward the biomedical model, as we have seen. Furthermore, psychology departments – which in recent years have started to carry out some psychotherapy-related research – do not systematically represent group analysis or psychoanalysis, nor have they established these fields academically.

Nonetheless, some initial efforts in recent years offer hope for the future (Giotsidis, 2013).

Regarding the approach of Greek group analysts to so-called evidence-based clinical practice, it can be said that it is not yet particularly widespread. The reasons for this include:

- Most clinical practice occurs in the private sector, often without formal diagnoses.
- Patients are rarely monitored by public institutions for symptom evolution, thus eliminating the need for such reporting.
- Analysts' fees are not covered by public or private insurance bodies (with very few exceptions), which means there is no external pressure regarding "effectiveness" measures.

Moreover, people who seek psychotherapy and commit to it are usually not solely seeking symptom relief and often show scepticism toward medication.

It is a common belief among Greek group analysts that Analytic Group Psychotherapy does not focus directly on symptoms. Instead, it focuses on:

- Relational aspects underlying symptoms.
- Treating therapy not as symptom elimination but as "ego training in action" toward new modes of relatedness.
- Offering a renewed sense of personal meaning for each analysand.

While on one hand, this could seem like an "uncontrolled" practice, on the other hand, it allows for alternative approaches against the pressures exerted by the biomedical model – which tends to focus exclusively on symptom control and elimination.

In general, Greek group analysts use research as part of their professional formation, incorporating international publications into their practice and cultivating a preference for qualitative research, primarily through case study analysis methods within their institutes.

Finally, it is very encouraging to note the gradual development of a body of Greek-language literature related to group analysis – through some translations (unfortunately, still not of Foulkes' works) and, more importantly, through original works by Greek authors over the past few years.

Challenges and Prospects

The challenges and perspectives for group analysis in Greece, as they have emerged from the dialogue among the institutes, can be summarized as follows:

- Consolidation of the network of institutes involved in psychoanalytic psychotherapy and group analysis.
- Formation of a legally established framework within which the training institutes can operate, aiming both to control the quality of education and to enhance the standards of group analytic clinical practice in general.
- Protection and official recognition of the professional title of Group Analyst or Group Psychotherapist.
- Integration of Analytic Group Psychotherapy into public mental health institutions.
- Connection of group analysis with university departments and development of a research culture.

"The Greek Group"

From the above, it is clear that there is no single, typical model of group analysis in Greece that can be identified with certainty. However, two tendencies can be distinguished in the coordination of groups: one more inspired by object-relations psychoanalytic psychotherapy, emphasizing analytic capacity; and a "communal" tendency that places greater emphasis on empowerment and is more closely associated with ego-psychology or relational models. It is also interesting to observe the coordination models that emerge. In the first tendency, the presence of the coordinator and their participation in the group's communication remains more distant and clearly distinct. For some, this reproduces social models of leadership, but in this way, it promotes personal responsibility and the self-determination of members regarding boundaries – a clearly democratic approach. In the second approach, the coordinator's stance is more "friendly" and participatory in communication, supporting permissiveness in the group, though at times they may exert their influence in a clear manner, especially when group communication tends toward destructiveness.

Although this distinction has previously been part of the theoretical conflicts that characterized the schisms of the institutes, it is possible that today it can serve as a subject of dialogue and exchange of experience.

But is there a typical model of the "Greek group"? Certainly, the culture of each country influences how communication within a group is shaped, but it would be naive to adopt a simplistic, scientifically unfounded, "national character" approach. Nevertheless, we can generally say that Greek culture is characterized by the historically rapid transformation of family structure. The Greek family functions as an extended urban family system, marked by a continuous flow of communication and contact within the kinship network (Mylonas et al., 2006). Many families are nuclear or "post-nuclear" in structure, but functionally they are extended, like traditional families, shaping the social identity of their members. Individuals often experience significant pressure. On one hand, they attempt to meet the needs of the family – which are governed by values of collectivism and interdependence – while also addressing their own needs for intimacy and connection; on the other hand, they seek personal success, privacy, and autonomy – values of modern individualism promoted in economic life, education, the media, and elsewhere. This conflict of values can take many forms.

When members of a group project this family culture onto the group, they display behaviours marked by high intimacy and solidarity in line with these typical values. To an outside observer, this might sometimes appear as a continual challenge to certain group boundaries (physical contact, gifts, shared treats, etc.).

At the same time, the group, functioning as a social field, must contend with a characteristic of Greek culture: a lack of trust in other communal institutions beyond the family. This often manifests as restrained, superego-driven "proper" behaviours of conflict avoidance, which lead to indirect challenges: fear of dependence on the group, managing family pressures related to therapy itself, the emergence of financial difficulties among others.

The contradictory values of Greek culture promote a "hypermodern", as Navridis and Christakis (2011) describe it, subjectivity that drives individuals toward over-adaptability in terms of psychology and identity. It pushes them toward a persistent pursuit of "personal" growth and pleasure, a compulsive responsibility for their physical, mental, and relational life – even the conditions of their reproduction – and a tyrannical race against time, overwhelmed by an unrelenting sense of urgency that can never be satisfied. Individuals seeking psychotherapy in Greece, whether presenting psychiatric symptoms, focusing on interpersonal issues, or facing life crises, ultimately negotiate this rupture of their internal cohesion and look to the group as a field of containment to reframe their existence and relationships.

References

Anargyros, K.P., Lappas, A.S., & Christodoulou, N.G., (2021). Community mental health services in Greece: Development, challenges and future directions. *Consortium PSYCHIATRICUM*, 2(4), 62–67. doi:10.17816/CP111.

Giotsidis, V. (2013). *Η αντίσταση στην ψυχοθεραπεία: Θεωρία, έρευνα και κλινικό έργο* [*Resistance to Psychotherapy: Theory, Research, and Clinical Work*]. Athens: Topos.

Karapostoli, N., Polyzos, N., & Tsegos, I. K. (2012). The cost of therapy services provided by a day psychotherapy unit. *Group Analysis*, 45(4), 515–535. doi:10.1177/0533316412453910.

Kolostasis, P. (2022). *Τι πιστεύουν οι νέοι* [*What youth believes*]. Athens: ΔιαΝΕΟσις.

Kotsis, K., Marchionatti, L.E., Simioni, A., Schafer, J.L., Evans-Lacko, S., Saxena, S., Kline, S., Kousoulis, A., Koumoula, A., & Salum, G.A., (2024). The state of mental health in Greece: An international comparative analysis using data from the Global Mental Health Countdown 2030. *International Journal of Social Psychiatry*, 71(4), 757–769. doi:10.1177/00207640241303029.

Loutsos, S. (2016). Maintaining group analytic training during the financial crisis in Greece. *Psychotherapy and Politics International*, 14(1), 38–47.

Mylona, D., & Moraitou, S.M. (2022). The paradox in the history of group analysis in Greece: Challenging and open-ended. GASI *Contexts*, 96, July. https://groupanalyticsociety.co.uk/contexts/issue-96/

Mylonas, K., Gari, A., Giotsa, A., Pavlopoulos, V., & Panagiotopoulou, P. (2006). Greece. In Georgas, J., Berry, J.W., van de Vijver, F.J.R., Kagitcibasi C., & Poortinga, Y.H. (Eds.), *Families Across Cultures: A 30-Nation Psychological Study* (pp. 344–352). New York: Cambridge University Press.

Navridis, K., & Christakis, N. (Eds.) (2011). *Το υπερνεωτερικό υποκείμενο* [*The Hypermodern Subject*]. Athens: Pedio.

Nitsun, M. (2001). Towards a group-analytic approach to individual psychotherapy. *Group Analysis*, 34(4), 473–483.

OECD (2021). *A New Benchmark for Mental Health Systems: Tackling the Social and Economic Costs of Mental Ill-Health*. Paris: OECD Health Policy Studies, OECD Publishing. doi:10.1787/4ed890f6-en.

OECD/European Observatory on Health Systems and Policies (2023). *Greece: Country Health Profile 2023, State of Health in the EU*. Brussels: OECD Publishing, Paris/European Observatory on Health Systems and Policies. www.oecd.org/content/dam/oecd/el/publications/reports/2023/12/greece-country-health-profile-2023_0d70aae7/5753e659-el.pdf.

Panagiotopoulou, N. (2021). *Ένας παράξενος ταξιδιώτης: Η ψυχανάλυση στους ελληνικούς θεσμούς* [*A Strange Traveller: Psychoanalysis in Greek Institutions*]. Athens: Armos.

Weinberg, H., Rolnick, A., & Leighton, A. (Eds.) (2024). *The Virtual Group Therapy Circle. Advances in Online Group Theory and Practice*. London: Routledge.

Chapter 12

Group Psychotherapy in Germany

An Overview That Includes Historical and Cultural Aspects

Karina Nahr and Ulrich Schultz-Venrath

History

Group analysis and group psychotherapy originated on the American East Coast in the first 30 years of the 20th century, long before the development of group analysis in England and German-speaking countries. Using the examples of Trigant Burrow, Paul Schilder, Louis Wender and others, previously little-known or even unknown sources are used to highlight both the theoretical concepts and the relevance and modernity of group psychotherapy in the United States in the 1930s (Schultz-Venrath, 2022a). In Germany, an interdisciplinary network developed from neurology (Kurt Goldstein), sociology and social psychology (Norbert Elias, Adhemar Gelb, Karl Mannheim) and philosophy and theology (Martin Buber, Franz Rosenzweig) – the so-called Frankfurt constellation, which enabled Siegmund H. Fuchs to establish group analysis in Exeter (Hermanns, 2009; Schultz-Venrath, 2008; Schultz-Venrath, 2022a).

In 1960, Siegmund H. Foulkes returned as emigrant for the first time to Germany to give a lecture on "Theoretical and practical foundations of analytical group psychotherapy" at the 10th Lindau Psychotherapy Weeks[1] with the topic theme: "Psychotherapy in the Group" as a milestone. He "specifically addressed his audience as general practitioners" and "presented his concept based on twenty years of experience with group analysis" (Hermanns, 2009, p. 112). Walter Schindler (London), the second emigrant and speaker on this Lindau Psychotherapy Week, was one of the pioneers or "classics" of group psychoanalysis, who founded the approach of "analytical group psychotherapy based on the family model" in intensive exchange with S.H. Foulkes in London (Mettauer, 2010, p. 32). The atmospheric problem was only that these Lindau Psychotherapy Weeks were organized by former psychiatrists with Nazi ties (Mettauer, 2010), which prompted Foulkes never to return to Lindau again. The training in group therapy and group analysis started 1960 in Lindau and Frankfurt with the foundation of the Institute and Training Centre for Psychoanalysis and Psychosomatic Medicine by Alexander Mitscherlich from Heidelberg, with two different training concepts: fractionated group work (Lindau) (Schindler, 2017) versus continuous self-experience in groups (Frankfurt a. M.).

DOI: 10.4324/9781003597674-12

The Institutionalization of Group Analysis and Group Psychotherapy

In the 1950s and 1960s, the beginnings of the application of group analysis in group psychotherapy were quite different in West and East Germany (Janssen, 2025b; Seidler & Misselwitz, 2014; Tändler, 2016). The East German Intended Group Psychotherapy differed from her western sister by inclusion of non-verbal and bodily communication as biographical network-printout. There was an increasing boom in methods in the 1970s and 1980s, which also led to the qualification of doctors, psychologists, theologians, educationalists, social workers and others in group therapy and group work. In 1967, the various movements were institutionalized as the German Working Group for Group Psychotherapy and Group Dynamics (DAGG) with six sections but without the East German Intended Dynamic Group Psychotherapy due to the political split between East and West. These sections represented the psychoanalytically based group methods in the so-called guidelines of psychotherapy as well as group dynamics, psychodrama and sociotherapy. Following reunification and the integration of the Intended Dynamic Group Psychotherapy, the DAGG was dissolved after lengthy discussions. What remained was the clinically and therapeutically oriented journal entitled *Group Psychotherapy and Group Dynamics*, which later received the subtitle *Theory and Practice of Group Analysis.*

In 2011, the German Society for Group Analysis and Group Psychotherapy (D3G) was founded (Döring & Knauss, 2013), which now represents the scientific interests of group analysis and psychodynamic group psychotherapy, whereas the professional interests are represented by the Professional Association of Licensed Group Psychotherapists (BAG), which was founded in 1999. The development of the concepts and methodology in group analysis and psychodynamic group therapy used in inpatient treatment differs significantly from outpatient therapy regarding the kind of patients, of institutions (psychiatry or psychosomatic medicine) and had also to be adapted for the treatment of children and adolescents.

For this reason, we organized a survey in 2024 among the members of the D3G in which 81 psychodynamic and psychoanalytic group therapists took part (15% of all members), 7.7% worked in inpatient settings and 5.1% in day clinics, with the remainder working in outpatient settings. Psychodynamic or psychoanalytic group therapy with children and adolescents was carried out by 14.1% of colleagues.

According to the survey, the most commonly used psychodynamic group therapy concepts are (multiple answers possible):

- Group Analysis (S.H. Foulkes): 71%
- Interactional Analytic Group Psychotherapy (Göttingen model, Heigl-Evers & Heigl), explained below: 61%

- Interactional group psychotherapy (Irvin Yalom & Molyn Leszcz): 58%
- Mentalization-based group therapy (Anthony Bateman, Sigmund Karterud, Helga Felsberger & Ulrich Schultz-Venrath): 44%
- Psychoanalytische Gruppentherapie (Wilfred Bion): 25%
- Intended Dynamic Group Therapy (Kurt Höck): 18%

Many group therapists use different concepts depending on the structural level and diagnoses of the patients or the specific group situation. The activity of the group leader also varies depending on the patient group and/or phase of group treatment. Most colleagues do not use one concept throughout. From a scientific point of view, one problem is that we do not know exactly how the different group psychotherapists really work.

After all, the theoretical approaches behind the concepts are not as different as they would like to be. In the survey, the differences relate more to the options for action: 80% of group therapists stated that they work psychodynamically; 60% work explicitly psychoanalytically (6% work by other methods). Janssen (2025b) emphasizes in accordance with *Psychotherapeutic Guidelines* by Faber & Haarstrick (Becker et al., 2025) that from an empirically based perspective there is hardly any methodological difference between psychodynamic and psychoanalytic group therapy. Only the length of funded treatment differs, which is historically based on psychodynamic and analytical individual therapy. For psychodynamic group psychotherapy, 80 double hours are fully financed for adults, while for analytical group therapy 160 double hours are fully paid by health insurance companies. For psychodynamic and psychoanalytic treatment of children and adolescents the number is identical (90 double hours), i.e. the same regardless of the method used. Due to the well-known concepts of Foulkes, Yalom and Bion, here is a brief explanation of the other models:

Mentalization-based Group Therapy

The breeding grounds of mentalization-based group therapy (MBT-G) were psychotherapeutic day hospitals, strongly influenced by therapeutic community ideology and group analysis (Bateman et al., 2009; Karterud et al., 2025), which started as a day treatment programme at St Ann's Hospital in London (directed by Anthony Bateman), at Oslo University Hospital (directed by Sigmund Karterud) and at the Clinic for Psychiatry, Psychotherapy and Psychosomatics at the Evangelical Hospital Bergisch Gladbach (University of Witten/Herdecke), treating patients with personality disorders, especially with borderline personality disorders (BPD). The outcomes of MBT (once a week) combined with high frequent MBT-G (four times a week) in a day treatment programme for BPD patients were so convincing that MBT was one of the empirical founding number one treatment concepts besides dialectical behaviour therapy (DBT), with a follow-up of eight years (Bateman & Fonagy, 2008; Storebo et al., 2020).

While psychodynamic group therapies usually took place once or twice a week, mentalization-based group therapies were used four to five times a week in day clinics – however, with differences in frequency, duration and treatment length. These treatment programmes were composed of a wide range of group therapies and the theoretical matrix that sustained them was influenced by authors such as S.H. Foulkes, Tom Main, Maxwell Jones, Wilfred Bion, Henry Ezriel, Pat de Maré and others. Unlike Germany, where these programmes remained primarily limited to hospitals and day hospitals, they were converted to intensive outpatient treatment programmes in other European countries in the early 2000s, composed of:

1 an introductory psychoeducational group;
2 weekly individual psychotherapy; and
3 weekly group psychotherapy.

It is noteworthy that the first practical MBT guidelines lacked any reference to group analytic theory (Bateman & Fonagy 2006; Karterud et al., 2025). This is reflected in the fact that the current MBT Group Curriculum of the global MBT network from the 23 June 2025 does not provide for the independent further development of mentalization-based group therapy or supervision by psychodynamic and trained analytic group psychotherapists, but exclusively by MBT supervisors who do not necessarily have to have undergone group therapy training with personal experience in the narrower sense.

> The relative lack of integrating the theoretical heritage has been paralleled by a lack of extensive training in MBT group therapy. On the advanced course of MBT at the Anna Freud Centre, minimal time (around one hour) is allocated to the MBT group component. There is no further training in MBT group therapy in the UK. It goes without saying that when MBT group therapists formerly trained in group analysis are dying out, MBT will be facing a rather large problem.
>
> (Karterud et al., 2025)

At the beginning of the establishment of MBT-G, "most of the MBT group therapists of that generation brought with them at least some kind of group analytic training" (Karterud et al., 2025). In the meanwhile, mentalization-based group psychotherapy (MBT-G) and the concept of mentalizing in group therapies is particularly suitable for inpatient or day treatment groups for patients with different diagnoses, e.g. post-traumatic disorders, autism spectrum disorders, somatoform disorders and others (Karterud, 2015; Krämer et al., 2021; Schultz-Venrath & Felsberger, 2016; Schultz-Venrath & Staun, 2025). In this respect, the German and Norwegian model differs from the British in that it uses disorder-specific mentalization-based psychoeducation models (e.g. ADHD). At present, MBT-G internationally appears to be more behaviour-oriented or, as in Germany, psychodynamically oriented, represented by the Institute of Group Analysis and Mentalizing in Groups (IGAM)[2].

Regardless of these difficulties in establishing a promising and empirically effective group therapy concept, mentalization-based group therapy is an integrative approach based on the mentalization theory, originally developed by Peter Fonagy and Anthony Bateman (Bateman & Fonagy, 2004, 2019; Fonagy et al., 2002). Focusing on pre-mentalizing modes (body, teleological, equivalent and pretend mode) and dimensions of mentalizing (affect vs cognition, internal vs external, self vs other, automatic-implicit-reactive vs controlled-explicit-reflective), it enables patients to understand their own and others' mental states, which leads to better social relationships and improved emotional self-regulation (Schultz-Venrath, 2025 [2013]). The therapists help to recognize and reflect on misunderstandings and emotional overreactions, enabling participants to learn to manage their relationships in a healthy and understanding way. The concept thus aims to promote patients' ability to recognize and understand their own mental states as well as those of others.

The Göttingen Model

Another important development within group analysis in Germany is based on the Göttingen model of psychodynamic group psychotherapy, primarily founded by Heigl and Heigl-Evers at the Tiefenbrunn Clinic near Göttingen, especially developed for patients with personality disorders (Heigl-Evers & Heigl, 1994; Janssen, 2025b; Staats et al., 2014). Heigl-Evers and Heigl developed a psychoanalytic based group psychotherapy that combined psychoanalytical, socio-psychological and group-dynamic approaches, which received little international attention or significance, which was due to a lack of English-language publications. This model distinguishes between three levels in group situations: the manifest action, the latent, unconscious action and the level of shared unconscious fantasies. Different approaches to group therapy are also differentiated according to these levels: psychoanalytic-interactional therapy (conscious interactions), psychodynamic therapy (preconscious interactions) and analytical group therapy (unconscious interactions). The analytic group therapy of the Göttingen model integrates approaches based on object relations theory. This makes it possible to work on re-enactments of early childhood relationship experiences in the transference. These transmissions often become apparent particularly quickly in group situations.

The psychoanalytical-interactional method became particularly important for the treatment of patients with a lower structural level or ego weakness (Janssen, 2025b). The group interactions themselves serve as a therapeutic medium. The focus is on the interactions between the group members and their significance for the therapeutic process. Central ego functions such as affect perception and differentiation of affects are promoted. The so-called "response principle" is preferred instead of interpretation. This means – according to Strauß (2022) – that the therapist specifically communicates their own countertransference reactions to the group process and to individual participants in order to support the maturation of ego functions. This special form of an auxiliary ego function also includes concrete explanations and model-based learning. Consciously experienced conflicts are placed in the foreground and given priority. Patients with ego structure disorders already reach their stress limits with these consciously experienced conflicts. Unconscious dynamics fade into the background; instead, the focus is on current behaviour and the immediate interaction between group members.

Intended Dynamic Group Psychotherapy

After the Wall was built in 1961, a separate treatment technique of psychodynamic group therapy was developed in East German Republic (DDR): a so-called Intended Dynamic Group Therapy (IDG) under the decisive influence of Kurt Höck (1976, 1967, 1982). It emerged from the debate around the Göttingen model with links to the Lindau Psychotherapy Weeks, in which 30 participants from East Germany took part in April 1960 (Geyer, 2011, p. 145). They were able to discuss their experiences with Foulkes, Raoul Schindler, Walter Schindler, Teirich and other renowned group psychotherapists (Heyne, 2019, p. 90). A special feature of psychodynamic intended group therapy is the conceptual integration of non-verbal, bodily communication in the group, called communicative movement therapy. Group therapists and co-therapists take on a more active role.

The Influence of Local Culture on Group Analytic Practice and Theory

Similar to Wolfgang Loch's diagnosis of post-war psychoanalysis in West Germany: "We were hopelessly behind, and yet there had once been a flourishing psychoanalytic movement in Germany" (Hermanns, 2022b; Loch, 1992, p. 226), the same was true of group analysis (Hermanns, 2022a). Most post-war group analysts learned the basics of group analysis from British and Dutch colleagues such as Siegmund Heinrich and Elizabeth Foulkes (Altaussee in Austria), Liesl Hearst (GRAS), Ilse Seglow (IGA Heidelberg), Hymie Wyse (GRAS) and Gregory van der Kleij (GRAS). This is well documented in two volumes (Hermanns & Schultz-Venrath, 2024; Hermanns & Schultz-Venrath, 2025), in which 28 group analysts (> 70 years) described their socialization and biography, and how they came to group analysis. In the 1960s, this corresponded with the radicalization of the student movement against petty bourgeois ideological fictions, which then took a political stand against the ruling establishment, especially the government, in various organizations, primarily in Berlin, Munich and Frankfurt on Main (Tändler, 2016).

Around 1969, a new function of psychotherapeutic practice emerged in connection with the disintegrating student movement. Psychological and psychotherapeutic methods, and group psychotherapy in particular, suddenly took on an instrumental political function, as they seemed suitable for remedying psychological impairments to such an extent that the individuals affected would become capable of revolutionary political work. This led to unruly and later sectarian group analysis-like therapy groups, including those led by Günter Ammon (1918–95) and his wife Gisela, who founded the German Group Therapy Society (DGG) in 1968 after his psychoanalytical training in Topeka in the Menninger-Clinic. Ammon was controversial in his role as head of the institute. He was heavily criticized by former colleagues, students and trainees. Ammon demanded unconditional loyalty, even in their private lives. Another shining light who attracted many students in large group therapy sessions in these years was the Austrian psychotherapist Josef Rattner (1928–2022), a student of Adlerian psychotherapy. Several times a week, publicly accessible therapy sessions and training courses took place at his home in Charlottenburg. During the therapy sessions, the problems of one person at a time were discussed in front of the group. The large group consisted of students, psychologists and other interested individuals. In addition to increasing self-awareness and knowledge of human nature, the therapy also aimed to impart cultural and historical knowledge. There are now 16 group analysis training institutes in Germany, which have joined forces under the umbrella of the D3G, but speak different dialects. Scientific exchange on this topic has only been successful to a limited extent so far, presumably because the professional integration of analytical group psychotherapies has been of greater importance.

Discussion on the Role of Group Analysts as Leader Versus Conductor

According to Schwartz (2006), the striving for hierarchy is not particularly pronounced in Germany. This can also apply to the leadership style of group therapy. The premise is often followed: as little leadership as possible, as much leadership as necessary. The activity of the group leader adapts to the structural level of the patients and the respective therapy phase of the group treatment.

However, the activity of the group leader also differs according to the concept used. With Foulkes, the leader tends to hold back ("trust the group"), and this concept is also more likely to be used with patients with a higher structural level. In interactional group therapy of the Göttingen model or in MBT-G, the group leader is much more active, integrating a mentalization-based dynamic administration (Staun & Schultz-Venrath, 2023b). However, both concepts are regularly used more frequently with patients of a lower structural level and with personality disorders.

The results of the survey showed the following attitudes among the group management (multiple answers possible):

- More active in patients with a low structural level, otherwise restrained: 80%
- More active at the start of a new group, more reserved as it progresses: 54%
- Always little active intervention: 10%
- Always active: 9%

But what does this mean in concrete terms? According to the survey, 65% of group participants in the outpatient groups have a structural level that is above the average structural level (medium to higher structural level or higher structural level). Most group leaders work rather cautiously with this patient group and a group that has been running for some time, often without actively opening the session. The group participants often begin to speak on their own and give each other their own interpretations. The group leader only intervenes in exceptional cases and then usually only gives a few interpretations. In groups of children and young people as in groups with personality disorders, the group leader generally has a more active role, especially if there are signs of destructive processes in the group.

Differences in the treatment technique therefore also affect the interpretations themselves, with the method fluctuating between the poles of always interpreting the group as a whole and always working individually in the group.

The survey revealed the following work in the group (multiple answers possible):

- The participants report on their individual problems in the group and interpret these among themselves: 69%
- Only in exceptional cases do I do individual work in a group: 65%
- Only in special group situations do I interpret the group as a whole: 58%
- I mainly interpret the group as a whole: 36%
- I mainly do individual work in groups: 21%
- I never carry out individual work in a group: 1%
- I never interpret the group as a whole: 1%

Current Group Analytic Practices in Private and Public Sectors

Since 1967, psychotherapy has been financed by health insurance companies in Germany on an outpatient basis. Since then, outpatient psychotherapeutic care has been constantly improving. Psychotherapy is accessible to everyone and fully funded. However, demand is very high. As a result, there are often long waiting times despite the number of psychotherapists having increased.

Around 90% of the population in Germany is covered by statutory health insurance. Every insured person has free choice and can go to any medical practice that is licensed by the Association of Statutory Health Insurance. This also applies to psychotherapy. There is a total of 39,627 registered psychotherapists in Germany who provide outpatient care under the statutory health insurance scheme (September 2024).

The remaining 10% of the population have private health insurance (permitted from an annual income of around €70,000). The insurance contracts vary greatly here, but psychotherapy is often paid for to a lesser extent than for those with statutory health insurance (e.g. a maximum of 50 hours per calendar year, or only 80% of the costs are covered).

Of 39,627 psychotherapists in their own practice in Germany, 5,912 are medical psychotherapists and 33,715 are psychological psychotherapists. There are 16,653 psychotherapists working in psychodynamic and psychoanalytic methods. Of these, 5,562 colleagues would be able to offer psychoanalytic or psychodynamic group therapy (587 of these are child and adolescent therapists). But not all of these colleagues are offering group therapy. Compared to the total number of psychotherapy patients, only 2.7% of all outpatient psychotherapies are group therapies (Christoffer et al., 2022), although improved funding over the last three years suggests an increase in group psychotherapy now. Group psychotherapy is currently estimated to account for roughly 10 to 15 per cent of all outpatient psychotherapy nationwide; depending on the approach and region, this figure is likely to be even lower. Some colleagues work on an outpatient basis, but only with privately insured patients or self-payers, or provide supervision/training therapy.

The exact number of colleagues who also work on an inpatient basis is difficult to determine. Group therapies of different kinds are the most offered therapies in clinics with low or missing standards. Psychiatric clinics work predominantly with behavioural therapies in contrast to psychosomatic clinics with a slight dominance of psychodynamic therapies. There are usually only a few fully qualified (group) psychotherapists working in clinics (often in management positions) and significantly more psychologists in training to become psychological psychotherapists. As a result, many trainee psychotherapists in clinics end up leading groups themselves. Inpatient and day treatment clinics are mainly used for stabilization and crisis intervention. Patients are often recommended to undergo outpatient psychotherapy afterwards.

Group Analytic Frameworks on Length, Frequency, and Payment

Outpatient patients with one or more F diagnoses according to ICD 10, International Classification of Diseases (ICD 11 is still not in use) are fully paid for psychotherapy by the statutory health insurance.

Individual Therapy for Adults

- Psychodynamic psychotherapy: up to 100 hours (usually once a week, up to two hours per week permitted).
- Analytical psychotherapy up to 300 hours (usually two to three or four appointments per week).
- Group therapy for adults: Psychodynamic psychotherapy: up two 80 double hours (usually 100 minutes once per week, 3–9 members).
- Psychoanalytic group therapy: up to 150 double hours (once or twice a week, 100 minutes, 3–9 members).

Individual and Group Therapy for Children and Adolescents:

- Individual psychodynamic therapy/psychoanalysis: up to 150 hours (children), up to 180 hours (adolescents).
- Psychodynamic/psychoanalytic group therapy: up to 90 double hours (3–9 members).

Group therapists often lead several groups. Our survey shows that between 1 and 4 groups are usually held each week. Long-term groups are predominantly offered (multiple answers possible).

- The length of the group is up to 150 double hours (usual psychoanalytic group according to statutory health insurance): 53%
- The length of the group is up to 80 double hours (usual psychodynamic group): 38.5%
- The group lasts more than 150 double hours (mostly self-awareness groups or self-pay groups): 30%
- I offer short-term groups (up to 24 double lessons): 9%

Janssen (2025b) deals with the question of why long-term group psychotherapies are preferred. He sees a connection with the group process. The specific effectiveness of group therapy only emerges after a participant has been accepted and fully integrated into the group. Only then can unconscious re-enactments be processed in the group. Groups are often put together heterogeneously in terms of gender, age and disorders. Of course, depending on the concept, there are also homogeneous groups. However, these are usually the exception rather than the rule.

According to the survey, the following disorders are predominantly treated in the group:

- Depressive symptoms: 96%
- Anxious/phobic symptoms: 86%
- Personality disorders: 64%

- Somatoform disorders: 60%
- Adjustment disorders: 55%
- Post-traumatic stress disorders: 50%
- Compulsive symptoms: 30%
- Eating disorders: 28%
- Self-awareness participants/teaching analysts: 23%
- Behavioural and emotional disorders in childhood and adolescence: 17%
- Gender identity disorders: 14%
- Developmental disorders: 14%
- Addictive disorders: 13%
- Sexual dysfunction: 13%

Training as a Psychological or Medical Psychotherapist

The basic requirement is a approval in medicine or a Master's degree in clinical psychology. The subsequent training must take place at a state-recognized training institute. A total of around 250 institutes in Germany are recognized for training as psychotherapists for adults and/or children and adolescents, of which around 100 institutes offer training in psychodynamic methods or psychoanalysis.

Only in a small number of these institutes is training as a group therapist offered. However, there are also around 20 institutes that are specialized in training psychodynamic/psychoanalytical group therapists.

The training as a psychological psychotherapist comprises a total of 4,200 hours and is divided into the following sections:

- Theory: at least 600 hours (for a combination of psychodynamic psychotherapy and psychoanalysis: at least 800 hours).
- Practical work (mostly work in clinics or day treatments): at least 1,800 hours.
- Training therapy/psychoanalysis: at least 120 hours (up to 600 hours required depending on the institute and training).
- Practical outpatient training: at least 600 hours of treatment (for a combination of psychodynamic psychotherapy and psychoanalysis: at least 1,000 hours of treatment).
- Supervision for outpatient work (at a ratio of 1:4).
- Other (varies depending on the institute, e.g. initial examinations, baby observation, group training, etc., must total at least 4,200 hours).

The training regulations have currently been revised. In future, more emphasis will be placed on the implementation of short-term therapies and group therapies. Thus, in the new training regulations, every prospective psychological psychotherapist will also be trained in group therapy.

Additional Qualification in Group Therapy

Prerequisite for billing with the Association of Statutory Health Insurance and private insurers: Training as a medical or psychological psychotherapist, additionally:

- Theory in psychodynamic group therapy: at least 48 hours.
- Self experience in the group: at least 80 hours (40 double hours).
- Group leadership: at least 120 hours of treatment (60 double hours).
- Supervision of the group leader: at least 40 hours.

For some training institutes, however, these minimum requirements are too low and they demand significantly more or even additional participation in Balint groups and casuistic-technical seminars or the leading of at least two treatment groups under supervision.

The payments for patients differ from €45–70 per group session (self payer or private patients) to €450–500 for a whole group session (100 min), covered by health insurance.

Combined or Conjoint Treatment (e.g. MBT, DBT, Others)?

Individual and group therapy may also be combined or even conjoint by two different psychotherapists, whereby individual or group therapy may predominate. A setting is often used in which, for example, a double hour of group therapy is combined with an hour of individual analysis, or even a fortnightly individual session. The main non-evidence-based argument of this is a much lower drop-out rate than with group therapy alone and the possibility of catching patients, especially those with a lower level of structure. However, various organizations rightly warn that additional individual therapy can undermine the group process and reduce participants' commitment. In our view, the group leader's epistemic trust in the group and in themselves determines whether a group member actually needs an individual session.

Outpatient groups are usually led by one therapist, whereas day-care and inpatient group therapies should, where possible, be led by two colleagues. A new development is that, in outpatient settings, groups of 6–14 participants can now be led by two group therapists, even though there is currently no training or empirical evidence to support this.

MBT-G for patients with personality disorders or with other specific disorders (e.g. eating, somatoform or autism spectrum disorders) should be started by mentalization-based administration for implementing epistemic trust (Staun & Schultz-Venrath, 2023b) and MBT-introductory, which is adapted to the specific requirements of the fault (Schultz-Venrath, 2025 [2013]).

Major Challenges Faced in Practicing Group Analytic Psychotherapy

Practicing group analytic or psychodynamic psychotherapy in Germany must face certain challenges, like:

1 Low Availability of Group Therapy

Of the 5,562 colleagues who have a licence in psychodynamic or psychoanalytic group therapy, only about 10% offer group therapy. The reasons are probably internal and external. The low uptake of outpatient group psychotherapy is due to various organizational obstacles, such as a lack of suitable premises. Other causes include insufficient demand from patients and a lack of interlocking between inpatient, day clinic and outpatient services, particularly following hospital or day clinic stays in psychiatric and psychosomatic outpatient clinics.

Against the backdrop of increasing waiting times for therapy places, politicians felt compelled to promote group psychotherapy more strongly. This led to a reform of the psychotherapy guidelines by the Joint Federal Committee in 2017, which included better financial framework conditions and the elimination of the review process for group treatments and was intended to facilitate the implementation of group therapies. As mentioned above, it is to be hoped that an increase of group therapy utilization will be observed at a later stage.

2 Repression of Psychoanalysis in Therapy and Research

Whereas in the 1970s and 1980s, university chairs in psychosomatic medicine and psychotherapy were generally psychoanalysts, today this is no longer the case. The holder of the only chair of psychoanalysis at the University of Kassel, Cord Benecke, sadly passed away in 2025. The development at clinics is not very different. Chief physicians at psychosomatic clinics also used to be psychoanalysts. Today this is hardly the case. Psychoanalysis and group analysis are losing influence and significance not only in absolute terms, but even more so relative to their environment.

3 Effects of the New Guidelines for Psychotherapy Training

This stipulates that group therapy is encouraged and that every candidate for further training must be trained in group therapy, even if they may have no interest in group therapy at all. In addition, the directive also stipulates that psychologists who are in further training after completing their studies at university will be paid properly (according to TVöD 14, Pay Group 14 of the collective Agreement for the Public Service). In some cases, however, senior psychologists in clinics only receive this salary level, while it is now to be given to new recruits. The financing of this salary level is still unclear, as neither clinics nor practices entitled to further training can justify hiring according to TVöD 14. Like some medical specialist training courses, financial support from politicians must be agreed, but this is not yet in sight. This means that psychologists who have recently completed a Master's degree only have the option of completing their degree in accordance with the old training regulations (further training to become a psychological psychotherapist must be completed by 2032 at the latest). As a result, there are currently more psychologists at training institutes than ever before, which will presumably lead to a glut of colleagues in the next few years, followed by a massive slump.

4 Overregulation

The general German desire to regulate precisely also affects psychotherapy and group therapy. This leads to German complaints about over-regulation, perfectionism and bureaucratic procedures.

As part of the agreements of the European Union, treatment by doctors (and therefore also by psychotherapists in Germany) is to become transparent for patients. A copy of the complete documentation should be made available to the patient on request (up to 10 years after the end of treatment). This documentation also includes the session protocols, including countertransference and hypotheses on psychodynamics. The therapist or psychoanalyst is therefore faced with a conflict. On the one hand, they should document in detail. This documentation would also be their evidence in the event of legal action due to an assumed treatment error. On the other hand, the communication of countertransference, but also of psychodynamic hypotheses, can be hurtful and even contraindicated for the patient.

The telematics infrastructure is also problematic, particularly regarding the confidentiality of sensitive health data. All health insurance companies, clinics, registered doctors and their staff, dentists, psychotherapists and pharmacies should connect with each other. Apart from pharmacies, all will have access to and the right to store all data entered. Laboratory findings, results of imaging procedures, all diagnoses and all discharge reports from clinics are to be stored on a mandatory basis. Discharge reports from psychosomatic and psychiatric clinics generally also contain the patient's biographical history. This puts psychotherapists, psychiatrists and psychosomatic colleagues in a tight spot. They are obliged to enter this information. Only an objection by the patient or their legal guardian can prevent this. In child and adolescent therapy in particular, interests can diverge widely here.

Review of Existing Research and Treatment Outcomes

Research and treatment outcomes are mostly published in "Gruppenpsychotherapie und Gruppendynamik – Zeitschrift für Theorie und Praxis der Gruppenanalyse" with an impact factor between 0.2 (2022–24) and 0.844

(2016) or in "Die Psychotherapie" with an impact factor of 0.6 (2024) by the research group of Bernhard Strauß (Barkowski et al., 2016; Bormann et al., 2011; Burlingame et al., 2013; Kösters et al., 2006; Kösters & Strauß, 2007; Schwartze et al., 2016; Strauß, 2009; Strauß, 2020a, 2020b) and by the research group of Ulrich Schultz-Venrath (Brand et al., 2013; Brand et al., 2016; Döring, 2013 [2015]; Hecke et al., 2016; Krämer et al., 2021; Pries et al., 2022; Reul et al., 2020; Schultz-Venrath, 2016, 2022b; Schultz-Venrath & Staun, 2025; Staun & Schultz-Venrath, 2023a). In addition, there is a range of significant conceptual research on inpatient and outpatient group psychotherapy in psychosomatic clinics (Janssen, 2025a, Janssen, 2025b; Janssen, 2010a, 2010b; Janssen, 2012, 2019). Bridging the science and practice of group psychotherapy is a constant challenge. "In order to establish a meaningful link between academia and practice, researchers must address the issues that practitioners consider important and useful" (Weber et al., 2013, p. 37).

Future Research Ideas and Perspectives on Evidence-Based Practices?

We believe it would be desirable to take a closer look at group psychotherapists in terms of their adherence to and competence in the respective procedures to identify the variables that distinguish good group therapists from less successful ones. It is highly likely that AI-assisted analysis of audio and video transcripts will be of great help in identifying specific factors that distinguish particularly effective group therapists from those who are less effective.

Another desirable aspect would be accompanying training research to find out what the individual obstacles are to implementing group psychotherapy in practice. As a third project, we believe it is important to compare the various psychodynamic group methods relating to disorder-specific groups, such as ADHD, anxiety disorders and depression, eating disorders and somatoform disorders, including also antisocial personality disorders, even though this appears to be a very challenging project.

Notes

1 Lindauer Psychotherapiewochen.
2 See www.igam-institut.com

References

Barkowski, S., Schwartze, Burlingame, G., Strauß, & Rosendahl, J. (2016). Wie wirksam ist Gruppenpsychotherapie im Vergleich zur Einzelpsychotherapie? *Gruppenpsychother Gruppendynamik*, 52(2), 142–155.

Bateman, A.W., & Fonagy, P. (2004). *Psychotherapy for Borderline Personality Disorder: Mentalization Based Treatment*. Oxford: Oxford University Press.

Bateman, A.W., & Fonagy, P. (2006). *Mentalization-Based Treatment for Borderline Personality Disorder: A Practical Guide.* Oxford: Oxford University Press.

Bateman, A.W., & Fonagy, P. (2008). 8-year follow-up of patients treated for borderline personality disorder: Mentalization-based treatment versus treatment as usual. *American Journal of Psychiatry,* 165(5), 631–638.

Bateman, A.W., & Fonagy, P. (Eds.) (2019). *Handbook of Mentalizing in Mental Health Practice.* Washington, DC: American Psychiatric Association Publishing.

Bateman, A.W., Fonagy, P., & Allen, J.G. (2009). Theory and Practice of Mentalization-Based Therapy. In G.O. Gabbard (Ed.), *Textbook of Psychotherapeutic Treatments* (pp. 757–780). Washington, DC: American Psychiatric Association Publishing.

Becker, M., Dieckmann, M., & Neher, M. (2025). *Faber /Haarstrick. Kommentar Psychotherapie – Richtlinien.* Munich: Elsevier GmbH.

Bormann, B., Burlingame, G., & Strauß, B. (2011). Der Gruppenfragebogen (GQ-D) – Instrument zur Messung von therapeutischen Beziehungen in der Gruppenpsychotherapie. *Psychotherapeut,* 56, 297–309.

Brand, T., Barzynski, E., Fuhrländer, S., Hecke, D., & Schultz-Venrath, U. (2013). Psychodynamische versus mentalisierungsbasierte Gruppenpsychotherapie – Versorgungsforschung in einer Tagesklinik. *Gruppenpsychother Gruppendynamik,* 49(4), 350–369.

Brand, T., Hecke, D., Rietz, C., & Schultz-Venrath, U. (2016). Therapieeffekte mentalisierungsbasierter und psychodynamischer Gruppenpsychotherapie in einer randomisierten Tagesklinik-Studie. *Gruppenpsychother Gruppendynamik,* 52(2), 156–175.

Burlingame, G.M., Strauß, B., & Joyce, A.S. (2013). Change mechanisms and effectiveness of small group treatments. In M.J. Lambert (Ed.), *Bergin and Garfield's Handbook of Psychotherapy and Behavior Change* (pp. 640–689). 6th Edition. New York: Wiley.

Christoffer, A., Hinrichs, J., Koch, R., Faldum, A., Knott, H., & Heuft, G. (2022). *Ergebnisbericht – BARGRU (Barrieren bei GruppenpsychotherapeutInnen gegenüber der ambulanten Gruppenpsychotherapie zu Lasten der GKV).* Klinik für Psychosomatik und Psychotherapie, Universitätsklinikum Münster.

Döring, P. (2013 [2015]). Mentalisierungsbasiertes Management. In U. Schultz-Venrath (Ed.), *Lehrbuch Mentalisieren – Psychotherapien wirksam gestalten* (pp. 351–382). 3rd edition. Stuttgart: Klett-Cotta.

Döring, P., & Knauss, W. (2013). Von der Sektion AG im DAGG zur D3G – ein Transformationsprozess. *Gruppenpsychother Gruppendynamik,* 49, 79–104.

Fonagy, P., Gergely, G., Jurist, E., & Target, M. (2002). *Affect Regulation, Mentalization and the Development of the Self.* New York: Other Press.

Geyer, M. (Ed.). (2011). *Psychotherapie in Ostdeutschland. Geschichte und Geschichten 1945–1995.* Göttingen: Vandenhoeck & Ruprecht.

Hecke, D., Brand, T., Rietz, C., & Schultz-Venrath, U. (2016). Prozess-Outcome-Studie zum Gruppenklima in psychodynamischer (PDGT) und mentalisierungsbasierter Gruppenpsychotherapie (MBT-G) in einem tagesklinischen Setting – Was verändert wen? *Gruppenpsychother Gruppendynamik,* 52(2), 175–193.

Heigl-Evers, A., & Heigl, F. (1994). Das Göttinger Modell der Anwendung der Psychoanalyse in Gruppen unter besonderer Berücksichtigung der psychoanalytisch-interaktionellen Methode. *Gruppenpsychotherapie und Gruppendynamik,* 30, 1–29.

Hermanns, L. (2022a). Geschichte der Gruppenanalyse in Deutschland. In G. Dietrich & F. Fossel (Eds.), *Gruppenpsychoanalyse: Theorie, Geschichte und Praxisfelder der gruppenanalytischen Methode* (pp. 188–196). Wien: Facultas.

Hermanns, L.M. (2022b). Die emigrierten Psychoanalytiker und ihre in Deutschland zurückgebliebenen Kollegen. Versuch der Rekonstruktion einer schwierigen Beziehung. *Psyche – Z Psychoanal*, 76(8), 671–706.

Hermanns, L.M. (2009). Über die Wurzeln der Gruppenanalyse in Nachkiegsdeutschland - ihre Rezeptionsgeschichte und Traditionsbildungen. *Gruppenpsychother Gruppendynamik*, 45, 104–127.

Hermanns, L.M., & Schultz-Venrath, U. (Eds.) (2024). *Gruppenanalyse in Selbstdarstellungen*. Göttingen: Vandenhoeck & Ruprecht.

Hermanns, L.M., & Schultz-Venrath, U. (Eds.) (2025). *Gruppenanalyse in Selbstdarstellungen – Teil 2*. Göttingen: Vandenhoeck & Ruprecht

Heyne, S. (2019). IDG – Ein Biotop im BIG. In C. Seidler, K. Albert, K. Husemann, & K. Stumptner (Eds.), *Berliner Gruppenanalyse – Geschichte – Theorie – Praxis* (pp. 89–112). Gießen: Psychosozial-Verlag.

Höck, K. (1976). *Gruppenpsychotherapie*. Berlin: VEB Deutscher Verlag der Wissenschaften.

Höck, K. (Ed.). (1967). *Gruppenpsychotherapie in Klinik und Praxis. Ergänzter Bericht des Internationalen Symposiums über Gruppenpsychotherapie in Berlin vom 20. bis 22.1.1966*. Jena: VEP Gustav Fischer Verlag.

Höck, K. (Ed.). (1982). *Gruppenpsychotherapieforschung* (Vol. 2). Leipzig: Johann Ambrosius Barth.

Janssen, P.L. (2010a). Gruppenpsychotherapie. Zur Geschichte und Theorie aus psychoanalytischer und psychodynamischer Sicht. *Ärztliche Psychotherapie*, 5(4), 221–227.

Janssen, P.L. (2010b). Stationäre und ambulante analytische Borderline-Therapie in Gruppensettings. In V. Tschuschke (Ed.), *Gruppenpsychotherapie. Von der Indikation bis zu Leitungstechniken* (pp. 221–224). Stuttgart: Thieme.

Janssen, P.L. (2012). Psychoanalytische Haltung und Gruppenanalyse. In *Tagungsband der DPV*. Frankfurt on Main: Geber und Reusch.

Janssen, P.L. (2019). Was bringt die neue ärztliche Musterweiterbildungsordnung (MWBO) für die Gruppenpsychotherapie? *Gruppenpsychother Gruppendynamik*, 55 (1), 2–7.

Janssen, P. (2025a). Übertragung-Gegenübertragungsprozesse zwischen Patientengruppe und Behandlungsteam. *Gruppenpsychother Gruppendynamik*, 61(1), 29–54.

Janssen, P.L. (2025b). Gruppenanalyse und ihre Anwendungen in der psychotherapeutischen Versorgung. *Forum Psychoanal*, 41(2), 149–163.

Karterud, S. (2015). *Mentalization-Based Group Therapy (MBT-G)*. Oxford: Oxford University Press.

Karterud, S., Gunnarsen, G., Kongerslev, M.T., Staun, L., & Schultz-Venrath, U. (2025). On the relationship between group analysis and mentalization-based group therapy. *Group Analysis*, 58(1), 115–129.

Kösters, M., Burlingame, G.M., Nachtigall, C., & Strauß, B. (2006). A meta-analytic review of the effectiveness of inpatient group psychotherapy. *Group Dynamics: Theory, Research and Practice*, 10(2), 146–163.

Kösters, M., & Strauß, B. (2007). Wirksamkeit stationärer Gruppenpsychotherapie - Eine kritische Betrachtung deutschsprachiger Studien. *Gruppenpsychother Gruppendynamik*, 43(3), 181–200.

Krämer, K., Vetter, A., Schultz-Venrath, U., Vogeley, K., & Reul, S. (2021). Mentalization-based treatment in groups for adults with autism spectrum disorder. *Frontiers in Psychology*, 12 (708557).

Loch, W. (1992). Mein Weg zur Psychoanalyse. Über das Zusammenwirken familiärer, gesellschaftlicher und individueller Faktoren. In L.M. Hermanns (Ed.), *Psychoanalyse in Selbstdarstellungen, Vol. 1* (pp. 203–236). Tübingen: Edition Diskord.

Mettauer, P. (2010). *Vergessen und Erinnern. Die Lindauer Psychotherapiewochen aus historischer Perspektive.* Munich: Vereinigung für psychotherapeutische Fort- und Weiterbildung e.V.

Pries, J., Niecke, A., Vetter, A., & Schultz-Venrath, U. (2022). More than one way home - Student raters' impressions of interventions and group processes in mentalisation based group psychotherapy and group analytic psychotherapy. *Research in Psychotherapy: Psychopathology, Process and Outcome*, 25, 314–326.

Reul, S., Schultz-Venrath, U., Vogeley, K., & Krämer, K. (2020). Mentalisierungsbasierte Gruppentherapie bei Erwachsenen mit Autismus-Spektrum-Störungen. *PiD – Psychotherapie im Dialog*, 21(3), 1–6.

Schindler, W. (2017). Fraktionierte Selbsterfahrungsgruppen. *Gruppenpsychother Gruppendynamik*, 53(4), 351–356.

Schultz-Venrath, U. (2008). Heute war ein historischer Augenblick der Psychiatrie, aber niemand weiß etwas davon: Zu den Anfängen analytischer Gruppenpsychotherapie durch S. H. Foulkes im Northfield Military Psychiatric Hospital. *Gruppenpsychotherapie und Gruppendynamik*, 44, 215–221.

Schultz-Venrath, U. (2016). Zur Wirksamkeit von Gruppenpsychotherapien. *Gruppenpsychother Gruppendynamik*, 52(2), 108–110.

Schultz-Venrath, U. (2022a). Es begann in Amerika …- die USA als Entstehungsort von Gruppenanalyse und Gruppensychotherapie. In G. Dietrich & F. Fossel (Eds.), *Gruppenpsychoanalyse – Theorie, Geschichte und Praxisfelder der gruppenanalytischen Methode* (pp. 151–167). Wien: Facultas.

Schultz-Venrath, U. (2022b). Mentalizing shame, shamelessness and fremdscham (shame by proxy) in groups. In O. Badouk Epstein (Ed.), *Shame Matters: Attachment and Relational Perspectives for Psychotherapists* (pp. 90–113). New York: Routledge.

Schultz-Venrath, U. (2025 [2013]). *Lehrbuch Mentalisieren. Psychotherapien wirksamer gestalten.* 4th edition. Stuttgart: Klett-Cotta.

Schultz-Venrath, U., & Felsberger, H. (2016). *Mentalisieren in Gruppen.* Stuttgart: Klett-Cotta.

Schultz-Venrath, U., & Staun, L. (2025). Wie kann die Umsetzung von Forschungsergebnissen zu mentalisierungsbasierten Gruppenpsychotherapien (MBT-G) das Behandlungsergebnis in psychotherapeutischen Tageskliniken und Kliniken verbessern? *Gruppenpsychother Gruppendyn*, 61, 58–89.

Schwartz, S.H. (2006). A theory of cultural value orientations: explication and applications. *Comparative Sociology*, 5, 137–182.

Schwartze, D., Barkowski, S., Strauß, B., & Rosendahl, J. (2016). Wirksamkeit von Gruppenpsychotherapie und ihre Bedeutung in Behandlungsleitlinien am Beispiel der Gruppenpsychotherapie von Angststörungen. *Gruppenpsychother Gruppendynamik*, 52(2), 128–141.

Seidler, C., & Misselwitz, I. (2014). *Neue Wege der Gruppenanalyse. Beiträge der Intendierten Dynamischen Gruppenpsychotherapie.* Leverkusen: Budrich UniPress Ltd.

Staats, H., Bolm, T., & Dally, A. (2014). Das Göttinger Modell der Gruppenpsychotherapie. In H. Staats, A. Dally & T. Bolm (Eds.), *Gruppenpsychotherapie und Gruppenanalyse. Ein Lehr-und Lernbuch für Klinik und Praxis* (pp. 47–56). Göttingen: Vandenhoeck & Ruprecht.

Staun, L., & Schultz-Venrath, U. (2023a). Epistemisches Vertrauen, Misstrauen und Leichtgläubigkeit in psychodynamischen Gruppentherapien. In P. Fonagy & T. Nolte (Eds.), *Epistemisches Vertrauen: Vom Konzept zur Anwendung in Psychotherapie und psychosozialer Beratung* (pp. 339–363). Stuttgart: Klett-Cotta.

Staun, L., & Schultz-Venrath, U. (2023b). Mentalisierungsbasierte dynamische Administration. Zur Förderung epistemischen Vertrauens in psychodynamischen Gruppentherapien. *Ärztliche Psychotherapie*, 18(2), 97–102.

Storebo, O.J., Stoffers-Winterling, J.M., Vollm, B.A., Kongerslev, M.T., Mattivi, J.T., Jorgensen, M.S., et al. (2020). Psychological therapies for people with borderline personality disorder. *Cochrane Database Syst Rev*, 5, CD012955.

Strauß, B. (2009). Evidenzbasierte Gruppenpsychotherapie: Ergebnisse der Gruppenpsychotherapieforschung. In D. Mattke, L. Reddemann, & B. Strauß (Eds.), *Keine Angst vor Gruppen. Gruppenpsychotherapie in Praxis und Forschung* (pp. 179–277). Stuttgart: Leben Lernen Klett Cotta.

Strauß, B. (2020a). Evidenz der Gruppenpsychotherapie – aktuelle Ergebnisse. *PiD – Psychotherapie im Dialog*, 21, 17–23.

Strauß, B. (2020b). Instrumente und Materialien zur Unterstützung gruppenpsychotherapeutischer Praxis. *Psychotherapeut*, 65, 277–284.

Strauß, B. (2022). *Gruppenpsychotherapie – Grundlagen und integrative Konzepte.* Munich: Kohlhammer.

Tändler, M. (2016). *Das therapeutische Jahrzehnt. Der Psychoboom in den siebziger Jahren.* Göttingen: Wallstein Verlag.

Weber, R., Ogrodniczuk, J., Schultz-Venrath, U., & Strauß, B. (2013). Zum Verhältnis von Forschung und klinischer Praxis – Ergebnisse der Mitgliederbefragung der Deutschen Gesellschaft für Gruppenanalyse und Gruppenpsychotherapie (D3G) zur Wahrnehmung von Psychotherapieforschung. *Gruppenpsychother Gruppendynamik*, 49, 47–63.

Chapter 13

French Perspectives

Psychoanalysis Extended to Groups, Families, and Institutions

Édith Lecourt, Almudena Sanahuja, Lila Mitsopoulou-Sonta, Aurélie Maurin Souvignet and Clarisse Vollon

Introduction

The role of small group work in mental health care has evolved over time, beginning with occupational groups, which were established in 1801 by the founder of French psychiatry, Philippe Pinel (1745–1826) (Pinel, 1801), and subsequently developed extensively in hospitals, particularly in the form of occupational therapy. Activity groups also had their place, particularly in psychosocial institutions. The anti-psychiatry movement, with psychoanalyst Dr Maud Mannoni (1923–98) (Mannoni, 1967) in France and, above all, the institutional analysis movement with Drs François Tosquelles (1912–94) (Tosquelles, 1967), Jean Oury (1924–2014) (Oury, 1965), and Félix Guattari (1930–92) (Guattari, 1972), and their "therapeutic clubs", brought about a profound revision of psychiatric care, including therapeutic groups. The latter should therefore be considered in the history of health care institutions. At the same time, the training of caregivers became more demanding and the person in charge of therapeutic groups, now neither a craftsman nor a facilitator, had to learn about group processes, first group dynamics and then, with the development of the psychoanalytic approach to groups, the unconscious psychic processes at work in and through the group setting. Clinicians were soon no longer satisfied with encouraging therapeutic results only; they had to reflect on the psychic processes involved in a group setting. Thus, on the initiative of Didier Anzieu (1984), then René Kaës (1993), several generations of group psychoanalysts participated in a major conceptualisation effort to produce a coherent set of theories on the preconscious and unconscious processes at play in group settings. This work was based on Freudian studies.

René Kaës showed that Freudian theory devoted to individual analysis itself includes group dimensions such as: the multiple identifications that constitute every individual, the plural instances of the individual psychic apparatus (Ego, Id, Superego), and fantasies, which constitute a form of internal groupality. The latter is analysed here in relation to the external group (therapy group, family, institution, social group). This led to the development of a coherent framework for understanding the unconscious psychic

DOI: 10.4324/9781003597674-13

processes at work in individuals, groups, families, and institutions. This theoretical construct is a distinctive feature of the development of French psychoanalysis, which extends to groups, families, and institutions.

Cultural Dimension

In its early development, group psychoanalysis in France was shaped by three major influences: social psychology, academic clinical psychology, and fidelity to Freud's work. This trajectory must be understood within a broader cultural framework. As emphasised by Shalom Schwartz (1992) in his theory of cultural value orientations, cultural dimensions shape and legitimise individual and collective beliefs, actions, and goals. Institutional arrangements, public policies, social norms, and everyday practices are concrete expressions of these underlying cultural value systems.

Two major thinkers from the late 19th century played a foundational role in articulating the relationship between individual psychology and the social sphere. Émile Durkheim (1858–1917), one of the founders of French sociology, argued that social facts could not be reduced to the sum of individual facts. Instead, they emerged from the fusion of individual consciousnesses, producing new realities irreducible to individual psychology. This position laid the groundwork for later interest in small groups as privileged sites for research and clinical experimentation, capable of revealing both social and therapeutic effects. Durkheim's seminal work on suicide (1897) offered a social interpretation of a psychological phenomenon, firmly linking social structures and psychic life.

On the psychological side, Gustave Le Bon (1841–1931), considered the founder of social psychology in France, exerted a decisive influence with his book *The Psychology of Crowds* (1895). This work had a major impact not only on psychology but also on political thought. Le Bon identified psychological processes specific to crowd situations, generated by the grouping of individuals into what he termed "psychological crowds". In doing so, he opened a field of reflection on the transformations of individual psychic functioning within collective contexts.

Twenty-six years later, in 1921, Freud published *Group Psychology and the Analysis of the Ego*, a work that can be read as a response to Le Bon. Freud acknowledged the relevance of Le Bon's observations and engaged with them explicitly, devoting part of his text to a critical discussion. However, in the midst of his theoretical elaboration of the ego, Freud attempted to trace the phenomena observed in groups back to individual psychic processes. The group, in Freud's view, did not constitute a separate psychic entity but rather a configuration shaped by identifications, libidinal ties, and ego processes.

Within this historical context, it is unsurprising that the founders of group psychoanalysis in France were clinical psychologists trained both in social psychology and in individual psychoanalysis. Didier Anzieu and his student

René Kaës exemplify this dual formation. Anzieu, already a practising psychoanalyst and a member of the Association Psychanalytique de France (APF), proposed to move beyond group dynamics by explicitly questioning the unconscious processes at work in group situations (1984).

It is important to recall that the APF emerged from institutional dissent linked to the work of Jacques Lacan (1966), whose theoretical innovations profoundly reshaped French psychoanalysis. This period was marked by intense debates concerning the respective roles of biology, society, and language in psychic life, as well as by institutional ruptures. Within this climate, Anzieu took the theoretical risk of introducing the unconscious into group analysis. He formulated this move through a striking analogy: "the group is like a dream … individuals enter the group as they enter a dream." He argued that unconscious, unfulfilled desires motivate the formation of groups, sustained by the illusion that these desires may find fulfilment there. This comparison with dreaming allowed Anzieu to remain firmly anchored in Freudian methodology, extending the analytic approach from individual dreams to group phenomena.

Anzieu further developed the concept of the "psychic group envelope", elaborating the processes of containment operating within groups and introducing the broader notion of unconscious psychic organisers. These concepts provided a framework for understanding how groups offer both protective and structuring functions for psychic life.

The question of a specifically group unconscious soon emerged. René Kaës extended this line of thought by proposing a transpersonal level of psychic functioning, theorised through the concept of the "group psychic apparatus" (1993, 2007). Drawing on Freudian metapsychology, Kaës moved from the individual psychic apparatus to a model capable of accounting for group-specific psychic processes. Through analogies of functioning, he developed a coherent set of concepts describing unconscious alliances, shared fantasies, and trans-subjective dynamics.

This work resulted in a highly coherent theoretical framework that integrated both French and international contributions. By articulating continuity and complementarity between individual psychoanalysis and group analysis, Kaës' conceptualisation enabled psychoanalysis to move beyond individual history toward an unconscious that resonates, circulates, and acts within groups. This theoretical shift opened access to the psychoanalytic study of institutions and to societal and cultural dimensions, notably through the work of Jean-Claude Rouchy (1998), Jean-Pierre Vidal (2008), and Jean-Pierre Pinel (2005). Psychoanalysis thus came to be practised and theorised at multiple levels: individual, family, group, institutional, societal, and cultural.

This expansion was supported by ongoing dialogue with British and Argentine traditions of group analysis, particularly the contributions of W.R. Bion (1961), Enrique Pichon-Rivière (1971), and José Bleger (1967). These international influences played a crucial role in consolidating the legitimacy and development of group psychoanalysis in France and continue to shape contemporary practice.

In the French context, group psychoanalysis was initially promoted by clinical psychologists who were not only trained in individual psychoanalysis and social psychology but also held university positions. This academic status conferred institutional authority and placed them in a position of transmission. René Kaës, in particular, was entrusted with developing a theory of group analysis consistent with Freudian metapsychology (1993, 2007). Despite the progressive reduction of institutional support due to the rise of cognitive psychology and neuropsychology, this model of transmission remains active. Research in group psychoanalysis continues through university-based training and supervision of students.

Today, several French universities—particularly in Paris, as well as Lyon, Besançon, Angers, Strasbourg, Aix-Marseille, Bordeaux, and Toulouse—still offer teaching and research programmes in psychoanalysis and group psychoanalysis.

A distinctive feature of French group psychoanalysts, compared with many practitioners trained in Foulkesian traditions, lies in their dual formation in individual and group psychoanalysis. Personal psychoanalysis allows the unconscious to be experienced not merely as a theoretical construct but as a lived dimension embedded in personal history and relational contexts. Consequently, the training of group psychoanalysts generally involves two personal analytic experiences: individual psychoanalysis and group psychoanalysis.

In clinical practice, group analysts must attend simultaneously to multiple levels of psychic functioning: intrapsychic, intersubjective, and group-level processes. This plural listening enables them to discern the level at which countertransference emerges and to evaluate the relevance of interpretation or intervention. They remain attentive to intrapsychic conflicts, intersubjective dynamics, and trans-subjective processes specific to the group.

The group analyst does not occupy the position of leader or facilitator but maintains an internally distanced stance that preserves this polyphonic listening. Such listening involves hearing multiple simultaneous discourses beyond spoken words: individual narratives, group dynamics, institutional resonances, conscious communications, and unconscious processes expressed through defences, identifications, transfers, countertransfers, and intertransfers. Intertransfer, conceptualised by Kaës, refers to the psychic reality emerging between analysts when group work is conducted collaboratively.

In practice, groups are often conducted by two analysts, allowing a division of roles adapted to individual styles and clinical needs.

The group psychoanalysis movement in France is institutionally represented by two main organisations: the Société Française de Psychothérapie Psychanalytique de Groupe (SFPPG), founded by Didier Anzieu in 1962, and the Fédération des Associations de Psychothérapie Psychanalytique de Groupe (FAPAG), founded in 1995, which brings together 12 professional associations encompassing diverse practices, including couple and family therapy and mediation-based group approaches. These institutions jointly support the *Revue de Psychothérapie Psychanalytique de Groupe* (RPPG), founded in 1985, which publishes two themed issues per year and holds recognised academic status.

More recently, the EFPPFrance has been established with four sections dedicated to group, couple and family, child and adolescent, and adult clinical practice.

Current Clinical Practices and Their Adaptations

The early links between Freud's work and social psychology help explain why Moreno's (1946) ideas, particularly psychodrama, rapidly gained recognition. However, when psychodrama crossed the Atlantic and reached France, it was quickly transformed into psychoanalytic psychodrama. This transformation was driven by the interest of psychoanalysts working with adolescents and young adults for whom classical individual analysis proved difficult to implement.

The psychoanalytic translation of psychodrama consisted in stripping it of its theatrical components—such as the stage, warm-up exercises, and directive intervention techniques—in order to focus on relational play and its interpretation. In this perspective, psychodrama became an analytic situation organised around transference and countertransference dynamics, much like play is used in child psychoanalysis. Psychoanalytic psychodrama thus made it possible to offer a clinical framework adapted to young patients who could not benefit from individual psychoanalysis.

Psychoanalytic psychodrama remains widely practised in France, where Morenian psychodrama as such is not used. It may take the form of individual psychodrama conducted within a group or of group psychodrama proper. These practices were developed and theorised within the CEFFRAP (French Study Circles for Training and Research in the Psychoanalytic Approach to Groups, Psychodrama and Institutions), founded by Didier Anzieu in the 1960s. Psychoanalytic psychodrama is also firmly established in public institutions devoted to care and specialised education. An intermediate Lacanian form has also emerged, namely analytical sociodrama, developed through the work of Liliane Goldsztaub (2009, 2024).

In contrast, group psychoanalysis centred exclusively on speech is now rarely offered. Instead, mediated group approaches have expanded significantly, particularly within institutions, though they are also present in private practice. These approaches have been the subject of extensive research, which has contributed to their clinical and institutional legitimacy. Mediation practices are diverse and often linked to artistic activities, including art therapy, dance, music, theatre, and visual arts. Other forms include photolanguage, modelling, storytelling, writing, and more recently digital mediation.

What all these approaches share is their reliance on a malleable medium that functions as an intermediary between the subject, the group, and the clinicians, mobilising creativity and sensory engagement. Each medium offers specific properties and therapeutic potentials, which must be carefully considered in relation to the clinical setting and indications (Lecourt, 2012; Lecourt & Lubart, 2017). Consequently, research has increasingly focused on sound, visual elements, and aesthetic emotion within groups, and on their effects on therapeutic processes.

In France, the vast majority of these clinical practices take place within public health care and educational institutions, where they are integrated into comprehensive care programmes covered by the social security system, thus ensuring largely free access for patients. From the state's perspective, group practices also present a clear economic advantage. Only very recently have a limited number of psychotherapy sessions in private practice been partially reimbursed by social security, usually around ten sessions per year. This remains insufficient and requires therapeutic frameworks to be adapted to short-term formats. Most psychoanalytic treatments in the private sector therefore remain at the patient's expense, with the exception of care provided by psychiatrists within the national health care system.

Group sessions typically last between 30 minutes and one and a half hours and involve small groups of three to eight participants, depending on clinical objectives and pathologies. They may be offered to children, adolescents, or adults and are facilitated by one or two therapists, sometimes with the presence of a clinical observer. Groups may be closed, open, or slow-open, the latter being the most flexible and therefore the most commonly used. Open groups, however, are particularly useful for working on group relational dynamics.

The group psychoanalytic approach is theoretically open to all pathologies, provided that the work focuses on relational processes and subjectivity. This broad clinical openness has been made possible largely through the development of therapeutic mediations. Nevertheless, in recent years, cognitive and neuropsychological approaches have been strongly promoted by health authorities, particularly by the French National Authority for Health (HAS), and have benefited from substantial research funding highlighting their efficiency and rapid outcomes.

Despite feeling increasingly threatened, group psychoanalytic practices—unlike individual psychoanalysis—have demonstrated a strong capacity for adaptation. In the current socio-political context, their main strength lies in their ability to respond to the search for meaning, relational depth, and humanity within an increasingly standardised and impersonal health care system.

In the private sector, the cost of a group analysis session is approximately €30 per participant. In the public sector, group practices are offered in hospitals, psychiatric and child psychiatry departments, and other specialised services such as psychosomatics and addiction treatment. They are also widely implemented in intermediate psycho-educational and psychosocial care structures under state authority, where they form part of integrated care programmes combining individual, group, and family treatments.

Finally, group psychoanalysts are frequently involved in institutional functioning through supervision, institutional analysis, and practice analysis. It is therefore rare, even in private practice, for group participants not to receive parallel medical or psychiatric care. Group analysts must be well versed in institutional psychological processes in order to understand individual suffering in relation to both the therapeutic group and the institutional context, while remaining attentive members of the clinical team.

Research

The place of the humanities and social sciences in contemporary society has evolved significantly, and universities now allocate dedicated funding to address major health and social issues through regional, national, and international calls for projects (the French National Agency for Research (ANR), regional funding schemes, etc.). Within this framework, researchers in group psychoanalysis are able to develop innovative research programmes supported by these funding opportunities. Such support enables them to strengthen their work at regional, national, and international levels, while also enhancing the visibility of their research through conference participation and the publication of articles, book chapters, and monographs.

Methodologically, research in group psychoanalysis draws on both qualitative and quantitative approaches. Studies may be cross-sectional or longitudinal and may include statistical analyses when appropriate. To explore psychic groupality, researchers often employ specific projective methodologies that articulate individual and group dimensions. These include group-based tools—such as observation groups inspired by Esther Bick's (1968) method and group projective tests (e.g., the "wonderful institution", the family tree, the dream house, or the wounded house)—as well as individual projective instruments for the subject, such as the Rorschach and the Thematic Apperception Test (TAT). Through these combined methodologies, it becomes possible to identify the presence of the group within the individual, both in terms of normative functioning and psychopathology. The results of such research contribute to the identification of new group mechanisms and to the improvement of clinical group care and institutional practices.

The study of preconscious and unconscious processes in groups is also facilitated by specific mediations, such as sound communication, analytical group music therapy, and the clinical analysis of sound recordings of group productions. These recordings provide a kind of "sound X-ray" of group functioning, offering access to rhythmic, tonal, and affective dimensions of group psychic life (Lecourt, 2021).

Beyond individual research projects, the vitality of the field is further demonstrated by the numerous "research groups" initiated by clinicians, which play a central role in sustaining the dynamic interplay between group, family, and institutional clinical practice. This scientific activity is reflected in a substantial body of publications, including books and journal articles. Most research in this field is published in the *Revue de Psychothérapie Psychanalytique de Groupe* (RPPG), complemented by journals such as *Connexions, Le Divan Familial, Dialogue*, and *La Revue de l'AIPCF* (Association Internationale Couple et Famille). Notably, all articles published in the RPPG from its inception until 2000 are now freely accessible via the PERSÉE and CAIRN platforms.

A significant proportion of this research is produced by doctoral students enrolled in the universities mentioned above, working in close collaboration with their supervisors, who are themselves university-based group psychoanalysts. Together, they contribute to the renewal and transmission of theoretical and clinical knowledge in this field.

Current research can be broadly organised according to several thematic axes.

General Perspectives on Group Functioning

Research in this area addresses the dialogue between group psychoanalysis and contemporary scientific approaches (Vidal, 2008), the atmospheres of therapeutic groups and institutions (Bittolo, 2015), and the countertransference of the group analyst in psychoanalytic family psychotherapy, including the analyst's dreams and hallucinations (Eiguer, 2004). Other studies focus on research methodologies applied to group mechanisms (Drweski, 2014; Brun, 2007; Gimenez, 2012), the mobilisation of figurability and symbolisation processes (Mitsopoulou-Sonta, 2016), the body and sexuality in groups (Lecourt, 2005; Mitsopoulou-Sonta, 2016), and the sound dimension in group analysis and, more broadly, the role of the senses (Lecourt, 2002, 2021). Additional work examines configurations of inter- and trans-subjective links (Gaillard, 2011; Maurin Souvignet, 2015; Mitsopoulou-Sonta, 2016), research and training clinics (Gaillard, 2011; Maurin Souvignet, 2015; Chatrousse & Pinel, 2022), the impact of family dynamics on institutional functioning through subjectal transference (Sanahuja, 2018; Sanahuja & Vidal-Bernard, 2023), psychic envelopes and group mechanisms (Mellier, 2010; Vollon, 2019), the psychopathology of group dynamics (Gimenez, 2012; Vollon, 2019; Caillet, 2020), and creativity and trauma treatment in groups (Brun, 2007; Gimenez, 2012; Vollon, 2019).

Societal Issues

Another major axis of research concerns the impact of broader societal phenomena on group life. This includes studies on migration and its effects on groups, couples, and families, particularly unaccompanied minors (Drweski, 2014; Benghozi (2010); Maurin Souvignet, 2015; Mitsopoulou-Sonta, 2016), the consequences of the ecological crisis on relationships and groups

(Drweski, 2014), narcissistic perversion and violence in groups (Sirota, 2006; Eiguer, 2004), sectarian dynamics (Diet, 2008), militant groups (Barrier, 2018), and support groups (Toupin, 2021).

Clinical Settings and Mediations

Research also focuses on specific therapeutic settings and mediations, including photolanguage groups (Vacheret, 2011; Mitsopoulou-Sonta, 2016; Ravit, 2014), psychoanalytic psychodrama groups (Mitsopoulou-Sonta, 2016; Riand, 2023; Drweski, 2014; Jacquet, 2018; Gimenez, 2014; Vollon, 2019; Caillet, 2020), group processes in art therapy and aesthetic emotion (Guénoun, 2016; Canet, 2016), bodily and sound experiences in adolescent art therapy groups (Brault, 2019), analytical group music therapy and sound communication (Lecourt, 2002, 2021; Lecourt & Julian, 2020), dance and movement as therapeutic levers in severe pathologies such as autism spectrum disorders (Lecourt & Lubart, 2017 ; Maurin Souvignet, 2015), body-based mediation groups for adolescents with obesity (Sanahuja, 2018; Picard, 2021), and group programmes for patients with schizophrenia (Gimenez, 2012; Vollon, 2019; Caillet, 2020).

Age Groups

Specific age-related perspectives include research on adolescence in groups and institutions (Duez, 2003; Maurin Souvignet, 2015; Brault, 2019), baby groups (Mellier, 2010), and groups in schools and educational institutions (Sirota, 2006; Nguyen Viet, 2018).

Groups and Institutions

Finally, a substantial body of work examines the relationship between groups and institutions. Topics include archaic and instinctual behaviours in institutions and the necessary "work of culture" (Gaillard, 2011), psychoanalytic work in institutions (Pinel, 2005; Gaillard, 2011; Vidal, 2008; Diet, 2008; Gratton, 2010; Vollon, 2019; Drweski, 2014; Maurin Souvignet, 2015; Mitsopoulou-Sonta, 2016; Dobrczynski, 2017), processes of deinstitutionalisation (Gomez, 2019; Ramirez, 2020), the analytical use of group effects in the clinical analysis of professional groups (Vidal, 2008), relationships between subjects, families, and institutions (Maurin Souvignet, 2015; Ramirez, 2020), and projective tools for evaluating institutional functioning, such as the "wonderful institution" (Sanahuja, 2018; Sanahuja & Vidal-Bernard, 2023).

Groups, Training, and Research

Research also addresses groups as spaces of training and knowledge production, including support groups for doctoral research (Robert, 2013, 2025), group-based training of future psychologists (Mitsopoulou-Sonta, 2016; Maurin Souvignet, 2015; Gaillard, 2011), and experiential groups within training processes (Gimenez, 2012; Vollon, 2019; Caillet, 2020).

Overall, the prominence of research on the relationship between groups and institutions reflects the French context, where most care is delivered within state or state-subsidised institutions covered by social security. This institutional anchoring helps to explain both the quantitative importance and the theoretical richness of this field of research.

We should also highlight some original areas of research, such as research on groups of babies in relation to nurseries, research on sensory experiences in groups, the body and sexuality, research on perversions, on sectarian groups, research on the countertransference of the group analyst, and research on new psychoanalytic approaches using art therapy.

Current research on groups unfolds across a wide and dynamic landscape, reflecting the complexity of collective psychic life and its contemporary challenges. We present the main research themes developed in France. It is extremely difficult to mention every colleague working on these topics, so we will refer only to some of them. Many of these researches are presented in the *Review of Group Psychoanalytical Psychotherapy* (*RPPG*). In the researches in psychoanalytical group psychotherapy interest in *group functioning*, some authors enter into dialogue with current scientific perspectives, such as J.-P. Vidal (2008). Others explore how groups create atmospheres (Bittolo, 2015), generate shared psychic spaces, and mobilise processes of symbolisation that allow what is initially unrepresentable to take form. Particular attention is paid to the sensoriality and sensory dimensions of group life like sound, movement, sexuality, and the role of the senses. The researches of E. Lecourt (2012, 2025), and many others reveal how the body itself becomes a medium of communication and transformation within the group. The analyst is not outside these processes, he/she participates in the group, studies countertransference, including dreams and hallucinations, which illuminate how the group resonates within the clinician's own psychic experience.

Beyond these foundational questions, research increasingly engages with *societal issues* that shape and disturb group dynamics. Migration, ecological crisis, violence, sectarian or militant affiliations, and narcissistic perversion are examined through their impact on couples, families, institutions, and vulnerable populations such as unaccompanied minors. Working with groups in a period of crises and often of social trauma emerges as crucial as the process of collective bonds can help metabolise trauma, loss, and social dislocation. Not surprisingly, a particularly prominent field of inquiry concerns *groups and institutions*. Psychoanalytic work examines institutional dynamics, archaic and instinctual behaviours, deinstitutionalisation processes, and the complex relationships between subjects, families, and institutional frameworks. The researches of Gaillard (2011) and Maurin Souvignet (2015) concern how to think of institutions not merely as structures, but as living psychic systems.

A significant body of work is devoted to *clinical and therapeutic settings*, where group processes are activated through diverse mediations. Photo-language, psychodrama, visual arts, music, dance, and body-based therapies provide innovative frameworks for care, particularly in severe pathologies, adolescence, schizophrenia, autism spectrum disorders, or obesity. These approaches highlight the creative potential of groups and their capacity to foster intimacy, emotional attunement, and psychic repair through aesthetic and sensory experience. For instance, the researches of L. Mitsopoulou-Sonta underlines the importance of this settings to the subjective appropriation of psychic trauma.

Psychoanalytic family therapies constitute another major axis of research. Sanahuja (2018), for example, investigates sibling relationships, couple and family dynamics, and the reverberations of trauma—migration, domestic violence, illness, foster care—within the family group. Projective tools such as the family tree, the dream house, or the spatiogram enrich clinical assessment and deepen understanding of both normal and pathological functioning. Countertransference remains a central concern here as well, revealing how family configurations affect the therapeutic space.

Finally, groups are explored as spaces of *training and research* in their own right. The research work of Gimenez (2012), Vollon (2019) with experiential groups, supervision groups, and support groups for doctoral students or future psychologists underscore the formative role of collective experience in professional development and knowledge production.

Overall, the prominence of research on groups and institutions reflects the French context, where care is largely delivered within state or state-subsidised institutions covered by social security. At the same time, several original and innovative lines of inquiry stand out: studies of baby groups, sensory and bodily experiences, sexuality in groups, perversion and sectarian dynamics, the countertransference of group analysts, and the growing integration of art into therapy into psychoanalytic practice. Together, these works testify to the vitality and diversity of contemporary research on groups.

Conclusion

Finally, the history of the development of group psychoanalysis in France can be seen as a condensation of numerous debates: individual/group, verbal/non-verbal, individual/subject (subject of the unconscious), family/group, group/institution, etc. Clinical practices and research based on these different approaches have also shed new light on the therapists and their counter-transference. Outside their consulting room, group psychoanalysts are challenged to contribute something to society, and not just to individuals. Wasn't that one of Freud's ambitions?

References

Anzieu, D. (1984). *The Group and the Unconscious*. London: Routledge.
Barrier, L. (2018). *Group Commitment and Militant Dynamics*. Paris: L'Harmattan.
Benghozi, P. (2010). *Psychoanalysis of Links: Family, Group, and Institutional Ties*. London: Karnac.
Bick, E. (1968). The experience of the skin in early object-relations. *International Journal of Psychoanalysis*, 49, 484–486.
Bion, W.R. (1961). *Experiences in Groups*. London: Tavistock.
Bittolo, C. (2015). Group atmospheres and institutional psychic climates. *Revue de Psychothérapie Psychanalytique de Groupe*, 64, 45–60.
Bleger, J. (1967). *Symbiosis and Ambiguity*. Buenos Aires: Paidós.
Brault, A. (2019). Body, voice and rhythm in adolescent group therapies. *Connexions*, 111, 89–104.
Brun, A. (2007). *Mediations and Symbolisation Processes*. Paris: Dunod.
Caillet, V. (2020). Group psychopathology and clinical dispositifs. *Dialogue*, 229, 71–85.
Canet, G. (2016). Aesthetic emotion and intimacy in art therapy groups. *Arts in Psychotherapy*, 49, 12–20.
Chatrousse, H., & Pinel, J.-P. (2022). Les enjeux cliniques de la prise en charge précoce des traumatismes psychiques partagés. *Revue de psychothérapie psychanalytique de groupe*, 78(1), 127–139. doi:2.fr/10.3917/rppg.078.0127.
Diet, E. (2008). Sectarian dynamics and psychic alienation. *Connexions*, 89, 25–40.
Dobrczynski, A.-C. (2017). *Institutional Transference and Professional Groups*. Paris: L'Harmattan.
Drweski, P. (2014). Migration, trauma and group processes. *Revue de Psychothérapie Psychanalytique de Groupe*, 62, 97–112.
Duez, B. (2003). *Adolescence and Institutional Frameworks*. Paris: PUF.
Durkheim, É. (1897). *Suicide: A Study in Sociology*. New York: Free Press.
Eiguer, A. (2004). *The Family Unconscious*. London: Karnac.
Freud, S. (1921). *Group Psychology and the Analysis of the Ego*. London: Hogarth Press.
Gaillard, G. (2011). Institutions as psychic systems. *Revue de Psychothérapie Psychanalytique de Groupe*, 56, 13–28.
Gimenez, G. (2012). Group creativity and trauma treatment. *Dialogue*, 198, 45–58.
Goldsztaub, L. (2009). *Analytical Sociodrama*. Toulouse: Érès.
Goldsztaub, L. (2024). *Sociodrame et psychodrame analytiques*. Toulouse: Érès.
Gomez, S. (2019). Deinstitutionalisation and psychic care. *Santé Mentale*, 241, 33–40.
Gratton, E. (2010). *Institutional Psychic Dynamics*. Paris: Dunod.
Guattari, F. (1972). *Psychoanalysis and Transversality*. London: Athlone Press.
Guénoun, T. (2016). Médiation thérapeutique par l'improvisation théâtrale. *Adolescence*, 34(1), 117–128. doi:2.fr/10.3917/ado.095.0117.
Jacquet, É. (2018). Psychodrama and group transferences. *Revue de Psychothérapie Psychanalytique de Groupe*, 70, 61–75.
Kaës, R. (1993). *The Group and the Subject of the Group*. Paris: Dunod.
Kaës, R. (2007). *The Psychic Apparatus of the Group*. London: Karnac.
Lacan, J. (1966). *Écrits*. New York: Norton.
Le Bon, G. (1895). *The Crowd: A Study of the Popular Mind*. London: Fisher Unwin.

Lecourt, E. (2002). Des liens sonores dans les groupes: une médiation méconnue. In C. Vacheret (Ed.), *Médiations groupales en thérapie, en formation* (pp. 33–42). Paris: Dunod.

Lecourt, E. (2005). Comment la question de la perversion peut introduire à l'étude de la dimension sexuelle du fonctionnement psychique en situation groupale. *Revue de Psychothérapie Psychanalytique de Groupe*, 43, 107–118.

Lecourt, E. (2008). *Introduction à l'analyse de groupe*. Toulouse: Erès (2nd edition, 2021).

Lecourt, E. (2012). Les thérapies médiatisées, médiations artistiques, musicothérapie. *Annales Médico Psychologiques*, 169, 685–689.

Lecourt, E. (2017). Frankreichs Situation hinsichtlich Gruppenanalyse. *Gruppenpsychother. Gruppedynamik*, 53, 357–368.

Lecourt, E. (2021). Bruits de groupe: du dieu Pan à la musicothérapie. In P. Laurent & D. Lhotellier, *La sensorialité dans les groupes* (pp. 101–116). Toulouse: Erès.

Lecourt, E. (2025). La communication sonore familiale et groupale, la traversée des codes verbal et musical. *Dialogue*, 3(249), 65–79.

Lecourt, E., & Julian, I. (2020). Résonances intergroupes et surdités groupales: L'écoute des groupes, son analyse, en musicothérapie analytique de groupe. *RPPG*, 75, 75–90.

Lecourt, E., & Lubart, T. (2017). *Les Arts thérapies*. Paris: Armand Colin.

Mannoni, M. (1967). *The Child, His Illness and the Others*. London: Tavistock.

Maurin Souvignet, A. (2015). *Institutional Links and Psychic Transmission*. Paris: L'Harmattan.

Mellier, D. (2010). *Psychic Envelopes and Early Groups*. London: Karnac.

Mitsopoulou-Sonta, L.-A. (2016). Figurability and trauma in therapeutic groups. *Revue de Psychothérapie Psychanalytique de Groupe*, 67, 83–98.

Moreno, J.L. (1946). *Psychodrama*. New York: Beacon House.

Nguyen Viet, C. (2018). School groups and institutional dynamics. *Dialogue*, 221, 59–72.

Oury, J. (1965). *Institutional Psychotherapy*. Paris: Minuit.

Picard, C. (2021). Body-based mediation groups for adolescents with obesity. *Psychologie Clinique*, 52, 101–116.

Pinel, J.-P. (2005). *Institutional Clinical Practice*. Paris: Dunod.

Pinel, P. (1801). *Treatise on Insanity*. Paris: Richard.

Pichon-Rivière, E. (1971). *The Operative Group*. Buenos Aires: Nueva Visión.

Ramirez, Q. (2020). Family–institution interfaces. *Dialogue*, 228, 91–105.

Ravit, M. (2014). *Photolanguage and Group Symbolisation*. Paris: Érès.

Riand, R. (2023). Le modèle théorico-clinique: apports et intérêts pour la recherche en psychologie clinique. *L'Évolution Psychiatrique*, 88(1), 91–99.

Robert, P. (2013). Doctoral support groups and research dynamics. *Connexions*, 100, 77–90.

Robert, P. (2025). *S'aventurer en thèse, des premiers pas à la soutenance*. Paris: Concept-Psy.

Rouchy, J.-C. (1998). *Group Psychoanalysis and Institutions*. Paris: Dunod.

Sanahuja, A. (2018). Family dynamics and institutional functioning. *Le Divan Familial*, 41, 45–60.

Sanahuja, A., & Vidal-Bernard, A. (2023). "L'institution merveilleuse" comme outil d'évaluation de la destructivité dans un groupe de professionnels. *Revue de Psychothérapie Psychanalytique de Groupe*, 81(2), 127–139.

Schwartz, S.H. (1992). Universals in the content and structure of values. *Advances in Experimental Social Psychology*, 25, 1–65.
Sirota, A. (2006). *Violence and Perversion in Groups*. Paris: Dunod.
Tosquelles, F. (1967). *Institution and Madness*. Paris: Maspero.
Toupin, K. (2021). Support groups and collective care. *Psychothérapies*, 41 (2), 87–95.
Vacheret, C. (2011). *Photolanguage and Clinical Mediation*. Paris: Dunod.
Vidal, J.-P. (2008). Group psychoanalysis and contemporary sciences. *Revue de Psychothérapie Psychanalytique de Groupe*, 51, 9–24.
Vollon, C. (2019). Experiential groups and psychic envelopes. *Dialogue*, 224, 63–78.

Chapter 14

What Happened to Group Analysis in the Successor States of the Former Yugoslavia after Its Dissolution

Tanja Frančišković, Esmina Avdibegović, Dolores Britvić, Elvir Bećirović, Maja Brkić, Tija Despotović, Ivanka Dunjić, Milijana Niskanović, Vladislava Stamos and Ljiljana Moro

Introduction

Looking at the development of group analysis (GA) in the Western Balkan countries, we cannot escape the impression that there is a deep connection between the work of group analysts and the cultural and historical specificities of the successor states of Yugoslavia (Slovenia, Croatia, Bosnia and Herzegovina, Serbia, Montenegro, Macedonia, and two autonomous provinces, Kosovo and Vojvodina). Until about 30 years ago, these countries were united in a single state that aimed to develop a common identity through various means, from motivational to repressive. The ubiquitous slogan "brotherhood and unity" symbolised this attempt to create a shared identity, accompanied by a strong suppression of dialogue, especially concerning historical traumas and conflicts (Lampe, 2000; Djokić, 2003).

The totalitarian socialist regime consistently upheld the authority – of individuals, groups, institutions. Questioning authority was almost a taboo, less so in some periods, more so in others. At the same time, language carried significant weight: "an inappropriate choice of words" could lead to a social penalty. In fact, there was a punishable "verbal offense". The ruling clique held power over nearly every aspect of life, which resulted in passivity and a constant expectation that all problems would be resolved by those in power. However, attitudes toward authority were shaped long before the Second World War and the socialist order – for centuries, these regions had occupied a somewhat colonial position in relation to powerful European kingdoms and states. This led to the development of a so-called "colonial mentality", where the stance toward authority extended in concentric circles from family to community, society, and external or foreign powers – without the habit or practice of questioning that position (Harris, 2024; Goldstein, 1999).

DOI: 10.4324/9781003597674-14

A significant change happened approximately 30 years ago, with the break-up of Yugoslavia, which resulted in bloody armed conflicts between certain member states of the former federation. This was followed by changes in the development of democratic processes, which took their own specific course in each of the successor countries. However, burdened by historical particularities, all these processes have, in fact, been slow, progressing step by step. Paradigm shifts are relatively swift only in a declarative sense; at the level of fundamental units such as society, community, organisations, and individuals, they actually go "two steps forward, one step back".

Historical Determinants

Group analysis was introduced to this region after the Second World War by individuals who had completed their education in Western Europe and wanted to apply the acquired knowledge in their own communities. Psychotherapy in the former constituent republics of Yugoslavia could only be practised institutionally (as private practice did not exist). It is no wonder that larger institutions such as psychiatric clinics and university faculties became the primary places for disseminating psychotherapeutic ideas, particularly those grounded in psychodynamic and group analytic approaches. In the 1970s, group analysis practices began to develop in the republic centres Zagreb, Belgrade, Ljubljana, and Sarajevo, and efforts were made to organise educational programmes for both psychiatrists and general practitioners (Klain, 2013, 2019).

Clinical institutions were the places that could provide space for both practice and education. Consequently, trainees were coming mostly from medical and psychological circles.

These groups in the republic centres began collaborating with one another, organising regular annual meetings and conferences, with a focus on expanding the theoretical knowledge and the practical application of group analysis. In addition, the journal *Psihoterapija*[1] was launched, which published primarily theoretical articles and case studies. With occasional interruptions, the journal has continued to be published to the present day. The circles of group analysis practitioners were of a somewhat insular nature, which reduced political suspicion toward psychodynamic theory and group analysis. Therefore, there were no major obstacles for further development. Other psychotherapeutic approaches gradually arrived from the West and developed as well; however, psychodynamic psychotherapy remained predominant in clinical institutions (Prevendar, 2021).

All this resulted in a need for more comprehensive training recognised by the London Institute of Group Analysis (IGA) and European psychotherapy associations. In the late 1980s, educational programmes were launched, in collaboration with the IGA educators from London, in Zagreb, Belgrade, and Ljubljana, taking the form of organised diploma courses.

These educational programmes had already begun when the war erupted in the region. The armed conflicts, primarily affecting Croatia and Bosnia and Herzegovina over a span of four years, led to changes in the social system and the organisation of nearly all societal aspects, including health care. Consequently, the position of psychotherapy within the health care system also underwent transformations. Group analysts, along with psychotherapists in general, gradually lost their space within clinical institutions and university settings. Just as the newly formed republics sought to establish and develop their own identities, psychotherapy and group analysts had to find a new "identity" in the society.

Group analytic practice in all the successor states of Yugoslavia has been based on the fundamental theoretical principles of group analysis, both in organising group analytic practice and in reflecting upon it. Group analysts have had a strong need for education, striving – and continuing to strive – to stay up-to-date with new findings and group analytic practices. On one hand, there is a constant struggle to survive in social circumstances that in no way encourage or support the development and initiative of individuals or groups. On the other hand, the "colonial" legacy in the mentality that "limits" the questioning of information and knowledge coming from authorities (i.e. from the West) has not allowed room for the development of specificities within group analytic work.

However, there are specificities that have developed in individual countries following the dissolution of Yugoslavia, which reflect both cultural characteristics and the post-war political context.

A Perspective on Group Analysis in Bosnia and Herzegovina

Bosnia and Herzegovina (BiH) is a post-conflict and transitional society marked by deep social, economic, political, and ethnic divisions. Post-war conditions have reinforced traditional cultural values, distrust, hierarchy, and patriarchal roles. To our knowledge, there has been no systematic research on the characteristics of group analytic practice in BiH. Therefore, the following text draws on our long-term experience in conducting and supervising small analytic groups, while acknowledging that other perspectives may differ.

Interest in group analysis in Bosnia and Herzegovina emerged in the late 1970s but increased significantly in the period following the 1992–95 war (Avdibegović et al., 2021). The first group analysts in BiH, trained by the Institute of Group Analysis in Zagreb (Croatia) and the Group Analytic Society in Belgrade (GASB) (Serbia), were individuals who themselves had diverse experiences of the horrors of war. Education in group analysis helped them to understand their own wartime experiences and to restore faith in their capacities, in other people, and in the world around them. Professionally, group analysis deepened their understanding of psychological trauma, the role of groups in fostering connection and deepening relationships, and the effects of shared social and cultural experiences. It also enabled them to learn new ways of communicating and understanding others by applying acquired knowledge and skills in group leadership, using the group's potential to facilitate healing. The practice of group analysis in BiH thus appears to be deeply rooted in war trauma, much like the group analysis of S.H. Foulkes, upon whose model it is based.

Group analysis is practised both in public health care institutions and private settings. The absence of legislation regulating psychotherapeutic practice poses challenges, particularly for private practitioners working outside the health care system. The framework of analytic groups follows the model developed by S.H. Foulkes: groups are heterogeneous in gender, socio-economic status, and psychological difficulties, with members approximately equal in ego strength, which is assessed during preparatory interviews. Ego strength refers to the degree of vulnerability and tolerance for frustration (Yalom, 2013). These interviews also explore previous experiences with change, failure, and loss, as well as individuals' ways of coping with them. Groups meet at the same time and place once a week for 90 minutes. Payment is based on the number of sessions held, not on attendance. Practice has shown that paying one month in advance helps maintain regular attendance among group members (Foulkes, 1986).

Maintaining the analytic framework poses challenges, particularly in preserving the consistency of meeting locations and group size. For group analysts working in public institutions and trainees, these challenges often arise from abrupt administrative decisions about repurposing spaces or cancelling previously agreed arrangements. Such "intrusions" into the analytic setting may evoke in members earlier traumatic experiences of loss and disappointment in authority figures who failed to protect them. The group may then regress into a state of helplessness and anger directed toward the conductor. By maintaining their work within institutions and resisting threats to the group's framework, group analysts can influence changes in the institutional culture itself.

According to Foulkes (1986), the ideal number of members for a small analytic group is seven; however, in clinical practice in BiH, groups often begin with fewer participants (typically three to five). The conductor initially works with three members, maintaining the group until new participants join and the group reaches five members. This is partly due to the limited availability of suitable candidates – individuals with strong paranoid tendencies, somatisation, or addictions are usually excluded – and partly due to participants' reluctance to join groups because of anxiety related to self-disclosure. This reluctance can be understood in the context of low generalised social trust in post-conflict BiH (Håkansson & Sjöholm, 2007). Due to the small number of members, the conductor and the group may experience fears of disintegration and disappearance, as if annihilation anxiety hovers over and within them. The therapist's task during this period is to contain and verbalise these anxieties appropriately, helping members recognise and articulate them rather than act them out or leave the group.

Practice has shown that individuals are more likely to accept group psychotherapy after a longer preparatory phase. Most often, participants join the group after six months or more of weekly individual sessions with the therapist. This increased need for individual work before entering the group indicates heightened anxiety related to sharing personal experiences with strangers. Most participants present with symptoms of anxiety, depression, personality disorders, and post-traumatic stress disorder accompanied by interpersonal difficulties.

Given the cultural norms surrounding relationships – particularly among the middle generation – considerable attention is devoted during the preparatory and early group sessions to establishing and maintaining boundaries, especially concerning contact outside the group, physical contact within the group, eating or drinking during sessions, and the exchange of gifts or invitations on birthdays or holidays. Although these behaviours can be viewed as forms of acting-in or acting-out, they also reflect cultural customs and relational patterns.

The predominant group dynamic is marked by the evacuation of content, feelings of being overwhelmed, and difficulties with reflection, suggesting a reduced capacity for symbolic processing. This corresponds to Tucker's (2011) observations on the loss of interpersonal trust and diminished symbolisation in group work with traumatised refugees and asylum seekers. Fear of self-exploration and distrust of others manifest through frequent absences, disregard for interpretations, and a tendency to keep discussions "on the surface". For most participants, group membership lasts up to two years. The therapist is often perceived as an idealised and omnipotent parent figure expected to provide safety and protection. Establishing stability is challenging due to absences and premature departures. These dynamics reflect the unstable social context in which the groups function, as well as fears of closeness and emotional contact. This corresponds with Bion's paradigm, in which groups are often dominated by the basic assumption of dependency (baD) – reflected in the idealisation of the therapist and passive participation – alternating with the basic assumption of aggregation/massification (baA/M), characterised by self-focus and fear of introspection, functioning as defences against annihilation anxiety (Hopper, 2003).

In public health care institutions, potential group members are referred to therapists by psychiatrists. Members do not pay directly; instead, they provide referral letters through which the health care system covers the service. This arrangement undoubtedly influences group dynamics and processes within the group. According to Grotjahn (1977), money in therapy represents a real, symbolic, transactional, psychodynamic, and value-related issue. In this context, the "referral letter" symbolically assumes the role of money. Patients tend to remain dependent on the group and the group conductor for extended periods, finding it difficult to enter phases of individuation and differentiation. Communication often remains focused on the present and on current issues, with pronounced resistance to change. Group members frequently struggle with unresolved traumatic experiences and the consequences of psychological trauma. Most undergo a combination of psychopharmacological treatment and group analytic therapy.

Serbia: Our Beginnings and Our Present Status

The "overseas" Group Analytic Training in Belgrade started in the late 1980s. When the previous plans of organising a joint Yugoslav training seemed to be utopian due to growing political tensions, the group of young professionals from Belgrade established contacts with IGA London and entered the Foundation Course in 1987, followed by the Diploma Course led by group analytic trainers from London. All five years of the course (1987–93) unfolded in an atmosphere of fear and uncertainty, due to the war, the disintegration of the country, the nationalist regime, increasing material poverty, and ultimately, international sanctions, but the training was fully completed.

It is also worth mentioning that all eleven candidates in the Diploma Course were distinctly anti-war and anti-regime oriented, actively participating in demonstrations, forums, and other events. It was extremely hard to establish a relationship with one's own national identity while simultaneously distancing oneself from aggressive nationalist propaganda.

The profound commitment of all candidates to group analysis education at that time can, to some extent, be understood through the fact that it was our only connection to the world during a period of isolation from the international community. It was an oasis of common sense, reflection, and deeper understanding of social and psychological processes in the environment of fragmentation and destruction.

Although group analytic training was the first internationally recognised training in Serbia, it coincided with the formation of the Psychoanalytic Study Group in Belgrade and its acceptance by the International Psychoanalytic Association (IPA) (Dunjić et al., 2023). The fact that several group analysts simultaneously became psychoanalysts probably contributed to a somewhat stronger emphasis on psychoanalytic thinking within Belgrade group analysis.

Possible Cultural Specificities

Gender ratio: In our generation, all founding members and current educators are women. Only in more recent generations have more men begun to enrol in the training (ratio 70/30). This raises the question: Is this a reflection of a general trend in psychotherapeutic professions, where women may be more skilful with verbal techniques, or is it reinforced by patriarchal prejudices (e.g., a certain devaluation of a profession centred on "talking" compared to more "powerful" active methods like surgery, cardiology, etc.)?

Acceptance of group analytic practice: Group analytic practice is highly represented in Belgrade, although even there, patients rarely seek out group therapy on their own, but can be relatively easily motivated, while in the small towns and rural areas it is almost non-existent – possibly due to traditionalism, conservatism, or fear of losing privacy.

Institutional and private practice: Group analytic psychotherapy was practised in the 1990s within psychiatric institutions, then gradually moved almost entirely into private practice.

Recently, through various forms of collaboration with the Institute of Group Analysis Belgrade, it has been increasingly returning to institutions, through applied groups, experiential groups, educational groups. Three years ago, when two independent shooting events occurred in Serbia within a month and caused social trauma, the collaboration between Group Analytic Society, mental health institutions, schools and other public health institutions were further strengthened. We will refer to this later in connection with group analytic work with trauma.

Cultural and political context: In an environment where a one-party system with pronounced cherishing of a personality cult prevailed for decades, and even later, when so-called free democratic elections were established, the citizens mostly elected individuals with autocratic and totalitarian tendencies (the one who was different – Prime Minister Đinđic – ended up being assassinated). In the therapy groups this was reflected in an emphasis on somewhat stronger unconscious tendencies to limit open expression, promote conformity of thought, and idealise the therapist as an all-knowing leader

Group analytic context in understanding and working with trauma (from isolation to international belonging): Although the Serbian territory was not as directly affected by war as other ex-Yugoslavian countries, the traumatic events were overwhelming – through fear, anxiety, poverty, mobilisation, hundreds of thousands of refugees, isolation through international sanctions (1992–2000) culminating with NATO bombing, due to the war politics of the Serbian government. The situation contributed to a deep split between two groups – metaphorically called "two Serbia's – one anti-war democratic and the other paranoid and nationalistic".

Group Analysis in Serbia started during this period of isolation as the first generation of group analysts established the GA Society and Institute for Training in group analysis in 1995. We think that the foundation matrix of the GASB was imbued with basic Fight–Flight and Dependence assumptions (Bion, 1948). At the same time the widely present group analytic practice was providing holding and containment for a large number of traumatised people (Dunjić, 2022; Varvin et al., 2022).

Only after 2000 did we start to connect and reconnect with the international group analytic world. We became qualifying members of the EGATIN,

EFPP, the GASi and over the years became a vibrant society (Despotović & Dunjić, 2014) with the desire to make stronger bonds with colleagues in the region and internationally. As a result, we organised the EGATIN Study Days in 2014 (Group Analytic Identity and Training), GASI Summer School in 2013 (Learning Across Boarders), the EFPP Conference of Group Analytic Section and Adult Section with the theme: Social Traumata (The inner world of outer realities) in 2018, and finally the 18th GASI Symposium (When Divided Worlds Meet: Confluences of Identities, Culture, Continuity and Change) in 2023.

New learning through a recent social trauma: After the tragic school shooting in May 2023, the GASB was invited by the Institute of Mental Health and the Ministry of Education to take part in a large psychosocial project – helping the traumatised community. The method of work was developed and created in action by Despotović and Dunjić (2014), through the hypothesis that the trauma was experienced in the group (classroom) and should be worked through in the group. So, the co-conducting couples were organised to work with different traumatised groups of children, parents, and teachers in the school setting for a whole year and more. Follow-up showed that post-traumatic syndrome disorder (PTSD) was prevented and that children were able to go through the mourning process and continue functional life (results are in preparation for publishing).

25 Years of the Group Analytic Society of Slovenia

Collaboration with the London Institute of Group Analysis in London (IGA) gave rise to the beginnings of systematic study of group analysis in Slovenia. Before that, some group analysts had already obtained full qualifications in Zagreb. The intense development in the field of group psychotherapy in Slovenia and the initiative of young, qualified group analysts led to the founding of the Group Analytic Society of Slovenia in 1998.

Organised education in group analysis declined during the dissolution of Yugoslavia and the rise of consumer society.

The Society organised regular monthly professional meetings focused on the study of group analytic theory, the presentation of group work, reports from conferences and workshops attended by members, and the presentation of students' theoretical and clinical papers. This professionalisation of the Society enabled better organisation and work in accordance with the regulations set by the state.

These developments ultimately resulted in the decision to form an independent institute – in 2011, the Group Analytic Society of Slovenia established the Institute of Group Analysis.

The Institute organised and conducted introductory, advanced, and graduate-level studies in line with the standards of the European Group Analytic Training Institutions Network (EGATIN).

Furthermore, the Group Analytic Society of Slovenia organised biennial workshops. These workshops also gathered foreign group analysts, and some of them were actively involved in the lectures. In these large groups with foreigners, discussions often began concerning the topic of language – an issue that had occupied us even during our studies. What language should be spoken in a group on Slovenian soil? Slovenian or English, or both? Who would translate? At these gatherings, we talked about traumatic experiences from the time of our studies, speaking almost entirely in a foreign language.

In 2018, in collaboration with the Group Analytic Society International (GASI), we co-organised an international summer school that connected members on an individual basis. The purpose of this workshop was to promote group analysis and support networking with foreign associations. The workshop, in which students and alumni of group analysis actively participated, was successful and resonated strongly in the international group analytic community. The theme was titled "Between Generations".

This marked the beginning of a generational shift in the leadership in both the Society and the Institute.

For years, the Society worked in the spaces of the Ljubljana Psychiatric Clinic, which had supported the development of group psychotherapy in the past. However, times changed. At a certain point, the Clinic withdrew its hospitality, and the Society practically ended up on the street. The Society hence became a nomad of sorts, and the matter of new premises brought some disagreements among the members.

One of the Society's great values is the median group. In Slovenia, it has a long tradition. The arrival of Patrick de Maré in Slovenia in 1994 helped establish an outpatient median group, which operated for two years, once a month, with two sessions per meeting.

After the establishment of the Institute for Group Analysis in Ljubljana in 2011, the median group was organised for the purposes of training and became part of professional meetings of Society members. Since then, this group has provided a space for communication among all members and those who occasionally join to experience the dynamics of a median group.

The purpose of the median group is to encourage the learning of dialogue, to transform frustration and hatred into positive energy necessary for reflection, and to create *koinonia*, the fellowship of fellowship. Such an atmosphere, where all kinds of content can be shared, where one can speak freely, listen, and reflect, allows for the formation of the group's microculture. That is why it is so important to hear the voices of all those involved. Especially now, when the older generation of group analysts is withdrawing and there is tension between the administration of the Society and the Institute.

This is the issue addressed by Harold Behr in his article titled "Why Is the Past Important in Group Analysis?" (2011). He argues that the past is a dynamic field surrounded by mystery and confusion, similar to what happens in the interpersonal field "here and now".

There is always an interest in what is transferred from "there and then" to "here and now" and how "what was there" affects "what is here".

In light of what has just been said, the past is not fixed and unchangeable. The next generation rediscovers it, re-examines its value, redefines its meaning in the context of the present and current preoccupations.

The Society is facing new challenges now. We must ask ourselves what we want to achieve together. The realisation of our objectives is possible only through continuous collaboration, which is based on fundamental respect and authentic interest in the other, in their ideas, and our differences.

From its beginning as a small analytic group to this day, the group analysis in Slovenia has come a long way, thanks to its members, group analysts, and others who are active in related associations and institutes both in Slovenia and abroad.

In Slovenia, group analysts are organised within the Institute for Group Analysis Ljubljana (ISAL), which offers training, supervision, and professional meetings in the field of group analysis. Training in group analysis has been present in Slovenia since 1991. Group analysis is practised in both hospital and extra-hospital settings, as well as in organisations, and the method is well-recognised and established within the Slovenian professional community.

The History of Group Analysis in Croatia

The initial impulse for the birth of group analysis was a visit by Prof. S. Betelheim to his friend S.H. Foulkes. Upon returning from London, he began working with groups. The first attempts at educational work in group analysis appeared in 1972 (Klain, 2019).

In 1973, the first postgraduate programme in psychotherapy was developed, where each technique was represented and theoretically analysed, and an introductory course in group analysis was organised for the candidates (Prevendar, 2021). This postgraduate programme is still held today as one of the postgraduate programmes at the School of Medicine of the University of Zagreb, and the introductory course in group analysis is part of psychiatry resident training within the psychiatry specialisation. The Centre for Mental Health of the University of Zagreb's Psychiatry Clinic offered group training in Balint groups for general practitioners and other professionals, as well as courses in interpersonal relations for teachers and similar professionals, led by group analysts (Klain et al., 2007).

In October 1988, the same year that the IGA Zagreb was officially established, the inaugural group analysis training programme organised by IGA London commenced.

In August 1991, the Yugoslav People's Army (JNA) launched an invasion of Croatia, marking the start of constant air raid alerts and prolonged stays in shelters. Soon, the first wave of displaced persons arrived from Eastern Croatia, causing work within institutions to be increasingly complex.

A significant effect of the war conflicts was the large number of psychologically traumatised individuals in need of psychological assistance. In Croatia, group analysts were largely engaged in working with those affected by psychological trauma, offering intensive group treatment during one or two weeks for acute stress disorders in refugees and soldiers and group treatment programmes lasting several months for refugees and war veterans suffering from PTSD (Bertović et al., 1992; Frančišković et al., 1992; Klain, 1992). Trauma-focused groups and sociotherapy groups were organised. Programmes were organised in mental health institution and a number of NGOs organised to help traumatised people (Arcel, 1998). This engagement provided both group analysts and psychotherapists from other approaches with sufficient confidence to develop the profession beyond the previous institutional frameworks. Through group analysis, we developed structured approaches for supporting newly formed groups, including refugees, displaced persons, combatants, and their aid providers. Our work focused on recognising and understanding the psychodynamics of the external reality by exploring aspects of the social unconscious (Klain, 1992; Diminić et al.,1994).

In their clinical work with the trauma survivors, they learned how to work through traumatic experiences and how to prevent burnout (Frančišković et al., 1998).

After the war ended, psychotherapy partially continued to operate within clinical institutions, but many therapeutic schools, including group analysis, continued their work in private counselling settings.

Following the war, the health care system underwent some reforms. Psychotherapy services were reduced to a minimum, the training was no longer conducted in clinical institutions, and each psychotherapeutic school started seeking legal status for educating the next generation through their European associations. Most psychotherapeutic approaches joined forces, and in 2017 psychotherapy became an officially recognised profession, and the Croatian Chamber of Psychotherapy was founded. Group analysis thus became one of the recognised psychotherapeutic schools, and the Institute for Group Analysis Zagreb became an educational centre for group analysis and group psychotherapy. The structure of the candidates also changed. Until 1990, candidates for training were doctors, psychologists, special education teachers, and social workers. Today, economists, lawyers, engineers, and teachers of various subjects are equally represented. Concerning the educators, some are retired, some work only in private practice, while some work in state institutions and once or twice a week in private offices.

The post-war years were a period of "assertion" of psychotherapy as an independent profession, which was not without conflicts within associations and groups themselves: between those who wanted to keep psychotherapy within the health care system and those advocating for the profession to expand and become independent, to break away from previously adopted working patterns.

Final Words …

One of the characteristics of psychotherapy is the lack of collaboration among different psychotherapeutic approaches. Collaboration occurs to some extent within institutions, but more thanks to a small number of trained professionals than out of a genuine need for collaborative work. One might say that the relationship with therapists from other modalities is mostly competitive. Psychotherapists trained in psychodynamic techniques, once institutionally privileged, now sometimes struggle in handling the market-driven competition for dominance, status, trainees, and clients alongside other psychotherapeutic approaches.

Research in the field of psychotherapy are already burdened with many difficulties, from the creation of instruments to the methods of their implementation. In the countries of the Western Balkans, research in the field of psychodynamic psychotherapy has struggled to find its place. Before the war, research in this field was mainly focused on specific group phenomena such as transference, somatisation, confrontation, and other (Klain & Moro, 1982; Moro, 1985; Nađ et al., 1987). During and after the war, using our knowledge of group analysis, we formed groups of war veterans and civilian war victims. We soon realised that this was a completely different population from those we had treated in groups before the war, which sparked our professional and scientific interest. Therefore, we conducted a series of studies on the effectiveness of group analysis and psychotherapy in treating war veterans, as well as on the effectiveness of group psychotherapeutic programmes (which included trauma-focused groups, sociotherapeutic, and psychoeducational groups), which were published in both domestic and international journals (Bertović et al., 1992, 1993; Frančišković et al., 1992; Vidović et al., 1993; Diminić et al., 1994; Kezić et al., 2016; Britvić et al., 2006, 2007a, 2007b, 2012; Urlić & Britvić, 2012; Gruber et al., 2013; Kekez & Britvić, 2009; Cvitanušić et al., 2022). The results mainly showed minimal or no changes in PTSD symptoms, but positive impact on quality of life, which was consistent with previous researches with Vietnam veterans.

The motivation of group analysts to research and reflect on their own work remains a task for associations of group analysts – a task that might add a significant qualitative dimension to their activities.

Note

1 See www.psihoterapija.biz.hr

References

Arcel, L. (1998). *War, Violence, Trauma and Coping Process.* Copenhagen: RCT/IRCT.

Avdibegović, E., Šošić, B., & Dobranić-Posavec, M. (2021). State of psychoanalytic psychotherapy in Bosnia and Herzegovina since the 1992–95 war. *Psychoanalytic Psychotherapy*, 35(2), 169–177.

Behr, H. (2011). Why is the past important in group analysis? *Group Analysis*, 44(4), 454–465. doi:10.1177/0533316411417380.

Bertović, G., Varenina, G., Frančišković, T., & Moro, L. (1992). Evaluation of short-term group psychotherapeutic treatment of soldiers suffering from psychical traumas. *Psychologische Beitrage*, 34, 280–288.

Bion, W.R. (1948). Experiences in groups: I. *Human Relations*, 1(3), 314–320.

Britvić, D., Radelić, N., & Urlić, I. (2006). Long-term dynamic-oriented group psychotherapy of posttraumatic stress disorder in war veterans: Prospective study of five-year treatment. *Croatian Medical Journal*, 47(1), 76–84.

Britvić, D., Antičević, V., Urlić, I., Dodig, G., Lapenda, B., Kekez, V., & Mustapić, I. (2007). Psychotherapeutic treatment program for post-traumatic stress disorder: Prospective study of 70 war veterans. *Group Analysis*, 40(4), 507–522.

Britvić, D., Antičević, V., Kekez, V., Lapenda, B., & Urlić, I. (2007). Psychodynamic aspects of adaptation and treatment of psychotrauma: Study results. *Društvena istraživanja: časopis za opća društvena pitanja*, 16(3), 497–513.

Britvić, D., Glučina, D., Antičević, V., Kekez, V., Lapenda, B., Đogaš, V., … & Frančišković, T. (2012). Long-term improvement in coping skills following multimodal treatment in war veterans with chronic PTSD. *International Journal of Group Psychotherapy*, 62(3), 418–435.

Cvitanušić, S., Britvić, D., Filipčić, I., & Frančišković, T. (2022). Predictors of chronic combat-related post-traumatic stress disorder group psychotherapy favorable outcomes: A prospective cohort study in Croatia. *Psychiatria Danubina*, 34(3), 455–463.

Despotović, T., & Dunjić, I. (2014). Vicissitudes of group analytic identity in search for democracy through training and clinical practice. Conference presentation. Group Analytic Identity and Training, EGATIN Meeting, Group Analytic Society Belgrade & IGA Belgrade, Belgrade, Serbia.

Diminić, I., Frančišković, T., Delić, B., Serdarević, I., & Moro, L. (1994). Traumatization of group leaders in their work with displaced persons. *Group*, 18(1), 46–54.

Dunjić, I. (2022). The echoes of social trauma in the consulting room. In C. Călărăşanu, U. Schultz-Venrath & H. Messner (Eds.), *A Psychoanalytic Exploration of Social Trauma* (pp. 67–77). Oxford: Routledge.

Dunjić, I., Jović, V., Jahović, S., Despotović, T. (2023). History of Psychoanalysis in Serbia (1), Lecture for IPA President and Board in Belgrade.

Djokić, D. (2003). *Yugoslavism: Histories of a Failed Idea, 1918–1992*. Madison, WI: University of Wisconsin Press.

Foulkes, S.H. (1986). *Group Analytic Psychotherapy: Method and Principles.* Oxford: Routledge.

Frančišković, T., Moro, Lj., & Palle-Rotar, D. (1992). Preparatory psychological programme for Croatian army officers serving in the Rijeka region. *Psychologische Beitrage*, 34(3–4), 295–301.

Frančišković, T., Pernar, M., Moro, Lj., & Rončević, I. (1998). Aggravating and mitigating factors in the development of the burn out syndrome. *War, Violence, Trauma and Coping Process.* Copenhagen: RCT/IRCT.

Goldstein, I. (1999). *Croatia: A History.* London: Macmillan Publishers.

Grotjahn, M. (1977). *Art & Technique of Analytic Group Therapy.* London: Bloomsbury.

Gruber, E., Rendulić, K., & Sušić, E. (2013). Grupna terapija bolesnika/zatvorenika oboljelih od posttraumatskog stresnog poremećaja i/ili trajnih promjena ličnosti na odjelu forenzičke psihijatrije zatvorske bolnice Zagreb. *Kriminologija & socijalna integracija: časopis za kriminologiju, penologiju i poremećaje u ponašanju*, 21(1), 139–149.

Håkansson, P. & Fredrik Sjöholm, F. (2007). Who do you trust? ethnicity and trust in Bosnia and Herzegovina. *Europe-Asia Studies*, 59(6), 961–976. doi:10.1080/09668130701489162.

Harris, R. (2024). *Croatia: A History: from Revolution to Independence*. Zagreb: Školska knjiga.

Hopper, E. (2003). *Traumatic experience in the unconscious life of groups: The fourth basic assumption: Incohesion: Aggregation/massification or (ba) I: A/M* (Vol. 23). London: Jessica Kingsley Publishers.

Kekez, V., & Britvić, D. (2009). Pacijentice s drugim anksioznim poremećajima u homogenoj grupi žena oboljelih od PTSP-a. *Socijalna psihijatrija*, 37(1), 37–42.

Kezić, S., Britvić, D., Caratan, S., Goršić, L., Ivezić, E., Matić, K., & Filipčić, I. (2016). Day hospital treatment as a missing link for single patients with posttraumatic stress disorder (PTSD): A preliminary study. *Psychiatria Danubina*, 28(2), 184–187.

Klain, E., Gregurek, R., & Praper, P. (2007). *Grupna psihoterapija za medicinske sestre i tehničare*. Zagreb: Medicinska naklada.

Klain, E. (2013). Povijesni razvoj psihoanalize i psihoanalitičkih psihoterapija. *Hrvatska psihoanalitička studijska grupa: Psihoanaliza u Hrvatskoj*. Zagreb: Medicinska naklada.

Klain, E. (2019). Kratka povijest. In Lj. Moro, E. Klain E., D. Josić, Z. Brumen Budanko, & S. Pavlović. 30 years of the Institute of group analysis. *Psihoterapija*, 33 (1), 46–122.

Klain, E., & Moro, L.J. (1982). What a patient can learn his narcissism in an analitycal group. In M. Pines and L. Rafaelsen (Eds.), *The Individual and the Group*, Vol. 2, *Practice* (pp. 87–92). New York and London: Plenum Press.

Klain, E. (Ed.) (1992). *Psychology and Psychiatry of a War*. Zagreb: Faculty of Medicine, University of Zagreb.

Lampe, J.R. (2000). *Yugoslavia as History: Twice There Was a Country*. Cambridge: Cambridge University Press.

Moro, Lj. (1985). Confrontation as intervention in the group. *Group Analysis*, 18(3), 194–198.

Nađ, M., Buzov, I., Josić, D., Klain, E., & Moro, Lj. (1987). *Psychodynamic Approach to the Patients Suffering from Breast Cancer* (pp. 2–3, 5). Zagreb: Liječnički vjesnik. Excerpta medica.

Prevendar, T. (2021). *Development of Psychotherapy in Croatia: From the Beginning Until 2018*. Zagreb: Medicinska naklada.

Tucker, S. (2011). Psychotherapy groups for traumatized refugees and asylum seekers. *Group Analysis*, 44(1), 68–82. doi:10.1177/0533316410390478.

Urlić, I., & Britvić, D. (2012). Group-based strategies employed in the wartime and post-war treatment of psychological trauma: Experience from the war in Croatia. *Clinical Social Work Journal*, 40(4), 421–428.

Vidović, V., Moro, L., Begić, N., Frančišković, T., Palle-Rotar, D., & Tocilj, G. (1993). Children in war and exile: Emotional reactions and signs of distress. *Medica Jadertina – Supplement*, 23(1–2), 13–20.

Varvin, S., Despotović, T., & Jović, V. (2022). Psychotherapy of posttraumatic conditions. In C. Călărăşanu, U. Schultz-Venrath, & H. Messner (Eds.), *A Psychoanalytic Exploration of Social Trauma* (pp. 133–154). Oxford: Routledge.

Yalom, I.D. (2013). *The Theory and Practice of Group Psychotherapy*. 5th edition. New York: Basic Books.

Chapter 15

Group Analysis in Finland

Taru Kaivola

Introduction

Interest in group psychotherapy emerged in Finland in the 1950s, and since then it has become a well-established and widely applied form of treatment. In recent decades, however, its position has been weakened by health policy decisions and broader cultural changes. Today, two major professional associations are active in the field: the Finnish Group Analytic Society and the Finnish Group Psychotherapy Association. In this article, I focus particularly on the position of group analysis in Finland.

I begin by outlining the development of group analysis and its distinctive characteristics in the Finnish context. In Finland, group analytic training has been organized entirely by domestic trainers and in the Finnish language—unlike in many other countries, where training is more strongly linked to international structures. This has certainly influenced both clinical practice and theoretical thinking on both a conscious and unconscious level.

I would like to highlight some cultural factors that are seen as specific to group psychotherapy in Finland. One feature that stands out as particularly characteristic of Finnish group psychotherapy is the role of silence. Secondly, I highlight the Finnish attachment to large groups. Even in these, silence has a special role to play.

In the second part of the chapter, I turn to the practice of group analytic psychotherapy. A significant recent change is that group psychotherapy has virtually disappeared from public health care. As a result, the focus has shifted to the private sector, where the clinical setting and patient population differ from those in the public system.

Finally, I discuss how recent changes in health care and psychotherapy training have affected the implementation of group psychotherapy, and consider the future prospects of group analysis in Finland.

DOI: 10.4324/9781003597674-15

Theoretical Foundations and Cultural Links in Group Analytic Psychotherapy

Group analysis was introduced to Finland by Dr. Heimo Salminen, a long-time educator and founding member of the Finnish Group Psychotherapy Association. This association implements the Tavistok tradition. He became increasingly drawn to group analysis during visits to London. His efforts to reform training in Finland based on group analytic principles faced resistance and internal disagreements, leading to a split from the existing structures. As a result, group analysis training was started under the leadership of Heimo Salminen in 1993 at the Finnish Mental Health Association. It should be mentioned that Heimo Salminen is the author of the Finnish textbook *Basics of Group Analysis* (1997).

In Finland, interest in group analysis emerged as a counterbalance to the dominant psychoanalytic training tradition, which was often perceived as hierarchical and authority-centered. Foulkes' (1964) ideas of equality and dialogue introduced a refreshing, participatory perspective on psychotherapeutic work. According to his theory, power and responsibility are not vested solely in the group conductor but are shared among group members. This view contrasted with the traditional therapist-as-authority model. Foulkes (1975) emphasized that the group itself functions as a therapeutic agent, and the conductor's role is to support rather than direct this process. In this way, the group becomes a dynamic space where multiple perspectives interact and evolve.

Teaching group analysis in Finnish has been of particular importance to us. This can also be understood in a historical context: centuries of subjugation under Swedish and later Russian rule created sensitivity to power imbalances and reinforced the value of collective responsibility. The struggle for independence and the affirmation of Finnish as a cornerstone of national identity made equality, self-expression, and being heard essential values. From the outset, Finnish group analytic training has emphasized dialogue and equality, both in content and format. Unlike many other European models, it has been conducted entirely in Finnish and led by Finnish professionals. While foreign trainers have occasionally contributed to large-group seminars, the core instruction has remained domestic. This deliberate choice helps to prevent asymmetrical power dynamics and cultural dominance, safeguarding the central role of local expertise. Finland's historical experiences of subjugation, along with the late official recognition of Finnish as an administrative language, have cultivated a national sensitivity to linguistic and cultural autonomy. These factors underpin the prioritization of local trainers and the Finnish language—forming the foundation for a culturally appropriate, independent, and sustainable system of group analytic training in Finland.

Psychotherapy is fundamentally rooted in language and interaction. In group psychotherapy, it is essential that participants can express themselves in ways that are understood, and that they, in turn, can understand others. As Foulkes and Anthony (1984, p. 245) note, language functions both as a teaching method and as a process in itself: "because words are old and carry layers of meaning … in a group their common meaning always exists between what they mean to the user and what they mean to the hearers." This linguistic dynamic is central to all group settings, and it becomes particularly significant in a multilingual and culturally sensitive environment such as Finland.

Group analytic training takes place within a group setting, reflecting its core: group dynamics and communal learning. All students read the assigned literature for the seminars, and each student takes turns presenting a theoretical article related to the training day. The topic is then discussed and reflected on together. Through dialogue, the aim is to foster a shared understanding and give students the opportunity to integrate new knowledge with prior learning, clarify ambiguities, and deepen their insight. Participants learn not only from trainers and literature but also from one another. The group's interaction creates a space where theoretical concepts come alive and are examined in practice. This communal form of learning allows for a multi-voiced and critical perspective in which different experiences and viewpoints enrich each student's understanding. Because group analysis emphasizes the social dimension of the human being, having a Finnish trainer ensures that the theory can be considered within the context of Finnish society and culture.

The training remains focused on core group analytic theory, with supporting influences from psychoanalysis, social psychology, existentialism, systems theory, and mentalization. Given the relatively short duration of training and the presumption of prior theoretical knowledge, the curriculum emphasizes essentials. This "orthodoxy" was also a conscious distancing from the Tavistock tradition, which had previously dominated group therapy training in Finland. Emphasis on core group analysis may explain why methods such as dialectical behaviour therapy (DBT) or mentalization-based approaches have not been fully integrated into Finnish group analysis, despite their popularity in the broader public sector.

Dr. Salminen and his colleagues aimed to assign training responsibilities to newly graduated group analysts as soon as possible. This was implemented with the support of mentoring from more experienced educators. They also encouraged students to form the Group Analytic Association, which was indeed established in 2003 by recent graduates and students.

While giving responsibility and freedom to new group analysts was inspiring and allowed for independent action, it also brought challenges. Senior trainers quickly withdrew to the background, leaving the newly qualified professionals without ongoing support from the previous generation. In hindsight, the situation resembled a family in which the parents leave the siblings to fend for themselves without guidance. As a result, some founding members have borne an unreasonable amount of responsibility and overcommitted themselves. Moreover, distributing power and responsibility equally has not been without issues. Envy, competition, and power struggles have simmered beneath the surface, and have not been easily resolved among themselves.

Regular large groups are an essential part of Finnish group analytic culture. The unique importance of language in Finnish culture provides a foundation for understanding the dynamics in large group settings, where language, silence, and authority converge in complex ways. These sessions have offered collective spaces to process historical traumas such as the 1918 Civil War and the Winter and Continuation Wars 1939–40, 1941–44. Large groups have made visible transgenerational effects and have helped connect personal dynamics with collective memory. However, when foreign conductors lead such groups, issues of authority and self-worth often surface. Finnish participants may idealize foreign experts, leading to feelings of inadequacy or shame, especially among those less fluent in English. Over time, more large or median groups have been conducted by Finnish professionals, reducing these dynamics.

Silence, another cultural hallmark, also plays a vital role in Finnish group therapy. Although language is important to us Finns, silence is also a national trait. Finns have a deep and meaningful relationship with silence, which is reflected in our culture, relationships, and connection to nature. Silence is not merely the absence of speech; it can signify presence, listening, and respect. In Finland, silence is not seen as uncomfortable but as a natural part of life. It relates closely to nature, self-reflection, and respect for others. Silence gives space for thoughts, feelings, and observations, and Finns are used to understanding much without words.

In conversation, pauses are not signs of awkwardness but may indicate contemplation or respect. A Finn does not feel the need to fill every silence with talk—sometimes the best thing is simply to be together without saying anything. Silence is not exclusionary; it creates space for others, for thoughts, and for oneself. It is part of the Finnish mental landscape, where words are not always necessary but still hold deep meaning. (Vatanen, 2021)

Although therapy often emphasizes the importance of speaking, silence can be just as significant a part of the therapeutic process. It offers space for reflection, emotional processing, and deeper connections between group members. In Finnish group psychotherapy, silence is not emptiness or resistance, but a space in which thoughts, emotions, and interactions can evolve. It can be a therapeutic force that enables profound reflection and the emergence of shared understanding. Silence can support growth, self-discovery, and the development of group dynamics—when it takes place in a safe and accepting atmosphere.

In Finnish therapeutic culture, where there is no need to fill every pause with talk, silence can serve as an invitation to introspection. It helps the client hear themselves better and recognize their emotions before putting them into words. The conductor can model an accepting and permissive attitude toward silence, making it feel natural rather than threatening. Through silence, the conductor can allow group dynamics to unfold without excessive direction. At the same time, they must recognize when silence becomes inhibiting or avoidant and help the group process it. Silence can create a protective space where group members feel safe without pressure to speak, but it can also reveal tensions or avoidance if difficult topics are left unaddressed.

Although Finnish silence is often seen positively, it can cause misunderstandings in international settings. In cultures where constant speech is seen as a sign of sociability and friendliness, Finnish reticence may seem distant or cold (Isosävi 2020). Many foreign large group conductors have observed that Finnish participants tend to be quiet and that group silences can last a long time.

Gerhard Wilke (2019) noted that Finnish group silences—sometimes lasting up to 40 minutes—reflect a cultural pact against shame and dependency. Silence becomes a communal ritual, avoiding social division and asserting equality. It can also mask fears of envy or superiority. For Finnish group analysts, understanding and working with silence is not optional—it is central.

Gerhard Wilke describes his experiences in Finnish large groups as follows:

> The frequent and long silences are the identity badge of the Finnish large group. In the role of the analyst, I was repeatedly put in the position of having to tolerate long silences of up to forty minutes. It was a unique experience to learn that silence could function as social glue through an unconscious pact—that it is the duty of every Finn to be proud by avoiding being shamed. The superego of many group members urged them on, to demonstrate to the community that they did not need to be dependent and could do without social chat and help. It was shameful to make yourself feel at ease through a sense of belonging achieved through an open exchange of feelings and thoughts in the service of a sense of communion. On the psychological level, the frequent silences, at least in my interpretation, were related to a fear of being envied and repression of the wish to be seen as superior in the eyes of your neighbor. In this way, silence functioned in this large group as a ritual of communion, where oneness without social division and beyond language and power differences could be held and maintained.
>
> (Wilke, 2019, p. 192)

Current Practice and Adaptation

Psychotherapy groups typically include men and women of varying ages and diagnoses. The most common diagnoses are anxiety, depression, and personality disorders. Each member commits to the group for at least one year. Groups may be either closed (where all members start and finish at the same time) or replenishing (where new members replace those who leave). Before the group begins, each participant undergoes an interview, and a therapy contract is signed. Sessions last one and a half hours and are held weekly.

The core of psychotherapeutic treatment lies in the interactions between group members. There are no predefined themes or turns to speak—members are encouraged to talk freely about whatever is on their mind. Through discussion, individuals realize they are not alone in their struggles and that others in the group face similar challenges. Over time, members recognize the value the group offers and begin to make progress. The way we relate to others in a group may mirror early childhood interactions or social patterns from outside the group. These relational styles are not always functional. Group therapy offers a chance to practice new, healthier ways of connecting with others and forming more satisfying relationships. While group therapy may not solve all life's difficulties, it can help individuals learn new ways of relating to themselves, others, change, and life's pressures.

Trust and open interaction within the group allow members to explore the roots and consequences of their problems. Group members offer each other new perspectives, and new solutions may emerge. It is often surprising how much support one can provide to others—and how much one can learn from them. The group's confidential and safe atmosphere creates space to express and work through difficult emotions. Over time, participants learn that all emotions can be expressed and managed.

Because people are often blind to their own behavior, the group provides valuable feedback, helping individuals see themselves through the eyes of others. Group therapy has been described as a "hall of mirrors," where one can view themselves from multiple perspectives. Others' stories also resonate with group members, helping them recognize their own experiences in those of others. This reflective process helps develop a clearer and more realistic self-image.

The Finnish term for group analyst is *ryhmänohjaaja* (group facilitator), which differs from the English "conductor." The former implies modest leadership and guidance, while the latter suggests orchestration and prominence. This semantic difference reflects cultural values: Finnish conductors are expected to enable, not direct. Their role is to support group processes organically, allowing space, silence, and multiplicity of voices. The role of the group therapist, or facilitator, is not emphasized. The facilitator is both outside and inside the group at the same time. The position of the facilitator at the interface allows them to see, experience, perceive and express what is beyond the reach of the other group members. It also gives the opportunity to join in. Sometimes the facilitator pays more attention to the individual and the issues they brings up, sometimes to the group as a whole, and sometimes to the relationships between group members. The group facilitator ensures the safety and functioning of the group. They keep to agreements, take care of boundaries and structures.

The Finnish psychotherapy field is currently in a state of flux. Until a few years ago, a shortage of psychotherapists meant that patients were frequently referred to group therapy. However, recent changes in health care have led to the opposite situation: psychotherapists—particularly those trained in psychodynamic approaches—are now experiencing a shortage of clients. Referrals to group therapy have declined, and therapists are increasingly accepting all referred patients, even those for whom group therapy may be unsuitable. This has led to poorer outcomes and increased dropout rates, discouraging referring doctors from making group therapy referrals.

Currently, group psychotherapy is available only in the private sector. Most group therapists operate in their own private practices or clinics. The public health care sector no longer offers traditional group psychotherapy. Instead, short-term or manualized group interventions—often run by nurses or psychologists without formal psychotherapy training—are more common.

Some patients pay for therapy themselves, but many receive financial support from social security. The Social Insurance Institution of Finland (Kela) is responsible for health insurance, student benefits, and rehabilitation services. Kela funds mental health rehabilitation, including psychotherapy, for individuals whose ability to work or function is at risk. Kela-supported rehabilitative psychotherapy is intended for individuals aged 16–67 whose work or study capacity has been reduced due to mental health issues. The primary goal is to improve functioning and prevent work disability. To qualify, a psychiatrist's statement and at least three months of prior mental health treatment are required. The need for therapy is reassessed annually through a new physician's statement and a therapist's evaluation report, including goal progress and ongoing treatment needs. Patients also complete the CORE-OM questionnaire before, during, and after therapy.

Kela sets rules for the provision of psychotherapy. For instance, a group psychotherapist cannot simultaneously provide individual psychotherapy. To deliver Kela-supported rehabilitative psychotherapy, a therapist must have a protected professional title granted by the National Supervisory Authority for Welfare and Health (Valvira), meaning a university-level psychotherapy qualification and an appropriate undergraduate degree. Kela must also approve the therapist's qualifications.

Kela covers part of the therapy cost, while the client pays the remaining co-payment. This amount varies depending on the therapist's fees. In group therapy, co-payments typically range from €5 to €20 per session. Kela typically supports group therapy for one to three years, up to 100 sessions. It cannot be combined with other therapies (e.g., individual therapy). After three years of Kela-supported therapy, a five-year waiting period is required before eligibility resumes.

In most cases, clients are referred to therapy through occupational health services. Finland's statutory occupational health care system aims to promote employee health and ensure a safe working environment. Employers must provide preventive occupational health services and may also offer general practitioner-level care. These services are employer-funded, with Kela contributing. Access to psychotherapy through occupational health is typically faster and simpler than through public health care, where patients often undergo several interventions before receiving the psychiatrist's statement required for Kela-supported therapy.

Over the past few years, the Finnish health care system has undergone substantial reforms. In 2021, the country was divided into 21 well-being services counties—a major administrative transformation aimed at equalizing access to services, reducing health disparities, and controlling costs. These changes have also impacted psychotherapy, shifting focus toward short-term treatments.

The "Therapies to the Frontline" initiative is a stepped-care model inspired by the UK's NHS Talking Therapies (formerly IAPT). It aims to expand access to psychosocial treatments, particularly in primary care. The model emphasizes short-term CBT-based interventions for common mental health issues like depression and anxiety but also includes other evidence-based approaches (Terapiat etulinjaan, 2024). In practice, "Therapies to the Frontline" offers limited, brief interventions—typically 1–7 sessions, possibly including online therapy or psychoeducational group programs. If needed, patients can be referred to short-term therapy of around 20 sessions. Recently, well-being counties have begun contracting private therapists to provide short-term psychotherapy, and public tenders have started to include group therapy options.

Specialized psychiatric care has also changed significantly. Treatment durations are shorter and service options more limited. Cognitive and biomedical approaches have largely replaced traditional psychodynamic or psychoanalytic therapies, reducing the variety and accessibility of treatments. Many trained psychotherapists have moved to private practice or changed careers. Only a few group analysts now work within the well-being services counties, and the status of group therapy has diminished.

Reforms have also impacted psychiatric inpatient care. The number of beds has decreased, and inpatient stays are now shorter, primarily for financial reasons. This has made implementing group psychotherapy in inpatient settings virtually impossible. Day hospital units have also declined, and the group interventions offered there are often not true group psychotherapies.

Challenges and Evidence-based Practice

Public mental health care has become more restricted and performance-oriented, which has particularly weakened the position of group analysis. This form of therapy emphasizes long-term, in-depth, relational work that takes into account both individual and sociocultural factors, but it requires time, trust, and flexibility—resources that are increasingly scarce in the current system. Client selection is often guided by work ability or productivity, leaving less room for exploring deeper inner experiences. In addition, due to historical developments, the service system has become fragmented and multi-actor, making it difficult to manage (Pirkola 2020). Structural reforms and the emphasis on short-term, measurable methods such as cognitive behavioral therapy have reduced referrals to group psychotherapy and diminished its visibility in treatment recommendations. However, this decline does not reflect a lack of efficacy, but rather systemic and ideological changes that favor quick, standardized interventions at the expense of long-term, in-depth therapeutic work.

Group psychotherapy—especially group analysis—remains relatively unknown in Finland and is often overshadowed by individual therapies, a tendency reflected both in health care structures and in psychotherapy training. One key challenge is the limited awareness and understanding of group analysis among referring professionals. General practitioners and psychiatrists are often unfamiliar with the method or hold outdated views. As a result, group therapy is rarely recommended to patients, who also tend to prefer individual therapy due to cultural norms of privacy and independence.

Another major shift occurred in 2011 when the responsibility for psychotherapy training was transferred to universities. This reform aimed to ensure quality and academic rigor but also introduced competitive bidding and stricter entry requirements. Group analysis, being a small and less visible modality, has struggled to secure a place in university-administered programs.

Psychotherapy training is offered as continuing professional education (not part of degree programs) and is formally provided by universities. However, universities collaborate with external psychotherapy associations or training institutes to deliver the actual training. Universities are the formal providers of psychotherapy training, issuing certificates and ensuring the training meets national (Valvira) standards. The actual training (lectures, supervision, clinical practice) is frequently outsourced to qualified external organizations, such as Group Analytic Associations: universities organize competitive bidding processes to select external training providers. The selection is based on criteria such as content quality, trainer qualifications, costs, and methodology. After winning the bid, the external provider delivers the training in collaboration with the university, but under the university's official umbrella. Students apply through the university, pay fees to the university, and receive a certificate from the university upon completion.

The increased role of universities has brought both benefits and challenges. While quality and oversight have improved, the reform has created particular difficulties for smaller and lesser-known therapeutic approaches such as group analysis. The reform of psychotherapy education has not sufficiently considered the diverse needs of the population or balanced representation of various approaches. While the current system has brought more quality and supervision, it has narrowed the possibilities for the survival, research development, and regional accessibility of smaller psychotherapy modalities (Lindfors, 2024).

Stricter admission requirements have reduced the number of applicants for group analysis training. Psychotherapy education is expensive, and group analytic training can cost the student as much as €30,000. This often limits participation to those with sufficient financial resources. Universities are not legally required to offer psychotherapy training, and state funding does not adequately support the programs. This hinders long-term development efforts and especially the survival of smaller approaches.

Only one university, the University of Helsinki, has offered training in group analysis. Since the reform, it has been very difficult to launch new training courses. Only a handful of students have completed group analytic training since the reform. In contrast, cognitive-behavioral and integrative modalities dominate admissions, accounting for over 40% of new psychotherapist licenses (Laukkanen, 2022 p 36-39). This imbalance raises concerns about the diversity of psychotherapeutic education.

The Finnish Group Analytic Society serves as an expert community for psychoanalytic group psychotherapy in Finland. Its mission is to maintain and develop expertise in group analysis, support training, and promote the field's recognition and appreciation. In recent years, however, the society has faced challenges that weaken its vitality and influence. The main issue is the lack of active members: the membership consists largely of senior professionals, many of whom are retired or nearing retirement. Recruiting younger members has proven difficult, leaving few people willing to take on responsibilities such as board work or event organization. Ultimately, much of the responsibility falls on a small group of active members: the board is expected to handle planning, execution, communication, and event organization. This overburdens the few and limits the society's ability to renew and develop its activities. For many, association activities feel like an extra burden in the midst of busy professional and personal lives. The society also lacks prominent representatives who could advocate for group analysis in public discussion or professional decision making.

The research foundation for psychoanalytic group analysis in Finland is still emerging. Although the method is widely practiced and clinically effective, stronger research evidence is needed to maintain its position in a health care system increasingly shaped by evidence-based criteria. This challenge is heightened by the fact that most group analysts work as independent practitioners without university affiliations or institutional employment that would support research as part of their professional duties.

To date, Finnish psychotherapy research has been dominated by qualitative and case-based studies (Kurri & Sampolahti, 2025). While these provide valuable insights into therapeutic processes, they fall short of the quantitative standards now emphasized in national treatment recommendations and funding decisions. No large-scale randomized controlled trials (RCTs) of group analysis have been conducted in Finland, and there is no national effectiveness study specific to this approach. Nevertheless, international meta-analyses (e.g., Burlingame et al., 2013) support the overall effectiveness of group-based therapies.

Current policy trends privilege RCT-level evidence, which is often unrealistic for complex, long-term, and flexible treatments like group analysis

(Lindfors & Keinänen, 2020). For this reason, many Finnish group analysts advocate for practice-based evidence, which reflects real-world treatment conditions, heterogeneous patient groups, and the therapeutic relationship. National reviews currently under way may help clarify the role and effectiveness of psychoanalytic group therapy within the broader mental health system.

Looking ahead, several priorities emerge:

- Securing funding and institutional support for smaller therapeutic modalities.
- Building national outcome studies that integrate qualitative and quantitative data.
- Strengthening collaboration across universities, training institutes, and professional associations.
- Enhancing the research readiness of practicing group analysts.
- Promoting awareness among referring professionals and the public.

By developing both methodological diversity and stronger institutional connections, psychoanalytic group analysis can consolidate its role as an evidence-informed, humane, and socially relevant treatment option in Finland's evolving mental health landscape.

References

Burlingame, G.M., Strauss, B., & Joyce, A.S. (2013). Change mechanisms and effectiveness of small group treatments. In M.J. Lambert (Ed.), *Bergin and Garfield's Handbook of Psychotherapy and Behavior Change* (6th edition) (pp. 640–689). Chichester: Wiley.

Foulkes, S.H. (1964). *Therapeutic Group Analysis.* London: George Allen & Unwin.

Foulkes, S.H. (1975). *Group Analytic Psychotherapy: Method and Principles.* London: Gordon & Breach.

Foulkes, S.H., & Anthony, E.J. (1984). *Group Psychotherapy: The Psychoanalytic Approach.* London: Karnac.

Isosävi, J. (2020) Cultural outsiders' evaluations of (im)politeness in Finland and in France. *Journal of Politeness Research*, 16(2), 249–280.

Kurri, K., & Sampolahti, T. (2025). Psykoterapiatutkimuksen politiikasta – onko tutkimus arvovapaata? *Perhe- ja pariterapialehti: Tutkimus & kliininen käytäntö -suhde*, 41(2), 112–138.

Laukkanen, E. (2022). Psykoterapiakoulutuksen nykytila ja haasteet ja tarvittavat toimenpide-ehdotukset. *Sosiaali- ja terveysministeriön raportteja ja muistioita*, 9. See https://urn.fi/URN:ISBN:978-952-00-9995-4.

Lindfors, O. (2024). Psychotherapy and Psychotherapists in Finland from the 1980s to 2020s: Reflections on changes as seen by a psychoanalytic practitioner-researcher. *Psychiatria Fennica*, 55, 18–27.

Lindfors, O., & Keinänen, M. (2020). Psychoanalytic psychotherapy in Finland. *Psychoanalytic Psychotherapy*, 34(2), 129–146.

Pirkola, S. (2020). Psykoterapiaa kaikille – mutta miten? In M.O. Huttunen & H. Kalska (Eds.), *Psykoterapiat* (pp. 466–474). Helsinki: Duodecim.

Salminen, H. (1997). *Ryhmäanalyysin perusteet*. Helsinki: SMS-julkaisut.

Terapiat etulinjaan. Therapies for the frontline (2024). Hankkeen verkkosivut. See https://terapiatetulinjaan.fi.

Vatanen, A. (2021). Co-presence during lapses: On "comfortable silences" in Finnish everyday interaction. In J. Lindström, R. Laury, A. Peräkylä, & M.L. Sorjonen (Eds.), *Action: Studies in language and social interaction* (pp. 251–276). Amsterdam: John Benjamins.

Wilke, G. (2019). Discovering the unconscious patterns of a national culture through a large group of psychotherapists and group analysts in Finland: An application of group analysis in an organizational context. In A. Novakovic & D. Vincent (Eds.), *Group Analysis: Working with Staff, Teams and Organizations* (pp. 183–196). London: Routledge.

Chapter 16

Social Applications of Group Analysis

Reflective Citizens Method

Marina Mojović

Beginnings and Work in Progress with 'Holes-and-Cracks on the Roads'

Since its conception, group analysis has brought us a new epistemology of relationships between the individual, group, and society. Its founder, psychoanalyst S.H. Foulkes, had, according to Dalal (1998), two theoretical masters – the founder of psychoanalysis, Sigmund Freud, and the sociologist Norbert Elias. In Germany, being a contemporary of Freudo-Marxists and Frankfurtians, having then as a Jew to flee from the Nazi regime, he was able in his new country to bring to reality his visions of interweaving psychoanalysis with sociology and to form his first groups.

Interdisciplinarity has always been a key feature of group analysis, but it requires a long time for higher comprehension – so now we are calling for transdisciplinarity. In his first book, *Introduction to Group-Analytic Psychotherapy* (1948) Foulkes emphasized the *deeply social nature of human beings.* 'The old juxtaposition of an inside and outside world, constitution and environment, individual and society, phantasy and reality, body and mind, and so on, is untenable. They can at no stage be separated from each other, except by artificial isolation' (1948, p. 10).

Although in his inauguration paper (Foulkes & Lewis, 1944) Foulkes emphasized that the vocation of group analysis is educating for *responsible citizens*, its social application, like the work with citizens outside of the consulting room, had a long 'below-the-radar' developmental journey. To become an established area, as is now the Reflective Citizens Koinonia Method (RC) and some 'sibling' methods, being easily transmittable and spreading across countries and globally, it seems that the fruition of group analysis was required. While RC was initiated in the mid-1990s in Belgrade with the first RC workshops in the early 2000s, there was no awareness of group analytic developments occurring in other realms, which were related and significant for RC.[1] These were like *parallel processes*, meaning isomorphism or patterns of similarity transmitted through channels of unconscious connectedness. Only now, after three decades of the RC journey, has this become clearer.

DOI: 10.4324/9781003597674-16

RC was born in a time of social trauma, thus often having to bear enormous uncertainty, painful, and even strange/uncanny experiences. The possibility of creating professionally designed, safe enough transitional reflective spaces, while also providing adaptable settings with 'nomadic movability', was also important. Additionally, nonlinear approaches that interlock group analysis with chaos and complexity[2] theories were also important (Schermer, 2012; Dodds, 2011), helping to cope more easily with the inevitable 'holes-and-cracks' along the way as a significant learning-through-experience.

* * * *

Foulkes considered *group matrix* as a cornerstone of group analysis:

> The matrix is the hypothetical web of communication and relationship in a given group. It is the common shared ground which ultimately determines the meaning and significance of all events and upon which all communications and interpretation, verbal and non-verbal, rest.
>
> (Foulkes, 1964, p. 292)

However, its conceptualization took time, with many milestones mapping that progress (Nitzgen, 2024). It was often not possible for steps in revisions to be either fully realized or appreciated by members of the group analytic community (Brown & Zinkin, 1994). Working and reworking, like spirals of resistance and progression, was sometimes dissociated, while at other times coming to more optimal relations – as if it were creating the DNA of the field. At the 1st European Symposium of Group Analysis in 1970, Foulkes introduced the advanced concept of matrix in terms of *dynamic* (DM) and *foundational*[3] (FM); in his last book Foulkes (1975) supplemented them by *personal*[4] matrix (PM), so that *tripartite matrix*[5] (TM) was established as the ultimate frame of reference of group analytic theory and practice (Nitzgen & Hopper, 2017). This defining feature of group analysis, its *insignia* (Hopper, 2024), continues to mature, especially within the field of social unconscious (SU), as the essence of group analysis through the ongoing international project led by Hopper and Weinberg (2011, 2016, 2017).

The idea of SU can be found in Foulkes' work from the very beginning. SU refers to:

> the social, cultural, and communicational constraints and restraints of which people are to varying degrees unconscious. The social unconscious emphasizes the shared anxieties, fantasies, defences, myths, and memories of the members of a social system … The field theory of the social unconscious encompasses its sociality, relationality, transpersonality, transgenerationality, and collectivity.
>
> (Hopper & Weinberg, 2017, p. xxii)

* * * *

With a higher conceptualization of SU, we may attempt to contextualize the mentioned parallel processes of RC within their time and social space using these theories. With some advances in understanding social constraints and restraints we might be able to see those complexities from wider perspectives within their dynamic intertwining and interpenetrating developmental spirals: in such cases, the phenomena of negative 'social-psychic-retreats'[6] (Mojović, 2011, 2019a, 2019b, 2020, 2023) or 'encapsulations' (Hopper, 1991)[7] would represent developmental 'stuckness', and their temporal/positive versions would help in the service of transitional spaces, enabling linking between developmental spirals – 'holes-and-cracks' transformed into process knowledge.

We now seem to be in the midst of a *paradigm shift* in our 21st-century approach to knowledge and science in general, shifting towards the *complexity turn* (Qvortrup, 2006), or the *paradigm of complexity* (Morin, 1992). If, for a moment, taking Deleuze and Guattari's (2003, pp. 372–373) call for more '*nomadic* and *ecosophy/ecosystemic*' moves, which oppose the dualisms nature/culture and natural/artificial, we might wish to explore new 'group analytic vehicles', for coming closer to *the edges of chaos* of the transformation zones of matrices. This becomes especially significant, if *attractors* (meaning points towards which a system tends to converge with a powerful pull) in trauma dynamics had swollen/pulled significant trauma contents or 'demonic creatures', which are threatening from within the 'black holes' of trauma matrices. RC has been described in the European Federation for Psychoanalytic Psychotherapy (EFPP) as such a 'vehicle' (Mojović, 2018b). Anticipations of involving complexity theory date back decades, as seen in dialogues between physicist Bohm and de Marè (de Marè et al., 1991), co-founder of the Group-analytic Society, whose concepts of 'transforming hate into dialogue' and 'Koinonia' are at the roots of RC. Perhaps only with the stronger establishment of group analysis were we able with our 'devices' to circulate 'craters' of traumas more freely – even return to some old ones, as in Northfield Hospital.

* * * *

Group analysis was born in the traumatic 1940s, with its earliest development at the Northfield War Hospital in Birmingham, alongside the beginnings of other analytic group-psychotherapy fields and therapeutic communities. Having the same origins, these fields continue to exhibit complex relationality among them. In post-war times, group analysis continued to grow, establishing the Group-Analytic Society (now GASi) in 1952 and its first training programme in 1971. How, then, do the developments and group analytic training that occurred in different countries and organizations shape the field's history, as well as some divisions? Retreats into binarization between individual and social as the primal juxtapositions still lurk, hiding in different clothes – our paranoid-schizoid positions[8] and basic assumptions are always there, waiting to 'rescue' us.

In Serbia, unfortunately, we shared a specific similarity in the beginnings of group analysis in wartime. Namely, the first war to happen in Europe after the Second World War was the Destruction of Yugoslavia throughout the 'Horrible Nineties', when by destiny group analysis in our country was conceived and established. This influenced us in many ways, such as 'conception trauma', which we reflected on and wrote about (Mojović et al., 2014). In 2007 Mojović founded the 'Study Group on Applied Group Analysis in Organizations and Society' with senior colleagues; then in 2010 the Psychosocial Section and Training in 'Applying Psychoanalytic and Group-Analytic Approach to Understanding Psychodynamics of Institutions, Organizations and Society', leading it throughout 15 years in cooperation with the '*Koinonia-Art* Learning Community'. Especially meaningful was the continuous internationalization of work-under-construction, which included over 20 international events for shared creativity in building our field of applied group analysis and fertile ground for RC.

Searching for some still missing links lost in old trauma, a fantasy was voiced in the 2nd Belgrade International RC-Conference 2014[9] ('Learning through Experience about Inclusion/Exclusion Phenomena in and between Traditions of Bion, Foulkes and Main') by a few senior staff members (Pines, Hinshelwood, Nitzgen, Penna) to continue that work in the Northfield Hospital. We brought that fantasy to reality for the 75th birthday of the Experiments as the 'Northfield Revisited' GASi Workshop in 2018 (Mojović, 2018a) with participation from 30 countries; listening to the 'ghosts' whispering during the group sessions in the old building, as a joint endeavour, rescuing some precious knowledge about the sibling fields from the trauma void at their birthplace. As a temporal international learning community in motion, we formed new connections and 'immunity cells'. Interestingly enough, it was in Northfield that Foulkes realized that the group-as-a-whole also 'symbolizes the community-as-a-whole' (Foulkes, 1984, p. 168). However, it appears that some cracks on further roads within the international group analytic community have still not been addressed or repaired, sometimes leading to pain and anger among group analysts. Traditions of group work, such as Bionian, with its group relation tradition (GR), Bridger's systems-psychodynamics, TC (therapeutic community), and group analysis, went their separate ways – unfortunately with insufficient relationality and transdisciplinarity.

Yet, the basic dichotomies between 'Orthodox' and 'Radical' Foulkes (Dalal, 1998) seem to have improved in the decades to come. RC experienced this, especially in collaboration with the SU project. Ongoing exchanges, jointly learning optimal flexibility, transformed some frozen, split, and disavowed splinters, related among others to conception traumas. Oscillating between rupture and repair, as if some orphan parts of matrices were contained, finding home and creative use. The 1st RC in Banja Luka (Bosnia &

Herzegovina) in August 2015 began with two artists singing Gershwin's 'Summertime', lullabies of black-slave-women in cotton-work holding their babies, one day '*you'll spread your wings and you'll take to the sky*'; in this song, we were able to make contact with the presence of a density of SU-meaning related to suffering in many wars in that region. At the same time, in the choice of the song, interwoven within the meaning was also the moment when a new RC branch was being born. There were also intercultural dimensions in the spiral dialectics of the tripartite matrices: this was, among others linked to the participant from Brazil, Carla Penna, which helped citizen-participants to soften their defensive shields and their usual numbness related to unresolved ethnic war traumas in the region. Unfortunately, this was mixed with fears of new wars – the trust and hope in the RC-space to be a helper in dealing with all those multilayered entanglements.

To understand the dynamics of RC-creation, it is helpful to look inwards and outwards, among other things, related to the simultaneous nature of projection and introjection in social systems, characterized by the paradox of inside-out and outside-in movements, akin to a Mobius strip (Hopper, 2024). In Banja Luka, layers of numbed anxieties in TMs were experienced and shared in circles of conversations during the RC sub-sessions. Significantly, it is also worth looking forward to further interconnectedness and backward to the origins – perhaps the unconscious group's knowledge that the initial RC spark occurred in Georgia, Atlanta, with Martin Luther King's '*I have a dream …*' (Mojović, 2022). Images of spirals for groups are helpful as social systems (Foulkes & Anthony, 1957). Pichon-Rivière's dialectic spirals, both their theory and practice, were brought directly to RC in person by Tubert-Oclander, Hernandez-Tubert, and Penna at the 1st Belgrade International RC Conference 'Large Groups and SU. Pichon-Rivière and Foulkes Meeting Citizens' 2013, unaware that on the very same days, June 26th–28th, Pichon-Rivière, in 1958, worked with citizen groups in Rosario, Argentina. Between the days of conference learning and reflection was an RC workshop with 180 participants from 32 countries. RC-theory and practice, both local and international, were experienced in shared creativity, with complex and challenging TM layers being revealed.

In other international events, RC-groups were moving in-between, as if in interstitial areas of more 'serious' professional meetings – as if a growing 'child', then 'adolescent' method. RC could be seen or unseen, but certainly impacted by lively processes – sometimes a 'personified' voice-of-hope. Surprises came with increasingly securing spaces for RC presentations and discussions, such as at SU panels of different conferences or for RC workshops on their margins; then even advancing to RC keynotes at esteemed professional organizations like GASi, EGATIN, ISPSO, OPUS, IAGP, EFPP, COIRAG, IIGA, Psych.E.In., and IGA-Slovenia.[10] As complex resonance, exchanges, and mirroring increased, the awareness of RC-identity slowly grew into a stable existence.

'Conception' of Reflective Citizens Koinonia in the Invisible Therapeutic Community

During the 1990s when group analysis arrived in Serbia, during my work in a therapeutic community (TC), where I spent the whole decade, the initial RC was conceived. It was named *invisible* due to the paradox of being embedded in the centre of Belgrade, part of the major Psychiatric Clinic, Clinical Center Serbia, over which the regime always had power; it was close to part of our Clinic, nicknamed 'bastion of pharmacotherapy' (where I worked before TC), and TC-work being rather *invisible*, despite a high professional level. I needed years to realize that *invisibility* meant safety in years of social terror, probably a conscious intention – part of a strategy. In material terms, TC was placed in a rather poor Day Hospital: a previous builder's house for the Clinical Center, as if they had forgotten to dismantle it, with low ceilings, easily burgled, and often was. We would bring carpets, curtains, and similar items from our own homes, and patients would bring items from their occupational therapy sessions – all *actions* aimed at creating a warmer place for us all. Sometimes, we used metaphors, such as 'orphanage', and we, staff and patients, jointly engaged in making a good enough place for psychological work; some appropriate actions included these:

'*TransformAction*' came to mind from the GASi Summer School 2024 title, as well as from 1993 with our IGA trainers, George Renton and Anne Mhlongo: when sanctions imposed on Serbia stopped our training, a joint decision was made to move the venue from the state hospital to a private house; or, when during a coffee break an officer told us 'we heard that bombing will start, we're responsible only for British citizens', our teachers decided to continue the training. Ways of maintaining good enough boundaries, even in a shattered and unstable setting, influenced RC-seeds.

In contrast to the material aspect, this TC was rich in professionalism, human-ness, shared creativity, and enthusiasm. It felt miraculous, including the invisibility, even to other wards in the same building, as if an invisible sign 'don't disturb – psychotherapy' had efficiently wrapped this oasis. When we asked Dr Kovačević, its founder and head for 30 years, how this was possible, he replied: 'We only carefully apply TC principles.' At the Serbian School, Dr Kovačević was among the senior training psychoanalytic psychotherapists; only later did I realize that he had probably been a visiting psychiatrist at the London Henderson Hospital TC, as well as possessing high skills in 'working-below-the-radar' of the regime. His non-communist orientation and family roots were invisible on the surface: stylish gentleman, stable psychoanalytic and ethical attitudes, shining liveliness, honesty, and humility, open to tactful-enough innovations.

Paradoxically, despite the serious abuse by the regime taking over our health system, the TC-micro-culture nurtured interdisciplinarity, democratic relationality between staff and patients, subsystems, etc. TC-members were heterogeneous in age, gender, class, ethnicity, religion, social attitudes, psychic disorders – refugees from different parts of Yugoslavia, even an 'ex-warriors-group'. Despite the devastation of the outer and inner lives of many people, we who worked there all had a place of psychological safety, containment, and freedom to express, learn, and think together. This included regular group spaces for staff to express and reflect on the complexity of transference and countertransference with clear boundaries of tasks and roles in various sub-sessions.

Even the 'homeless'/movable Study Group Klein/Bion/Neoklein (led by psychologists from London and Belgrade, Branka Pecotić, and me, its participant and manager for 18 years), which had to be hidden at the previous ward, was able to feel accepted and learn the field's relatedness to TC-culture. Interweaving this area of knowledge into RC became visible only later.

I started conducting my first group analytic sessions twice a week in this TC. The large psychoanalytic group, which had already been established for years, three times a week, slowly shifted towards a group analytic style, supported by Dr Kovačević. In this special oasis, the matrix enabled hope to be alive, and to spread a similar culture of group matrices.

Being socially traumatized at the same time as other citizens, ideas emerged of making oases areas of psychoanalytic and group analytic reflections with 'ordinary citizens'. The meaningful experience of working on social trauma even in such poor and difficult circumstances, in the midst of horrendous social destruction, initiated actions of making reflection groups with citizens: first on the margins of Belgrade Peace Protests, then in shelters during NATO bombing, in parks, river banks, shipwrecks, gardens, schools … It was on this ground that RC-creation began. Maturation, of course, needed a long process.

'Koinonia' Relating to RC-Roots, RC-Method, and RC-Community of Communities

There is a contrast between a lengthy creation process with numerous refinements and the opposite being true for RC transmission (Mojović, 2026; Mulasso, 2022, 2026). Once it was made, RC became an easy method to learn! Training is easy, but necessary!

As part of TC-experience, trainings in psychoanalytic psychotherapy and group analysis, psychiatric work with 'difficult patients', the special mission of psychologist Branka Pecotić and her '*London Link* – Society for Psychoanalytic and Psychodynamic Psychotherapy Klein/Bion/Neo-Klein and Organizational Consultancy', of which I was a director, was significant. Over 25 years, Branka persistently introduced knowledge from London: Kleinian and group relations with their organizations OPUS and ISPSO, Listening Posts Method (LP);[11] child, couple, and family psychoanalytic psychotherapy, endeavouring to link with membership in EFPP (now three EFPP sections from Serbia) and with Gordon Lawrence, founder of social dreaming. Yet, without the wise embrace and synergy within TC, the process of bridging psychoanalytic areas would probably be unimaginable. The presence of EFPP as another tactful and wise authority was meaningful.

The term 'Koinonia' is used by de Marè (de Marè et al., 1991): *koine* meaning common language belonging to everyone in classical Greek times of

> ascendance of democracy, the large groups and citizenship over small group oligarchy and aristocracy .... Koinonia is linked to democratic exchange, referring to impersonal fellowship rather than personal friendship, of spirit-cum-human participation in which people can speak, hear, see, and think freely – a form of togetherness and amity that brings a pooling of resources.
>
> (p. 2)

RC-Koinonia is both the method and the community of RC branches practising this method in free cooperation. RC has become a shared journey with many citizens, colleagues, and helpers – a *shared/social creativity* among people and among fields. Bridging of psychoanalytic fields is in 'RC-DNA': between traditions of group analysis, group relations, TC, Pichon-Rivière, complexity theories, social dreaming, and LP – in practice and theory. Surviving various attacks, rooted in social and organizational disruptions, required making a home for the emerging new area of work that was at the same time secure enough *and open enough*. This is built into the RC-matrix – keeping it continuously *open for learning from each other, appreciating ancestors' fields in group work, and shared creativity for new ideas to emerge.*

RC-basic principles, values and culture – all in RC, including training, is free of charge: democratic principles of keeping the flame of liberal and cosmopolitan ideals in fields-of-citizenship; free floating discussion, reverie, freedom of exchanging ideas, fantasies, feelings, dreams, new thoughts; allowing difficult feelings and defences from them to be seen/understood; trusting in the capacity of raw human exchanges; freedom of diversity learning-through-experience of true dialogue-culture and citizens' responsibility; opening up minds to the chaotic and uncontrollable unconscious of communities within safe dialogue situations; not aiming to arrive at any sort of homogeneous conclusion; learning to listen and to be heard, opening up new themes and perspectives; learning about others and oneself in relation to others, including also the hosts, participants, without any assumed privileges to own the 'Truth'; opening minds for the variety/diversity of discourses/paradigms and curiosity for interactions; RC-learning of the '*art-of-listening*' and the '*art-of-dialogue*' (Mojović, 2019b); *transforming hate into a culture of dialogue.*

Techniques at RC-workshops serve as basic building blocks: in the RC-workshop, all can be done by one person alone, similar to an analytic group, both organizing (dynamic administration) and convening. The Koinonia aspect of doing things together often prevails, although some people like to do everything themselves. Supporting any other colleague or citizen in conceiving a new local RC branch is part of RC culture and technique.

Parts/program of RC-Workshop:

1. *Entry* with an introduction.
2. *Social dreaming* (SD)[12] has been regularly included since 2012 – a method developed by Gordon Lawrence: it takes place in a collective of dreamers telling of dreams and associations to dreams as an access to the unconscious knowledge of the dreams in relation to their social context (in RC we host in Lawrence's style).
3. *1st RC-large group.*
4. *RC-small groups* are similar to LP-leaderless group in which 'task-is-the-leader' of jointly finding a few emerging themes from previous sub-sessions, eventually joint drawing or other artwork. In longer events, this can be enriched with inter-group visiting events in GR-style, meetings among groups, 'market-events', and creative methods keep emerging.
5. *2nd RC-large group* has aspects of LP in serving contents and/or artwork from SGs, to it, if people wish, and continue *dialoguing in Koinonia style.*
6. *Exit-event* has two parts: review & application mini-groups in threes (RAGs in GR-tradition), and all participants coming together at the last closing and planning session.

The number of participants is flexible, ranging from a few dozen to 180. Duration is assessed before creating the RC-flyer with a precise programme, typically ranging from 90 minutes to two/three days, with most RC-workshops lasting 3 to 4 hours. It is adaptable to resources and needs: after the tragic Belgrade School Shooting in 2023, we held a series of two-day thematic RCs, as did Kavita Avula, who hosted the USA's 'North-East Pacific RC' following the 7th October 2024 Israeli tragedy.

One or more persons are *hosting* the event (term taken from SD): the *host-organizer* and *host-convenor* can be the same person, or tasks are divided among the RC-hosting group. Pre- and post-event meetings for reviewing in Bridger's 'double task' frame (systems-psychodynamic parallel reflections on practical and dynamic aspects, with suggestions for improvement); major themes noted, and in a few sentences archived for local/country/global RC-branches. How much RC-archive is communicated is freedom-of-choice.

RC is essentially group analytic, drawing on Foulkesian, Latin American (Pichon-Rivière), and Serbian traditions. GR-RC aspects relate mainly to techniques, including disciplined changing of settings and tasks within and between sub-sessions, RAGs, inter-group visiting, and ways of shaping SGs and organizational roles. SD is significant, but not essential (relationality between SD and the group analytic world continue to be explored; RC has become a rich source).

With SD in RC, we come into contact with universal realms, their meaning, and this helps foster cohesion – deep content from SU can emerge, enabling encounters even with ugly, demonic, or evil content without being overwhelming. All levels of TMs occur, but the major focus is usually on FM, sometimes even 'cosmic matrix' (Hopper, 2024). Moving to 1st RC-LG is a perceptual shift, entering another realm of various citizenship roles (parental, neighbourhood, sports, work ...) with distinct names and identities, with DM and PM being the major focus, while keeping an eye on FM as well. It is similar in SGs, but for some participants in that 'niche', sharing is easier. Again, in the 2nd RC-LG, coming together. In RAG, the focus is on PM – what each citizen takes away. Those RC-specific shifts of paradigms within sub-sessions also enable the potential richness of perspectives in a short time, with shared *creative turbulence* among them. This partially explains how new levels of understanding the world and ourselves within it often emerge. In this joint endeavour, destructive spirals can turn in a different direction, with disentanglements.

RC-Community of Communities

Now endeavouring to recontextualize the RC-community in relation to other professional and social realms, it is interesting to trace particular dimensions throughout TMs. In years of social trauma, social fields and systems were, certainly, flooded with 4th ba I:A/M (Hopper, 2003) – social defences, such as forms of negative 'social-psychic-retreats' spread. Oases, such as TC and RC, being kinds of positive 'social-psychic-retreats', were able to offer new ways for the survival of trust in community dialogue – a hope for democratic and responsible citizenship.

With the transpersonality, relationality, transgenerationality, and collectivity of the RC communities, its '*matrix-of-hope*' and other properties became available throughout RC fields. As an illustration from the 3rd Banja Luka RC: Bosniak/Muslim citizen-participant: '*Don't know where-from I found trust to come ... in Srebrenica I lost father and two uncles ... we can't move without finding forgiveness*'; a participant from Belgrade, deeply touched, openly shared his prejudice, crying at his own trans-generational trauma stories, as were many others in the wave of sharing; interweaved with collective memories in an up-and-dawn spiral process through trauma knots, malignancy dissolving, encapsulating pain experienced; the presence of the 'social third' and human-ness enabling revisions. As if when touching/sensing destructive areas, 'RC-matrix-of-hope-and-wisdom' gets attracted, rushing through vessels in the fields. Encounters of multicultural/postmodernist dimensions with local ethnic ones often bring capacities of multivision. An almost infinite resource of positive potentials from the multiverse may arrive, facilitating lively transformation. A desire was voiced for RC to travel to other ethnic areas (applied-RC-project for 'young leaders in multi-ethnic schools' included almost 400 schools, Mojović, 2016).

RC-oases are disseminated, branches keep growing (a few hundred events): parts of Belgrade, many Serbian towns, villages, regionally (Bosnia & Hercegovina, Slovenia, Montenegro); other countries: Greece, the USA, the UK, Italy, Ireland, Sweden, Turkey, preparing in Germany, the Netherlands, Belgium, Armenia, Lebanon, Romania … Local hosts can become hosts in International-RC (IRC), which we established during the COVID-19 pandemic online – so far there are nine IRC workshops (often having 180 participants from six continents – now limited to 100). The IRC Steering Team holds pre- and post-IRC meetings; RC training; prepares webinars, the RC book, and further RC conferences (Belgrade 2025,[13] Italy 2027); and nurtures relationships with sibling methods, including the 'Sandwich Model', 'Social Dreaming Hubs', 'Voices after Auschwitz', 'Large-Group-Dialogues', and the 'Trilogy Model'.

RC-adaptability and sensitivity to the soil of local communities, their *genius loci*, allows diversity to keep flourishing: the Polish tradition in RC-workshops has developed since 2014, within the project *Poland-on-the-Couch* led by Anna Zajenkowska and Tomasz Wyrzykowski, initiated by the concern of '*fear of the other*' in Polish SU, endeavouring to build relationality. It begins with SD, presentations, or a Trilogy-event, starting with 'what does it means to be a Polish citizen?' The 1st Greek RC branch in Thessaloniki, with Francesca Bascialla, adapted to the pandemic by going online and has continued thus. 'All-Island RC-Koinonia Ireland' emerged in 2023 from IRC, organized by O'Byrne-Maguire within GR-Ireland, and continues online to include the diaspora. The last Serbian village-RC in Visibaba (spring flower) established connections with the diaspora in Chicago, eager to spread Visibaba-RC throughout Western Serbia. A newborn baby-RC on Crete, May 5, 2025, with Konstantinos Liolios at the Chania school, already has five branches. Children and parents, as well as schools, museums, and galleries' representatives, travelling, ecology, and other thematic RC-representatives have been presented at international events and continue to be.

'*Flourishing of RC in Italy across Cities from Turin to Sicily*' was presented at the International Congress in the Serbian Medical Society in 2025 by Alice Mulasso (with voices of Italian-RC-hosts, 2022), starting with Alice's dream after the 1st RC 2019 in Chieri:

> San Vito Bay in Sicily … family is with me, people practicing underwater fishing with spear-guns, told not being true guns. Marina arrives wearing a long dress with ethnic patterns … We dance towards RC, people joining in, forming a sort of human dancing train, a feeling of involvement in something great.

The dance goes on: from Chieri to Padua (2021), Rivoli (2022), Cinisi (2023), Pachino (2024), Palermo (2024), and Crotone (2025), with plans to reach Milan and Genoa in 2025, and Rome and Trento awaiting the right moment. The Italian national RC-network has 38 hosts, 7 branches, and 36 workshops, reaching out to citizens of different generations, social and professional backgrounds; some citizens may consider RC not their cup of tea, but there is freedom to join, freedom to leave. Here are a few testimony illustrations from citizen-participants follow:

> Due to its *method* .... RC bridges personal and collective experiences without division. Mandela's approach to preventing civil war in South Africa ... was a similar practice that transformed strong emotions into ways to address potential intra-ethnic violence. RC helps find hopeful words, moving from dystopia to utopia.
>
> Reflective-citizenship meetings lighten my burdens. Sharing concerns, ideas, and hopes with others gives me confidence about the future. It's a unique chance for everyone to express their opinions respectfully, enriching me each time.
>
> Through listening, solicitations and silences reach access to knowledge that inhabits each of us. Flexible and fluctuating connections are created where everyone contributes to the community and to expanded thinking, where conflict can be one of the crossings that lead to integrated and inclusive thinking while maintaining the identity and authenticity of the individual.

Ending ...

If the migrant-citizen from Africa in Pachino-RC liked being there, perhaps mirroring human-ness and engaging in 'access to knowledge inhabiting us all', like Nikola Tesla's access to 'the core from which all our strength comes ... beauty and humility in the harmony-of-the-whole' ([1899]1952), from where he (while reciting poetry to a friend in a park), conjured up his major invention of alternating current, which would become the world's electrical lighting system (Mojović & Satarić, 2024, 2025), we should continue co-creating these and similar oases of human-ness.

RC might be like those 'live fireflies dance ... sparkling lights of understanding and thinking to face darkness ... representing community of survival and community of resistance' from Penna's book (2023, p. 216). Today, as citizens and professionals, we often feel lost at the edges of total ecological and war catastrophes, paralysed, looking into the eyes of shocking evil. May RC-vehicles, with their ecosystemic and nomadic equipment, designed for quick shifts in paradigms, temporal creative turbulence, and safe landing, help us reconnect the disjointed/compartmentalized matrices of our societies and minds. Sometimes, even brief moments of hope can bring freedom of thought and inspire visions for some transformative actions. In the current crises of humanity, *keeping the flame of group analysis and its social applications alive* seems a meaningful endeavour to take seriously.

Notes

1 Especially important were some areas, which were initiated by Foulkes, but waited for their evolution to come later, as those of the social unconscious, social trauma, incohesion theories, tripartite matrix, large groups, and field theories. *They were theoretically holding the RC practice*, even at times when they did not know enough of them from those practising RC. The existence of such parallel processes is explored in group analysis, usually relating to projective and introjective processes throughout group matrices.

2 Chaos theory focuses on the sensitive dependence of deterministic, nonlinear systems on initial conditions, leading to unpredictable, complex behaviour like the '*butterfly effect*'. Complexity theory expands on this, examining the dynamics of systems with many interacting, semi–independent parts that exhibit emergence, self-organization, and global patterns arising from local interactions. While chaos describes the unpredictability within such systems, complexity theory provides a broader framework for understanding the structure and behaviour of these dynamic, interconnected wholes.

3 Originally Foulkes described matrix having two aspects: Foundation Group Matrix created by past familiar, cultural, social, and lingual experiences and one Dynamic Group Matrix emerging through the interactions and the relationships growing during the group process.

4 Personal matrix refers to the unique network of relationships, past experiences, and emotional templates an individual brings to a group, influencing their interactions and resonating with the group's dynamics.

5 Tripartite matrix, developed by Earl Hopper, Dieter Nitzgen, and colleagues, extends Foulkes' ideas to explore the '*social unconscious*' within individuals, groups, and societies by examining the interacting forces of the personal, foundation, and dynamic matrices.

6 Social-psychic retreats are a concept developed by Mojović since 2005. '*Social-psychic-retreats*' are complex and obscure psycho-social phenomena, which originate in people's experiences of despair during extreme and cumulative social traumas. Mojović conceptualized them (Mojović, 2007, 2011, 2012, 2015, 2017, 2018), developing the psychoanalytic concept of 'psychic retreats' (John Steiner, 1993) through her group analytic and psychosocial work. According to Steiner, psychic retreats, as spaces of withdrawal from human contact which are experienced as threatening, are internal 'pathological organisations' involving highly-structured and closely-knit systems of defences and object relations. Formed initially out of desperation, these sabotaging, self-protecting, and self-organizing internal subsystems provide alternative shelters for human relationships and for reality in general. In their very essence lies a paradox: they both protect and imprison the vital parts of the self.

As equivalence phenomena of internal psychic retreats, social-psychic-retreats are formations of social systems co-created by recursive externalization and internalization processes between psyche and society, which simultaneously occur in both directions. *The social unconscious operates extensively through these figurations,* which involve highly structured systems of social defences and object relations, creating alternative shelters to the social mainstream. They indirectly influence the dynamics of social discourses and power relations significantly. They are being discussed in both their positive forms – as survival manoeuvres – and their negative forms, as obstacles to development. The latter underlie much of the social pathology aggravating with time and trans-generational transmission, becoming vicious psychosocial spirals and causing unforeseen troubles.

7 Encapsulations is defined as a defence against annihilation anxiety usually caused in early traumata. Hopper conceptualized it as an introjective process through which attempts are made to fuse and confuse parts of the self with parts of the lost and abandoned object.
8 The paranoid-schizoid position, a concept from Melanie Klein's object relations theory, describes a primitive stage of infant development (0–6 months) characterized by a splitting of the ego and a fear of annihilation. Infants experience an '*all-good*' or 'all-bad' world and defend against frightening, aggressive feelings by projecting them onto the outside world, leading to paranoia, while simultaneously splitting off good experiences to protect themselves from overwhelming anxiety.
9 2nd Belgrade International Conference 2014, organized in the Koinonia-Art Learning Community together with the Psychosocial Section of the Group Analytic Society Belgrade was co-convened by Bob Hinshelwood and Marina Mojović. Its aim was to work jointly with senior and younger colleagues from many countries on bridging a few psychoanalytic fields as is Bion's tradition with group relations, Foulkes' group analysis, and Tom Main's and Herold Bridger's therapeutic community traditions. It has had long-lasting waves of influence both locally and internationally in the spiraling dialectics of the tripartite matrices (49th Foulkes Lecture Carla Penna, response Marina Mojović).
10 GASi – Group Analytic Society International; EGATIN – European Group Analytic Training Network; ISPSO – International Society for Psychoanalytic Studies of Organizations; OPUS – Organization for Promoting Understanding of Society; IAGP – International Association for Group Psychotherapy and Group Processes; EFPP – European Federation for Psychoanalytic Psychotherapy; COIRAG; IIGA – Israeli Institute of Group Analysis; Psych. In. – Psychological Early Intervention in Trauma; IGA – Slovenia Institute of Group Analysis Slovenia.
11 Listening Posts is a method developed in OPUS: regular meetings that take a 'snapshot' of society at a particular moment in time. It explores the underlying dynamics in society as a piece of social science research, with data now available from over 30 countries around the world. Serbia joined regularly since 2004 (Mojović the national representative).
12 Social dreaming is a method developed by Gordon Lawrence in the 1980s. *It takes place in the SD Matrix*, 'where a collective of dreamers gives voice to the continuous dreaming activity of the mind. Dreams, dreamwork, and free associations are the object of its inquiry, not the dreamer. It is a methodology for transforming thought and fostering the emergence of new ideas. It taps into a creative core. The practice fosters free and open minds, allowing them to think. In SD, dreams are not viewed as personal; rather, they are seen as interconnected and become meaningful narratives for the collective. I have a dream, we say in English; in many languages, the same concept is expressed by I see a dream, underlying the fact that dreams are experienced as a given to the dreamer rather than created by them. SD opens to spiritual dimensions and to existential questions (Franca Fubini, 2025, International Conference in Belgrade Medical Society) Belgrade SD-hosting training is conducted by Angela Eden with Mojović (in-person and online), and an additional branch has recently been established for RC. *Only if a trained SD host is not available*, RC goes without SD.
13 Jubilar '10th International Belgrade Conference of Reflective Citizens and on Invigorating Bridges among Psychoanalytic Fields' took place in October 2025 in the *Learning Community and School for Integrative Group Analysis Koinonia-Art* in person and online with participants from 20 countries.

References

Brown, D., & Zinkin, L. (1994). *The Psyche and the Social World: Developments in Group-Analytic Theory.* London: Routledge.

Dalal, F. (1998). *Taking the Group Seriously. Towards a Post-Foulkesian Group Analytic Theory.* Philadelphia: Jessica Kingsley Publishers.

Deleuze, G., & Guattari, F. (2003). *A Thousand Plateaus: Capitalism and Schizophrenia.* Minneapolis: University of Minnesota Press.

de Marè, P., Piper, R., & Thompson, S. (1991). *From Hate, Through Dialogue, to Culture in the Large Group.* London: Routledge.

Dodds, J. (2011). *Psychoanalysis and Ecology at the End of Chaos. Complexity Theory, Deleuze, Guattari and Psychoanalysis for a Climate in Crisis.* London: Routledge.

Foulkes, S.H. (1948). *Introduction to Group-Analytic Psychotherapy.* London: Karnac.

Foulkes, S.H. (1964). *Therapeutic Group Analysis.* London: Karnac.

Foulkes, S.H. (1975). *Group Psychoanalytic Psychotherapy: Method and Principles.* London: Karnac.

Foulkes, S.H. (1984). *Therapeutic Group Analysis.* London: Karnac.

Foulkes, S.H., & Lewis, E. (1944) *Group Analysis: A Study in the Treatment of Groups on Group Analytic Lines.* In S.H. Foulkes, 1984 (pp. 20–37). London: Karnac.

Foulkes, S.H., & Anthony, E.J. (1957). *Group Psychotherapy: The Psychoanalytic Approach.* London: Karnac.

Hopper, E. (1991). Encapsulations as defence against the fear of annihilation. *International Journal of Psychoanalysis*, 72(4), 607–624.

Hopper, E. (2003). *Traumatic Experience in the Unconscious Life of Group.* International Library of Group Analysis. Philadelphia: Jessica Kingsley Publishers.

Hopper, E. (2024). *The Tripartite Matrix in the Developing Theory and Expanding Practice of Group Analysis: The Social Unconscious in Persons, Groups and Societies: Volume 4.* London: Routledge.

Hopper, E., & Weinberg, H. (2011). *Social Unconscious in Persons, Groups and Societies, Vol. 1: Mainly Theory.* London: Karnac.

Hopper, E., & Weinberg, H. (2016). *Social Unconscious in Persons, Groups and Societies, Vol. 2: Mainly Foundation Matrices.* London: Karnac.

Hopper, E., & Weinberg, H. (2017). *Social Unconscious in Persons, Groups and Societies, Vol. 3: The Foundation Matrix Extended and Re-configured.* London: Karnac.

Mojović, M. (2011). Manifestations of psychic retreats in social systems. In E. Hopper & H. Weinberg (Eds.), *Social Unconscious in Persons, Groups and Societies* (pp. 209–234). London: Karnac.

Mojović, M. (2005). *Rad sa psihičkim skloništima u maloj analitičkoj grupi* [Work with psychic retreats in a small group analytic group]. Belgrade: Group Analytic Society Belgrade.

Mojović, M., Despotović, T., & Satarić, J. (2014). 'Conception trauma' of group analysis in Serbia. *Group Analysis*, 47(2), 111–127.

Mojović, M. (2015). Disrupted matrices. Challenges and changes. *Group Analysis*, 48 (4), 540–557.

Mojović, M. (2016). Serbian reflective-citizens flourishing in the leaking containers. *Group Analysis*, 50(5), 370–384.

Mojović, M. (2017). 'Untouchable Infant Gangs' in group and social matrices as obstacles to reconciliation. In G. Ofer (Ed.), *A Bridge Over Troubled Water. Conflicts and Reconciliation in Groups and Society* (pp. 119–139). London: Karnac.

Mojović, M. (2018a). Introduction and welcome for the Winter Workshop 2018, 'Northfield Revisited'. *Group Analysis*, 51(4), 426–433.

Mojović, M. (2018b). Social Traumata 'Black Holes' in Matrices and Ghostly Creatures at Event Horizons as Helpers in Transformation. Presentation at EFPP Conference, May 10 to 13, 2018, Belgrade.

Mojović, M. (2019a). Totalitarian and post-totalitarian matrices: Reflective-citizens facing social-psychic-retreats. In B. Huppertz (Ed.), *Approaches to Psychic Trauma: Theory and Practice* (pp. 159–177). London: Rowman & Littlefield.

Mojović, M. (2019b). Serbian reflective-citizens and the art of psycho-social listening and dialogue at the caesura. *Journal of Psychosocial Studies*, 12(1–2),81–95.

Mojović, M. (2020). The Balkans on the reflective-citizens couch unraveling social-psychic-retreats. In A. Zajenkowska and U. Levin (Eds.), *The Psychoanalytic and Socio-Cultural Exploration of a Continent* (pp. 175–187). London: Routledge.

Mojović, M. (2022). Thinking together in reflective citizens. In M. Ringer, R. Gordon, & B. Vandenbussche (Eds.), *The Collective Spark: Igniting Thinking in Groups, Teams and the Wider World* (pp. 211–224). Gent: Grafische Cel.

Mojović, M. (2023). Trauma and social-psychic retreats: Facing and transforming in group analytic groups – clinical and applied. *Gruppi*, doi:10.3280/gruoa2-2021oa15815.

Mojović, M., & Satarić, J. (2024). Tesla and the social unconscious of Serbs: The dance of science with poetry–the earthly with the heavenly. In E. Hopper (Ed.), *The Tripartite Matrix in the Developing Theory and Expanding Practice of Group Analysis: The Social Unconscious in Persons, Groups and Societies: Volume 4*. London: Routledge.

Mojović, M., & Satarić, J. (2025). Concept of transformer: Tesla in the social unconscious of Serbs and music of the universe in tripartite matrices. Online, July. doi:10.1177/05333164251348891.

Mojović, M. (2026). TrasformAzioni con il Metodo di Cittadinanza Riflessiva Koinonia. *Gruppi-Nella Clinica, Nelle Instituzione, Nelle Societa*. Milan: Franco Angeli.

Morin, E. (1992). From the concept of system to the paradigm of complexity. *Journal of Social and Evolutionary Science*, 15(4), 371–385.

Mulasso, A. (2022). Reflective-citizens koinonia matrix in movement. *Group Analysis*, 55(4), 516–522a

Mulasso, A. et al. (2026). *Il Fiorire della Cittadinanza Riflessiva in Italia: Da Torino alla Sicilia. Gruppi-Nella Clinica, Nelle Instituzione, Nelle Societa*. Milan: Franco Angeli.

Nitzgen, D. & Hopper, E. (2017). The concepts of the social unconscious and of the matrix in the work of S.H. Foulkes. In E. Hopper & H. Weinberg (Eds.), *The Social Unconscious in Persons, Groups and Societies:* Volume 3 (pp. 3–26). London: Karnac.

Nitzgen, D. (2024) The cornerstone once more. In E. Hopper (Ed.), *The Tripartite Matrix in the Developing Theory and Expanding Practice of Group Analysis: The Social Unconscious in Persons, Groups and Societies:* Volume 4 (pp. 19–34). London: Routledge.

Penna, C. (2023). *From Crowds Psychology to the Dynamics of Large Groups: Historical Theoretical and Practical Considerations*. London: Routledge.

Qvortrup, L. (2006). Understanding new digital media: medium theory or complexity theory? *European Journal of Communication*, 21(3), 345–356.

Schermer, V. (2012). Group-as-a-whole and complexity theories: Areas of convergence. Part II: Application to group relations, group analysis, and systems centered therapy. *Group Analysis*, 45(3), 275–288.

Steiner, J. (1993). *Psychic Retreats: Pathological Organizations in Psychotic, Neurotic and Borderline Patients.* London: Routledge.

Tesla, N. ([1899]1952). Interview with Nikola Tesla. In *From Colorado Springs to Long Island: Research Notes, Colorado Springs, 1899–1900, NY, 1900–1901.* Belgrade: Nikola Tesla Museum, 2008: 244.

Chapter 17

Modern Group Analysis

Sigmund Karterud

What do I (or we) mean by linking, in the heading of this chapter, the word "modern" to group analysis? It is not in the meaning of fashionable, although I would have liked that group analysis was more present in social media. Group analysis is poorly known to the public. It is not discussed on popular radio stations. People do not have any informed opinions on group analysis. Partly this is due to the secretness of group analysis. One should not speak to others about one's experiences because of confidentiality for other group members. Consequently, the public seldom hear success stories about "how group analysis changed my life." The advertisement is also quite modest. On the homepage of the Norwegian Institute of group analysis and psychotherapy (IGA), as of July 2025, we learn that "group psychotherapy is a kind of treatment where a (small) group of people meet, led by a professional group therapist, to help oneself and each other." One can hardly say this is eager marketing!

This is not my main concern, although I would have liked group analysts and group analytic institutes to be more engaged in public affairs with the perspectives that group analysis can offer. I am more concerned with "modern" meaning being in dialogue with developments in neighboring fields like philosophy, evolution theory, developmental and personality psychology, psychoanalysis, social psychology, neuroscience, etc. All these disciplines have something to say about what it is to be human and what is the nature of social reality and all of them are *social* disciplines in constant movements. Their developments indeed impact upon the theory and practice of group analysis (Karterud, 2024).

Some few examples: It was crucial for the pioneers of group analysis (e.g., S.H. Foulkes) to emphasize that man was "a social animal." Today, we will regard this as almost self-evident. However, during the 1950s and 1960s, this was important to state because of the individualistic psychic-apparatus model of the mind inherent in the psychoanalysis of those days. Today, we will say, of course, but in which way? What do we *mean* by "social animal"? In what sense? Chimpanzees are also social animals. Evolution theory was quite primitive in the 1950s. Thus, Foulkes (1964, p. 235) could state that when people

DOI: 10.4324/9781003597674-17

overcome initial resistances, as in an analytic group, they will be overridden by an almost irresistible need for contact and reestablish old and deep-seated modes of group behavior. Previously isolated individuals will be affected by "*ancient tribal feelings*" and these forces will penetrate the individuals to their innermost core and all later interaction between them will invariably be woven into this common matrix.

This is not exactly how we see it today. Firstly, we would specify "ancient tribal feelings." What kind of feelings are they? We would start with replacing "feelings" with "*emotions.*" There are some basic facts which constitute human beings. One of them is that we are equipped with emotions. Some of them are primary and those are: seeking (exploratory/expectant behavior), fear, rage, sexual lust, separation anxiety, care/love, and (joyful) play (Panksepp & Biven, 2012). Next, we would maintain that *attachment* is a feature of being human and that attachment comes with the mammals, when mothers start to take care of their offspring who signals separation anxiety (Bowlby, 1988). Subsequently there will be families and tribes, often lead by an alfa-male. All primary emotions are involved in tribe formation and tribe maintenance. However, it is not correct to state that these forces will penetrate the individuals to their innermost core. These forces, the primary emotions, emanate from the individuals but are shaped by the encounter with similar emotions and cultural adaptations from their tribal fellows. The question is how the individuals succeed in living together without killing each other. Some kind of domestication takes place during evolution, e.g., whereby male aggression towards tribe members is tamed.

However, the big issue is the development of *human* groups. Human groups are different from all other animal groups in one respect which is that they are founded upon a linguistic capacity that enables human groups to be organized through a "common ground" which constitutes rules and codes of behavior that can be verbally transmitted and reflected upon. Thus, to cite the Canadian philosopher Charles Taylor (2016), humans are not foremost social animals, they are *linguistic animals.* And with that capacity, they can create groups that are constituted by verbal declarations (speech acts) which are accompanied by so-called *deontic powers* (Searle, 2010). Deontic powers are those rules, commitments, obligations, etc. that come with group membership. It concerns all types of groups (or social institutions), be it a football club, a school class, a therapeutic group, a university, a national state, etc. It is crucial for social groups that they are dependent on social recognition. If nobody believes in them, they will cease to be social realities and dissolve. If the football players don't show up for matches and the public don't pay for tickets, the club will die. As will the therapeutic group if no patient turns up for the group meetings, or the university that doesn't attract any students.

Groups in General versus Clinical Groups

The group analytic literature has been preoccupied by a general theory of a group matrix, expanding on Foulkes original ideas (Foulkes, 1948, 1964, 1973). These ideas do, in my opinion, lack clarity. They are somewhat vague and rely heavily on *mechanical metaphors.* The matrix is described as a communicational "web" which transmits "massive forces" which "pass through" the individuals which can be likened to "knots in this web." The emphasis is upon what "the group" does with the individual, not with what the individual does with the group. From the outset, the concept of the group matrix was plagued with flirting with a concept of a group mind. This tension is still there in the literature on the social unconscious (Hopper, 2024; Nitzgen, 2024). The debate about these concepts have been quite confusing. Are the individual members of a group to be likened to puppets that are being played with by an agent with the name of Group?

Instead of a general theory of a group matrix (and how could clinical studies alone, of therapeutic groups, generate a general theory of groups?), one should pay more attention to what constitutes clinical groups; e.g., how do they come about? Following Searle (2010), we would say that an analytic group comes into being by the group analyst's speech act of declaring it: "I hereby create an analytic group."

> By my analytic group I mean a group that meets each Wednesday at 3 pm at my office and consists of nine members, me included. People can attend this group for years if they want, if they pay their fee and if they attend to the basic obligations of the group. The purpose of the group is self and personality development of the individual members.

This declaration comes with a lot of deontic powers. If the therapist declares the project to be "group analytic psychotherapy," they place themselves in a certain professional position that obliges them to follow certain rules, e.g., advising the group members not to socialize outside the group. By advertising "group analytic psychotherapy" the therapist connects to a tradition which is recognized by local, national, and international authorities. They appeal to be recognized as a member of this professional community. It is not a totally private project organized by e.g., a certain Jim Smith in Delaware who is free to act upon his impulses. If the therapist is a training candidate of group analysis, they are obliged to follow certain standards set by the teachers and supervisors of the local group analytic institute.

The members of the group must also follow a range of more or less explicitly stated (deontic) obligations. They must meet regularly and on time, prioritize the group above other activities, pay their bills, not meet outside the group, don't be friends on Facebook, etc. But most important is what follows from the *purpose* of the group. That is not as clear as the above-mentioned behavioral issues. They have signed in as members of a group which is supposed to promote self and personality development. What is that? What is the self? What is personality? What kind of group can provide such development? Notably, the members do not get any manual for creating such a group and the therapist is not exactly helpful with pedagogy or modeling appropriate group behavior. This does not mean that the therapist is blank in their head. To the contrary. They have an ideal model in their head about what counts as a "group analytic discourse," which is certain modes of speaking, listening, understanding, and relating. What is set in motion is not so much "ancient tribal feelings" as trial and errors by the group members of finding out and living up to the expectations of what might be a good group according to the supposed standards of the therapist. They will notice that the therapist, lights up when people start to tell stories with an emotional content, when they open up, when they respond with eagerness and empathy to each other and with similar stories or experiences (resonance), and when they point out corresponding ways of behaving in the group. They will also notice that he/she seems to dislike monologues, scapegoating and victim scenarios, advice-giving, intellectualizations, and boring café-style chat.

They will realize that they must cooperate in this foggy landscape to find a direction. However, what does such cooperation mean?

> It is said that we should become a group but what does that imply when it comes to the purpose of the group. It's much easier to be a member of a quiz club. There I know the rules and my position. But what are the rules when it comes to understanding self and others and our personalities? And besides, the guy over there semes rather rigid. How can we cooperate? We are told that we should be aware of emotions and to be honest, he irritates me a bit. Should I say so? I don't want his anger upon me …

Such are the typical dilemmas in a new therapeutic group. They are different from dilemmas in other kinds of groups. They stem from the discrepancies between high ambitions on behalf of the therapist about a kind of group analytic discourse which is free and associative, and group members' more rigid states of mind, which might be avoidant, detached, fearful, distrustful, non-cooperative, angry, resentful, envious, and the like.

Thus, the tensions within the group do not come from activation of "ancient tribal feelings" that penetrate the individual members, through the matrix, to their innermost core. The tensions come from the fact that (1) the purpose of the group is quite difficult to realize and, (2) the individuals in the group differ with respect to their capacity for emotion consciousness, for closeness and intimacy, for mentalizing, and the very ability for cooperation – in short, with respect to their different personalities. If all group members were alike when it comes to personality, there would be no problem with group cooperation.

These basic facts have been somewhat ignored by group analysis. Rightly, the modern conception of the matrix consists of a tripartite matrix: a foundation matrix, a dynamic matrix, and a personal matrix (Hopper, 2024; Nitzgen, 2024). However, the literature on the topic deals mainly with the foundation and the dynamic matrix (Karterud, 2011; Karterud et al., 2019), discussing the dynamic forces within and between groups as observed from the outside, i.e., taking *the group as object*. There has been less interest in *the group as subject*, i.e., the effort at structuring ways of speaking, listening, understanding and relating that we, in the group, struggle with, to make sense of our being together, here and now, for this particular purpose. The group as subject concerns the experiential field of *we-ness* (Karterud, 2023).

In the history of group analysis, the emphasis of the group as object was strengthened by the work of Morris Nitsun, around the turn of the century, with his popular notion of the anti-group (Nitsun, 1999). It represented a kind of climax of object-relational thinking about group analysis. Foulkes himself was not adherent to any of the object-relational schools. He considered himself a "strictly Freudian," an adherent of ego psychology. After his death, there surfaced a debate about future directions for group analysis (e.g., Brown, 1994). Malcolm Pines was the primary spokesperson for integrating theoretical and therapeutic principles from self psychology (Pines, 1990; Karterud, 1998). However, his efforts failed. We should remember that these discussions happened in the UK, the homeland of object relations. Pines had actually few chances to succeed with his flirting with self-psychology. The problem with Nitsun's approach was that the individual got lost in the anti-group. The topic of personality disorders was absent in his book (Nitsun 1999), except for some derogatory remarks about the very concept. According to Nitsun, destructive forces resided not in certain personalities, but in the metapsychological concept of the death drive, with references to Melanie Klein and Wilfred Bion. This unhappy development was mainly due to the conceptual flaws in Bion's famous volume "Experiences in Groups" (1961). Bion conceptualized the dynamic core in groups as the fluctuating relationship between the so-called work group versus the so-called basic assumption (BA) groups of fight/flight, dependency, or pairing. By labeling concerted rational deliberations a "group" (i.e., the work group) and shared emotional mental states also being a "group," the *very notion of what is a group was mystified*. The road was opened up for wild speculations, which included metapsychological speculations about the paranoid-schizoid versus the depressive position.

My PhD dissertation (Karterud, 1988, 1989a, 1989b) was about Bion's theory of groups. Not from a metapsychological perspective but from an empirical one. What actually happened in groups replete with basic assumption phenomena? I rated approximately 33,000 verbal statements in therapeutic groups with respect to their emotional content (Karterud, 1988). Yes, we could observe how rational deliberations in the groups were influenced by shared emotional states, sometimes to an extreme degree. However, this was not surprising, taking into account the general contradiction between rationality and emotional arousal. This is one of the central tenets of mentalizing theory, that when emotional arousal increases, after a certain threshold, mentalizing capabilities go down (Fonagy et al., 2002). That this relationship is also at work in groups should be no big surprise. And today, after much research, there is no big surprise that this contradiction between emotional arousal and rationality/mentalizing is strongly dependent on the personality makeup of the individual. Bad thinking creeps in when this contradiction becomes assigned to "groups," be it basic assumption groups or anti-groups.

Morris Nitsun was the most explicit manifestation of this trend in group analysis that neglected the significance of personality. However, the same trend is also visible in the work of Schlapobersky (2016) and Barwick and Weegmann (2018). Therefore, group analysis lost terrain when competing group therapies entered the scene, such as the group components of dialectical behavior therapy (DBT) (Linehan, 1993), mentalization-based treatment (MBT) (Karterud, 2015a, 2015b) and schema therapy (Farrell & Shaw, 2012). The popularity of these approaches was linked to:

1 the more modern, empirical and non-metapsychological conception of personality and personality disorders (Karterud & Kongerslev, 2019);
2 the emphasis on measurements of treatment efficiency;
3 a pragmatic attitude to the combination of individual and group psychotherapy (Karterud 2015a, 2015b); and
4 the supplement of pedagogic measures (Karterud & Bateman, 2011).

Pedagogic Measures in Group Analysis

In classical group analysis, as in psychoanalysis, pedagogical measures have been regarded "un-analytic." The pathological core of the individual should manifest itself spontaneously in the transference, not being contaminated by theoretical explanations which inevitably would enhance intellectualization as a defense mechanism. However, this attitude encountered problems when it came to people with severe personality disorders, like borderline personality disorder (BPD). Due to their vulnerability and emotional dysregulation, transference phenomena became so intense and unmanageable, that a majority of these patients dropped out of psychodynamic therapies. Malcolm Pines was an early pioneer with respect to theory and group analytic practice with borderline patients (Pines, 1990). He maintained that analytic groups might contain one borderline patient, but that several of them, or in worst case the whole group consisting of borderline patients, was not possible. This opinion has proven to be wrong. We have demonstrated that conjoint group–individual therapies with mostly borderline patients might have very low dropout rates and very high effect sizes on crucial variables (Kvarstein et al., 2015).

Our clinical experiences tell us that part of this success has to do with the supplement of pedagogic measures. The patients in the study mentioned above attended 11 sessions of a psychoeducational group in addition to the conjoint group and individual psychotherapy according to the principles of Karterud & Bateman (2011). The psychoeducation involved topics like what are primary emotions (including guilt and shame), how is my emotional profile, how can I regulate my own and others' emotions, what is attachment and what is my attachment pattern, what is mentalizing and what is it good for, what are mentalizing failures and how can I identify them in myself and others, what is personality and what are personality disorders, how is my personality profile, what is mentalization-based treatment and what is expected of me, what should be my main targets in treatment and what should I be aware of for the group therapy component. It is our strong belief, supported by some research (Ditlefsen et al., 2021), that attending such groups enhances the alliance and thus prevents early dropouts.

Defining Clinical Group Analysis

One may object that what is referred to above is not group analysis. Rightly so, but it is not that far from group analysis. At this point we need to qualify what group analysis really is. One formal definition might be a group psychotherapy format performed by a professional who is trained by one of the institutes of the European Group Analytic Training Network (EGATIN). However, since such a professional might conduct other kinds of groups as well, one could add that it should concern therapeutic groups conducted according to the principles of *psychotherapy through the group process*, whereby the main activity of the group analyst is that of *analyzing* (not leading or instructing or advising) for the aim of qualifying the group to perform and reflect upon intersubjective scenarios that promote self and personality development of the individual members of the group. One could also say that an analytic group is a group where the therapist has succeeded in creating an analytic discourse which is characterized by modes of speaking, listening, understanding, and relating that promote self and personality development (Kalleklev & Karterud, 2018; Karterud, 2018).

No definition will be very precise and accordingly not appropriate for categorization as to "this is definitely group analysis," in contrast to "this is not." In real life there will be a lot of intermediaries since most psychological phenomena are of a dimensional character. Groups will be *more or less analytic*. Less so in the earlier phases of the life of the group, more so in mature stages. And there are groups conducted by qualified group analysts that are stuck in atmospheres of passivity or distrust or fight. They never or seldom reach the stage of a proper group analytic discourse. And once there, they might soon relapse. Are those groups group analytic? If not, should e.g., the group analyst do other things than just analyze, to promote development of their group? Should they be more pedagogic, more helpful, kinder and more supportive, more individually oriented, more alert to insults and withdrawals in the group, etc.?

Groups that are "less analytic" are typically composed of members with more severe personality disorders (Karterud et al., 2024). It follows logically from what a personality disorder is all about (Karterud & Kongerslev, 2021). Above all it is about emotion consciousness, attachment pattern, and mentalizing abilities. The more disordered, the more emotion dysregulation, the more insecure attachment strategies and the less capacity for intuitive mind-reading and reflective functioning – altogether this implies poorer cooperative abilities, more misunderstandings, being more sensitive to perceived insults, more withdrawal or anger, and less trust.

Applied Group Analysis?

Consequently, there are several dimensions here to consider which are important for the notion of *applied group analysis.* Applied group analysis can be contrasted to standard or *classical group analysis* which will typically take place in a private practice setting where the therapist is in full control of the boundary conditions; in particular, with respect to duration and selection of suitable group members. In this long-term group with higher functioning patients, the analyst may cultivate a predominantly analyzing therapeutic style. Applied group analysis will typically take place in a public sector where the stakeholders have a choice of duration and selection. Maximum treatment length will be shorter, and the patients come with more severe symptoms and personality disorders and less favorable motivation for change. If the therapist behaves as they typically would do in classical group analysis, they would most probably soon end up in trouble due to poor group cohesion: poor attendance, reluctance to speak, distrust, complaints about too little support from the therapist(s), withdrawal and restricted interaction. If the therapist were to expand their repertoire, besides analyzing, what should they do (Karterud, 2015a)? And will it still count as group analysis?

Let me try to answer this question by introducing another group therapy format which is not group analysis: mentalization-based group therapy (MBT-G) (Karterud, 2015a, 2015b). MBT-G is designed for slow-open groups where the maximum treatment length for the individual is in the range of 1.5–3 years. The average patient will have a personality disorder, most typically BPD, and often with co-morbid disorders like bipolar-II, substance use disorders, eating disorders, mood and anxiety disorders. At the beginning of treatment, some will be in a miserable condition with little social support and a self-destructive lifestyle which includes self-harm and suicidal gestures. Some will be heavily medicated. The level of emotional pain is high, often almost unbearable, but the motivation for change might nevertheless be low.

These patients need a structured and supportive therapeutic environment – in particular in the initial stage. A MBT program provides that. In addition to the dynamic MBT group, the clients receive 11 group session of psychoeducation (as already described) and weekly individual psychotherapy for the first year, later to be declined. These additional components are noteworthy. In the history of group analysis, when the early pioneers found out that a once-a-week group was not enough for certain clients, they introduced twice-a-week groups as standard (Kreeger, 1991). That is not what we recommend for poorly functioning patients today. We add something different and supplementary: pedagogy and individual therapy. In earlier days, this was regarded as "taking something out of the group." Earlier generations of group analysts thought that this "something" should be kept in the group by adding one more session a week. Unfortunately, the benefits of twice-a-week groups have never been proven by research evidence.

Today we have good evidence of the usefulness of a more pragmatic stance. In 1992 I founded with some colleagues the Norwegian Network of Personality Disorders, a clinical research network, which today consists of 21 different group therapy units located all over Norway (Pedersen et al., 2022). The database of this network counts today around 15,000 cases, whereof around 4,000 borderline patients, and is presumable the largest database in the world on the (mostly group) treatment of personality disorders. Later I founded the state-supported Norwegian Competence Center for Personality Psychiatry with its Psychotherapy Laboratory which offered services to local group therapy units, whereby they could send video-recordings of their group (and/or individual) sessions and have them rated and commented on according to an MBT adherence and quality scale (Folmo et al., 2017). Today, we are involved in a project to develop a generic group psychotherapy scale that rates (1) level of group functioning and (2) therapist intervention profile. These rating experiences together with a lot of video-based group supervisions have demonstrated that there is no sharp demarcation between group analysis proper and group psychotherapy according to e.g., MBT principles.

Oh yes, there are clearly distinct prototypes, but most importantly there are a lot of intermediary groups, we might call them hybrid groups, that are more or less analytic, or more or less mentalization based. Sometimes our advice to poorly functioning analytic groups would be to adopt some MBT principles, and more often our advice to rigid MBT groups would be to set the group more free, to stimulate more group-relevant discussions, and trying to trust the group (Karterud et al., 2024; Schulz-Venrath & Felsberger, 2016). Both poles, the analytic and the MBT-ish, should attend to the basic principles of "psychotherapy through the group process." Both poles should regard *symptoms as unmentalized emotions.* In group analysis, the therapist will follow the principles which are so well described by Foulkes on how to listen to and tune into resonance in the group, stimulate and translate the communication in the group, and thus help the client(s) to find words, concepts, and narratives for the formerly painful and wordless parts of the self. What Foulkes describes so well, is *mentalizing processes in groups* (Karterud, 2026). By partaking in such processes, the reflective capacity of the individual will increase. That's what Foulkes formulated into the slogan: *Group analysis is ego-training in action*. In MBT-G similar processes will optimally take place, although directed more by the therapist(s) who actively encourage group members to explore social events together, in their present life or in the past, where something happened that overstimulated the members' emotions and left experiences to be unintegrated and thereby without meaning, or attributed by false, or even reality-distorting meaning.

Challenges for Training Institutes

With these fleeting boundaries between classical and applied group analysis, it is important in my view that institutes of group analysis extend their curricula and also provide training in applied versions. That means psychoeducational groups as well, and even the combination with individual psychotherapy which has hitherto been considered a taboo. We must accept the fact that some patients need conjoint individual–group psychotherapy. This combination is a challenge. Where can training candidates learn this combination? They don't learn it at psychoanalytic or traditional psychotherapy institutes. The integrational work I am suggesting means that we take personality disorders, with their range from light to moderate to severe, seriously. Personality theory and assessment will therefore need more space in the course of training. I am confident that group analysis, at least in the long run, will prosper with an expansion along these lines. Group analysis will get a better hold in the public mental health services with all the positive implications that follow from that. It is worth mentioning that in the year 2023 Norwegian mental health leaders regarded group therapy as the most successful way of organizing treatment in the public sector (Karterud et al., 2025). This positive view reflects experiences with an increasing number of group units at Norwegian Community Mental Health Centers (CMHC), led by competent group analysts. This public recognition is open for more power, more money for training, more therapists, and hopefully more enthusiasm which is necessary for the thriving of a professional field.

Summary: For the Decade to Come

1 Group analysis as a clinical discipline should be more visible in the media.
2 Group analysis should advertise itself as a long-term treatment option for self and personality development that also alleviates symptom disorders and prevents relapse.
3 The theory of group analysis should be modernized, in particular with respect to evolutionary perspectives on primary emotions, attachment, and mentalizing/self-consciousness. These perspectives, in concert with social ontology based upon speech act theory (Searle, 2010), will expand our understanding of what is the nature of human social groups.

4 The history of group analysis has been overly preoccupied with the notion of the group as object (Bion/Nitsun). We should be more concerned with the group as subject: e.g., what does it mean to be "a we."
5 The category "group analysis" is dimensional. Concrete groups exist on a continuum between "classical group analysis" and "applied group analysis."
6 The most important variables for this continuum are (1) level of personality functioning, and (2) duration.
7 Most groups in the public mental health sector are composed of people with considerable personality pathology.
8 Applied group analysis might be supplemented with psychoeducational groups as well as individual psychotherapy and these combinations should be taught at group analytic institutes.
9 The curriculum of group analytic institutes should also be modernized and include more of personality theory and assessment.
10 Norwegian experiences indicate that public mental health leaders might hold applied group analysis in high respect and support CMHC group units with power, prestige, money, and positions, which is necessary for a professional community to thrive.

References

Barwick, N., & Weegmann, M. (2018). *Group Therapy: A Group-Analytic Approach.* London: Routledge.

Bion, W.R. (1961). *Experiences in Groups.* London: Tavistock Publications.

Bowlby, J. (1988). *A Secure Base: Clinical Applications of Attachment Theory.* London: Tavistock/Routledge.

Brown, D.G. (1994). Self development through subjective interaction. A fresh look at "ego training in action". In D.G. Brown & L. Zinkin (Eds.), *The Psyche and the Social World.* London: Routledge.

Ditlefsen, I.T., Nissen-Lie, H.A., Andenæs, A., Normann-Eide, E., Johansen, M.S., & Kvarstein, E.H. (2021). "Yes, there is actually hope!" A qualitative investigation of how patients experience mentalization-based psychoeducation tailored for borderline personality disorder. *Journal of Psychotherapy Integration*, 31(3), 257.

Farrell, J.M., & Shaw, I.A. (2012). *Group Schema Therapy for Borderline Personality Disorder.* New York: Wiley-Blackwell.

Folmo, E.J., Karterud, S. W., Bremer, K., Walther, K., Kvarstein, E., & Pedersen, G. (2017). The design of the MBT-G adherence and quality scale. *Scandinavian Journal of Psychology*, 58, 341–349.

Fonagy, P., Gergely, G., Jurist, E.L., & Target, M. (2002). *Affect Regulation, Mentalization, and the Development of the Self.* New York: Other Press.

Foulkes, S.H. (1948). *Introduction to Group-Analytic Psychotherapy.* London: Wm. Heinemann Medical Books.

Foulkes, S.H. (1964). *Therapeutic Group Analysis.* London: Allen & Unwin (Reprinted London: Karnac Books, 1984).

Foulkes, S.H. (1973). The group as matrix of the individual's mental life. In L.R. Wolberg & E.K. Schwartz (Eds.), *Group Therapy: 1973 – An Overview.* New York: Intercontinental Medical Book Corporation.

Hopper, W. (2024). *The Tripartite Matrix in the Developing Theory and Expanding Practice of Group Analysis.* London: Routledge.

Kalleklev, J., & Karterud, S. (2018). A comparative study of a mentalization-based versus a psychodynamic group therapy session. *Group Analysis*, 51(1), 44–60.

Karterud, S. (1988). The valence theory of Bion and the significance of (DSM-III) diagnosis for inpatient group behavior. *Acta Psychiatrica Scandinavica*, 78, 462–470.

Karterud, S. (1989a). A study of Bion's basic assumption groups. *Human Relations*, 42, 315–335.

Karterud, S. (1989b). A comparative study of six different inpatient groups with respect to their basic assumption functioning. *International Journal of Group Psychotherapy*, 49, 355–376.

Karterud, S. (1998). The group self, empathy, intersubjectivity and hermeneutics: A group analytic perspective. In I. Harwood & M. Pines (Eds.), *Self Experiences in Group: Intersubjective and Self Psychological Pathways to Human Understanding.* London: Jessica Kingsley Publishers.

Karterud, S. (2011). Constructing and mentalizing the matrix. *Group Analysis*, 44(4), 1–17.

Karterud, S. (2015a). On structure and leadership in MBT-G and group analysis. *Group Analysis*, 48(2), 137–149.

Karterud, S. (2015b). *Mentalization-Based Group Therapy (MBT-G): A Theoretical, Clinical and Research Manual.* London: Oxford University Press.

Karterud, S. (2018). A high-quality mentalization-based group therapy session. *Group Analysis*, 51(1), 18–43.

Karterud, S. (2024). *Group Analysis: A Moderne Synthesis.* London: Routledge.

Karterud, S. (2026). *Mentalizing and Group Analysis.* London: Routledge.

Karterud, S., & Bateman, A. (2011). *Manual for mentaliseringsbasert psykoedukativ gruppeterapi.* Oslo: Gyldendal Akademisk.

Karterud, S., & Kongerslev, M.T. (2019). A Temperament, attachment and mentalization-based (TAM) theory of personality and its disorders. *Frontiers in Psychology*, 10, 518. doi:10.3389/fpsyg.2019.00518.

Karterud, S., Folmo, E., & Kongerslev, M.T. (2019). Personality and the group matrix. *Group Analysis*, 52(4), 503–519. doi:10.1177/0533316418824210.

Karterud, S., & Kongerslev, M.T. (2021). Psychotherapy of personality disorders needs an integrative theory of personality. *Journal of Psychotherapy Integration*, 31(1), 34–53.

Karterud, S., Gunnarsen, G., Kongerslev, M.T., Staun, L., & Schultz-Venrath, U. (2024). On the relationship between group analysis and mentalization-based group therapy. *Group Analysis*, 58(1), 115–129. doi:10.1177/05333164231218694.

Karterud, S., Bjerke, S.N., Normann-Eide, T., & Ulland, A. (2025). Group treatment is favoured by Norwegian mental health leaders. *Group Analysis*, 1–17. doi:10.1177/05333164241300693.

Kreeger, L. (1991). The twice-weekly groups. In J. Roberts & M. Pines (Eds.), *The Practice of Group Analysis.* London: Routledge.

Kvarstein, E., Pedersen, G., Urnes, Ø., Hummelen, B., Wilberg, T., & Karterud, S. (2015). Changing from a traditional psychodynamic treatment program to mentalization-based treatment for patients with borderline personality disorder. Does it make a difference? *Psychology and Psychotherapy: Theory, Research and Practice*, 88(1), 71–86.

Linehan, M. (1993). *Skills Training Manual for Treating Borderline Personality Disorder*. New York: Guilford Press.

Nitsun, M. (1999). *The Anti-Group: Destructive Forces in the Group and Their Creative Potential*. London: Routledge.

Nitzgen, D. (2024). The cornerstone, once more. In E. Hopper (Ed.), *The Tripartite Matrix in the Developing Theory and Expanding Practice of Group Analysis*. London: Routledge.

Panksepp, J., & Biven, L. (2012). *The Archeology of Mind: Neuroevolutionary Origins of Human Emotions*. New York: W.W. Norton & Company.

Pedersen, G., Wilberg, T., Hummelen, B., & Kvarstein, E. (2022). The Norwegian network for personality disorders – development, contributions and challenges through 30 years. *Nordic Journal of Psychiatry*, 77(5), 512–520. doi:10.1080/08039488.2022.2147995.

Pines, M. (1990). Group analytic psychotherapy and the borderline patient. In B.E. Roth, W.N. Stone, & H.D. Kibel (Eds.), *The Difficult Patient in Group*. Madison: International Universities Press.

Schlapobersky, J. (2016). *From the Couch to the Circle: Group-Analytic Psychotherapy in Practice*. London: Routledge.

Schultz-Venrath, U., & Felsberger, H. (2016). *Mentalisieren in Gruppen*. Berlin: Klett-Cotta Verlag.

Searle, J.R. (2010). *Making the Social World: The Structure of Human Civilization*. Oxford: Oxford University Press.

Taylor, C. (2016). *The Linguistic Animal: The Full Shape of the Human Linguistic Capacity*. Cambridge: The Belknap Press of Harvard University Press.

Chapter 18

Integrative Approach to Research in Group Analytic Psychotherapy

A Narrative Survey

Steinar Lorentzen

A Short History of Group Research

Group psychotherapy has been practiced for more than 120 years and researched for about the last 80 years. Early reports of *outcome* were at first anecdotal, describing single groups. Then reviewers started to add up numbers of studies with positive, negative, or no effects, the so-called *box score method* (Burchard et al., 1948; Thomas, 1943). Eventually, Smith and Glass (1977) introduced a new review strategy, called *the meta-analysis*: The sum of scores from several outcome measures was averaged, allowing for direct comparisons with other studies. Results from studies including control groups were presented from the 1970s (Bednar & Kaul, 1978; Emrick, 1975; Lieberman, 1976; Luborsky et al., 1975; Meltzoff & Kornreich, 1970; Fuhriman & Burlingame, 1998, pp. 14–20; Burlingame et al., 2016).

The Handbook of Psychotherapy and Behavior Change

This book has been a rich source of research methodology and results, appearing with seven editions between 1971 and 2021. Especially important for this presentation is the chapter on *group psychotherapy research*, the last one by Burlingame and Strauss (2021). Space only permits a few samples of the contents of the group chapter to be presented here: the *five-factor model* (see Figure 18.1), a recent *meta-analysis* of outcome studies, and samples of *updated process studies.*

A quick look at a simple five-factor model (Burlingame et al., 2004), demonstrates how it is possible to conceptualize small-group treatments. Therapy outcome is placed in the center, and the model identifies potential variables influencing treatment outcomes (directly as predictors, or in interaction with others, as moderators or even possible mediators). The variables are grouped under headings such as structural factors (length, frequency), patient and therapist variables, small group processes (aspects of interaction, group development, cohesion), and formal change theory (Group Analysis, CBT, Systemic, etc.).

DOI: 10.4324/9781003597674-18

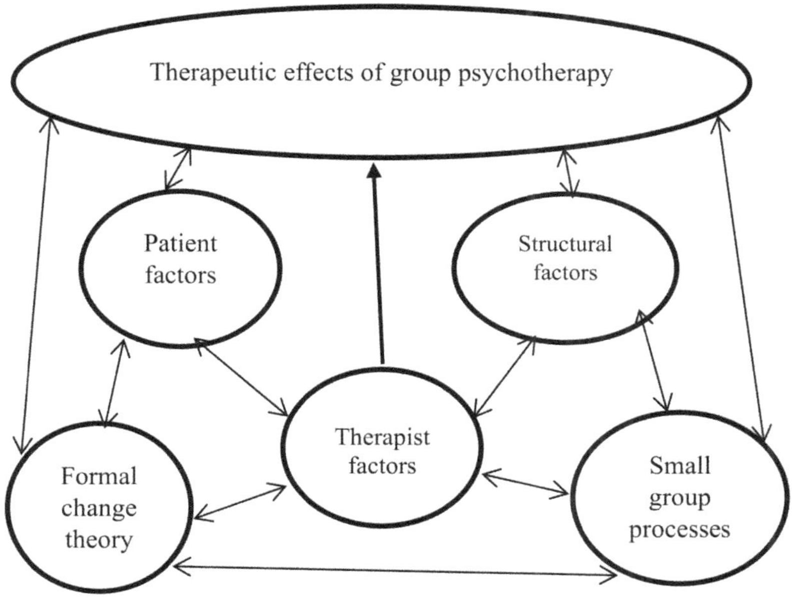

Figure 18.1 Factors contributing to change in group psychotherapy. Reworked from Burlingame, MacKenzie, and Strauss (2004).

When it comes to *outcome studies*, the number of randomized clinical trials (RCTs) included in the chapter has increased over the years, and the methodology used in meta-analyses has improved. In the last edition (Burlingame & Strauss, 2021) ten meta-analyses are reviewed, summarizing 329 RCTs comprising 27,000 patients, from the last 30 years. The main conclusion is that group psychotherapy is effective compared with non-active treatments and equivalent to other active treatments (including individual psychotherapy), for various mental disorders. Most of the studies are on group cognitive-behavioral therapy (CBT), but next to that the psychodynamic/group analytic models have the longest tradition and are found in studies of the treatment of patients with Borderline PD (15), eating disorders (12), and post-traumatic stress disorders (PTSD) (14). The number of psychodynamic studies is noted in parenthesis. Most of the efficacy studies have been conducted in *outpatient settings* and are mainly focused on *short-term groups.* The last summary of *inpatients* (Kösters et al., 2006) demonstrated a small and large effect size for *controlled* and *observational* studies, respectively.

Process studies include measures of *cohesion* that intend to measure the sense of connection or closeness among group members, while *therapeutic alliance* as a relational factor traditionally has been studied in individual psychotherapy. More recently, however, the alliance between the therapist and the individual patients has attracted more interest, also in group research.

One such study found a significant weighted average correlation (r=0.17) between member–leader alliance and treatment outcome in a meta-analysis of 29 studies including 3,628 group patients (Alldredge et al., 2021). This is low compared with the correlation (r=0.28) found for alliance in individual treatment (Flückiger et al., 2018; Rosendahl et al., 2021: 57). One relatively recent meta-analysis included 55 studies and more than 6,000 patients and demonstrated a significant correlation of moderate effect size (r=0.26) between cohesion and improvement (Burlingame et al., 2018a). This is about the same value reported above for the therapeutic alliance in individual therapy (r=0.28). A fairly recent process measure, the Group Questionnaire, has created much interest. From the patients' point of view, cohesion consists of *three structural components*: the patient–patient relationship, the patient–group relationship, and the patient–therapist relationship. Johnson et al. (2005) sought to achieve a conceptual clarification of cohesion and carried out a factor analysis of the items in the four most commonly used cohesion measures (group climate questionnaire, cohesion, therapeutic alliance, and empathy). This resulted in three qualitative factors encompassing two affective aspects (positive emotional bonds and negative relationships) and one work-based facet of group relationships (positive work). These qualitative factors were then intersected with the three structural patient factors mentioned above to capture the diversity of the group relationships. The factors have been partially validated in follow-up studies (Bormann & Strauss, 2007; Bakali et al., 2009). A user-friendly cohesion measure, the Group Questionnaire (GQ), was arrived at by reducing the number of underlying items (Krogel et al., 2013; see also Lorentzen, 2022, p. 150). There has been an increase in the use of GQ in clinical practice, and the following two studies demonstrate that continuous feedback to therapists on patients' experience of group relationships resulted in significantly better treatment outcomes and fewer premature terminations (Burlingame et al., 2018b; Gleave et al., 2017).

I will end this section with a few words about *attachment, a patient characteristic* that may influence group therapy outcomes, and that has gradually come more into focus (Marmarosh, 2017). It has also become clearer that interaction with responsive and supportive leaders and cohesive groups beneficially alters a person's attachment patterns and psychological functioning (Marmarosh et al., 2013). This personality characteristic may very well be a mechanism of change and should therefore be the target for increased and specific group analytic research in the future.

Research on Studies of the Clinical Effectiveness of Group Analysis and Analytic/Dynamic Group Psychotherapy

I will now turn to more specific studies of GA research, consisting of the Sheffield report (Blackmore et al., 2009) and a recent literature search covering the last 15 years, bringing us up to date.

The Sheffield Report (Studies up to 2009)

This review came about because GA seemed to gradually lose its position compared to CBT within the National Health System (NHS) in the UK, possibly because group CBT offered shorter therapies and produced more empirical data supporting its efficacy/effectiveness. Consequently, the Institute of Group Analysis (IGA) and the Group Analytic Society (GAS), London commissioned the University of Sheffield (Centre for Psychological Services Research, School of Health and Related Research) to evaluate the evidence base for Group Analysis (GA) and Analytic/Dynamic group psychotherapy (A/D).

The mandate was to provide a systematic review of the efficacy and effectiveness of these therapies, to look for factors that influenced the results, and there was also a wish for a clearer description of the patients who underwent GA, including the duration of their therapies.

Results and Conclusions

Data searches of the literature gave a total of 34 primary studies by sifting the literature from 2001 to 2008 (Blackmore et al., 2009, 2012). In order to catch all previous studies, 19 reviews of outcome studies carried out before 2001 were also included. Five of the studies were randomized controlled studies (only one GA study), and there were seven other controlled studies, 21 observational studies (ten GA), and one qualitative study. *The results* showed that all the studies, including earlier reviews, supported the use of psychodynamic group psychotherapy as an *effective approach across diverse conditions, participants, groups, and settings.* Several predictor and moderator analyses demonstrated that there might be important effects of age, sex, self-efficacy, psychological mindedness, and quality of object relationships (QOR) on outcomes (Lorentzen & Høglend, 2008), and attachment style and interpersonal distress had a bearing on group attendance.

Limitations and Recommendations

There were also several *limitations in the literature*: the data search gave no information as to the types of patients for whom GA and A/D group therapies were most effective. The different indications for group vs. individual psychotherapy, and the comparable cost-effectiveness, had not been studied. There was no data on the degree to which the aspects of heterogeneity vs. homogeneity of group membership impacted the outcome. The methodological quality of studies varied, and the Sheffield group had the following *recommendations* to the field: It is urgent to do trials of GA and A/D group therapies compared with group CBT. It is also important to make a review of the service users' personal testimony. To improve *reporting* (publishing) of research, authors were encouraged to use structured abstracts, to give clear definitions of interventions and use agreed keywords in titles and abstracts, and develop (and use) a consistent set of outcome measures.

Many group analysts were surprised by the scarcity of quality research studies. I was especially struck by the fact that only one of the five RCTs and ten of the observational studies were on GA. The Sheffield group argues convincingly that it is impossible to declare a winner when GA and AD group therapy are compared to each other as to efficacy, based on the existing data. Lack of space makes it difficult to give too many details from the different studies in this review, but readers are recommended to read the original reports (Blackmore et al., 2009, 2012). I will briefly present a few facts from the only group analytic RCT that appeared in the report and one of the observational studies, which I find to be typical for a clinical pre-post research study.

Example of RCT in the Sheffield Study: Outcome of Systemic and Analytic Group Psychotherapy for Adult Women with a History of Intrafamilial Childhood Sexual Abuse – A Randomized Controlled Study (Lau & Kristensen, 2007)

One hundred and fifty-one women were randomly allocated to systemic or slightly modified (more support) analytic group psychotherapy. Quality of life, psychosocial functioning, psychological distress, and flashbacks were assessed before and after treatment. Results: 82 patients completed therapy. Both therapies led to improved quality of life, fewer symptoms, and better overall functioning, but the systemic therapy had a better outcome than the analytic group therapy. Longer-term follow-up data are required for conclusions on the maintenance of therapeutic gains.

Example of an Observational Study in the Sheffield Study: Long-term Analytic Group Psychotherapy with Outpatients – Evaluation of Process and Change (Lorentzen et al., 2002)

This is an observational study of 69 outpatients with the diagnoses of mostly depression and/or anxiety disorders on Axis I, and 68% with one or more personality disorders (PDs). The *research questions* were: What is the effectiveness of long-term group analytic psychotherapy? What factors predict change or moderate change? The patients were treated in three slow-open groups, and the mean duration of therapy = 32.5 months, 90 min/week (range 6 months to 8 years). The therapy approach was group analysis, as developed by Foulkes and successors (Foulkes, 1977; Foulkes, 1986; Foulkes and Anthony, 1984; Pines, 1983). The patients were evaluated pre-post, and each patient also had a follow-up interview with the therapist and an independent evaluator, one year after the end of therapy. *Results*: only two patients dropped out; 61–86 % of the patients improved or moved into a non-clinical part of the population (recovered) as to symptoms, interpersonal problems, and/or psychosocial functioning. Eight patients remained unchanged in psychosocial functioning, and no patients deteriorated.

My work with this study clearly demonstrated a need for more high-quality clinical research on group analytic psychotherapy, and shortly after the publication of this project (Lorentzen, 2003), I got a position at the University of Oslo, which made it possible to plan a larger research project: short- and long-term group analytic psychotherapy. A randomized clinical trial (Lorentzen et al., 2013, 2015a; For more references, see below). The study has resulted in about 25 papers in peer-reviewed journals, two books, several book chapters, and two doctoral theses (Bakali, 2013; Fjeldstad, 2019). These papers appeared after the Sheffield report had been published, and the time was ripe to check whether the field had changed, 15 years later!

A New Search for Studies of the Clinical Effectiveness of Group Analysis and Analytic/Dynamic Group Psychotherapy (from 2009 until March 14, 2025)

Assisted by the library of the University of Oslo, we did a systematic search of the research literature, covering the last 15 years since the Sheffield report was published. We were primarily interested in outcome studies of short- or long-term groups based on group analytic or A/D theory that included subjects with a clinical diagnosis, had a description of the group interventions, and were published in English. The following three databases were searched: Scopus, APA PsycINFO (via Ovid), and PubMed. After removing duplicates and sifting according to the criteria described above, we were left with *24 papers* that describe group analytic (explicitly characterized as such) and/or A/D groups (i.e., other analytic and/or dynamic) treatments. As mentioned, we only found *one randomized clinical trial* based on group analytic theory (Lorentzen et al., 2013), and it was one of *nine* papers in the search, all covering diverse aspects of the same project (outcome, moderators, process, etc.). The study was carried out by a research group I have administered for some years, and the main results and references will be presented in the section below. Further, we found *six* randomized trials based on A/D theory (one on perfectionism and five on complicated grief) and *five* observational studies (one based on GA theory; Østergård et al., 2022, and one with patients randomized to A/D or Group CBT; Zajenkowska et al., 2019). We also identified *a protocol* of an RCT, intended to compare potential differences in efficacy between group CBT and A/D or GA therapies (Suszek et al., 2015), which will be briefly described under the RCTs. The last *three* studies consisted of one qualitative study (Pingitore & Ferszt, 2017), an ultra-brief integrative approach (Whittingham, 2018), and finally, the search revealed my book on a newly constructed group analytic therapy: *Focused Group Analytic Psychotherapy* (Lorentzen, 2022). The GA projects mentioned above will be described in some depth, while the rest will be mentioned cursorily.

References in the following text will, however, enable the reader to localize and study these papers further. The main part of *the excluded papers* dealt with studies with another theoretical background (than GA or A/D group psychotherapy), the great majority being group CBT, followed by the existential, systemic, mentalization-based group, dialectical, behavioral therapy, art groups, etc.

Short- and Long-term Group Analytic Psychotherapy: A Randomized Clinical Trial

This trial (Lorentzen et al., 2013) is represented by nine papers in the search, which are all among the references presented under the sub-heading *Results* below. The main *objective of this project* was to study the significance of treatment length for outcomes during and after short- and long-term group analytic therapy (STG and LTG). It was also to study the development of group processes in therapies of different lengths. *Methods*: 167 outpatients were recruited from three urban sites in Norway. Inclusion criteria were at least one diagnosis on Axis I (symptom disorder) or II (personality disorder) (DSM-IV), self-perceived interpersonal problems, motivation to work on these problems in a group, and agreement to randomization. The patients were randomized (stratified on gender) to short- or long-term GA and allocated to 18 groups, with 7–8 patients in each group. There were nine therapists who each conducted both a short-term and a long-term group. The duration of the treatments was 20 versus 80 weekly sessions of 90 minutes each (altogether 6 or 24 months). The sample consisted of 62% women and 38% men. The mean age was 38.7 (9.4) years. As to diagnoses, 80% had mood disorders and 60% had anxiety disorders. The number of axis 1 diagnoses was mean = 3.3; 45% had one or more personality disorder(s), mostly mixed and avoidant PD, and 65% had been in previous treatment. Symptoms and interpersonal problems were measured repeatedly until 7 years after the start of therapy, and Global Assessment of Functioning and self-esteem were measured at the therapy start and after 3 years (see Table 18.1). Patients were interviewed at follow-up three years after therapy started.

Linear mixed models for repeated measures were used to analyze longitudinal data. Both intragroup and between-group differences were calculated. Outcomes were studied both for the typical (average) patient and for patients with or without personality disorders.

Manuals and Treatment Fidelity

The therapies were *manualized*, describing theory, methodology, and techniques and giving clinical examples within the two formats (Lorentzen, 2014). Both therapies were group analytic, but the short-term group therapy differed in a few respects: more time was used on pre-therapy preparation and to

Table 18.1 Duration of short- and long-term groups and time points for data collection

Months	**0**	**6**	**12**	**18**	**24**	**36***	**84****
Duration of groups							
Short-term groups (S)	Start	End					
Long-term groups (L)	Start				End		
Measures (data collection)							
SCL-90-R Symptoms	SL	SL	SL	SL	SL	SL	SL
IIP-C Interpersonal problems	SL	SL	SL	SL	SL	SL	SL
GAF Symptoms & functioning	SL					SL	
SCID-II Criteria of PD	SL					SL	
SASB Introject	SL					SL	

Note: * Follow-up interview; ** Follow-up by mail.

negotiate a therapy focus, the therapist was more active, worked more in the here-and-now, and was more alert to specific stages in the group process (opening, differentiation, interpersonal work, and termination). Treatment fidelity and therapist competence were checked for details (see Lorentzen et al., 2013: 283).

Results

Both short- and long-term group analyses demonstrated efficacy. The *typical* (average) patient changed quickly and more during STG (6 months) than in LTG, but the change was equal in the two treatments after 3 years (Lorentzen et al., 2013). The initial effect was sustained in STG for up to 7 years, while LTG patients also had a *delayed effect* (patients continued to change after termination (Lorentzen et al., 2015a)). Patients with one or more *personality disorders* (PD) did equally well in STG and LTG during the first 6 months (STG). However, LTG patients with PD also demonstrated a delayed effect up to 7 years of follow-up, while the early effects in the STG groups were sustained after 7 years (Lorentzen et al., 2015b; Fjeldstad et al., 2016). Patients without PD also changed faster in the STG, and LTG patients took a couple of years to catch up. Another important point is that the LTG patients never exceeded the improvement in the STG patients during the last 5 years of the follow-up period (Fjeldstad et al., 2016). The fact that the degree of personality pathology moderates the outcome of short- and long-term group analytic psychotherapy may have important implications for the type of group (short- or long-term) these patients should be primarily allocated to. This underlines the importance of a thorough evaluation of the patients' personality organization before therapy starts. We found a significant association between cohesion and improvement in symptoms and interpersonal problems in STG, but not in LTG (Lorentzen et al., 2018). To see more details about differences in outcomes and development of therapy processes, in the two therapies, the original studies should be consulted (Fjeldstad et al., 2017; Lorentzen et al., 2015c; Bakali et al., 2009, 2013; Lorentzen et al., 2012). *Deteriorations* are often not reported in psychotherapy studies. In this study, 5.8% deteriorated across all outcome measures and treatment lengths at 3-year follow-up. There were no serious adverse events (suicide or suicide attempts).

RCTs about Perfectionism and Complicated Grief and a Research Protocol

Perfectionism

Kealy et al. (2025) compared the efficacy of dynamic *relational* group therapy (DRT) relative to group psychodynamic *supportive* therapy (PST) in improving perfectionism-related attitudes and components of the perfectionistic self-relationship. The first therapy is more focused on group process and insight, the other on support. Eighty highly perfectionistic persons were allocated to 12 sessions of either. Results revealed significant decreases in dysfunctional attitudes, concern over mistakes, self-criticism, self-esteem problems, and an increase in self-reassurance in both DRT and PST. Moderate-to-large between-group differences favoring DRT over PST were found for dysfunctional attitudes and self-assurance.

Complicated Grief

Five papers reported from studies involving outpatients suffering from *complicated grief* (and a variety of DSM-IV Axis I and II diagnoses), who were treated at the psychiatry services of two university hospitals in Canada (University of Alberta Hospital and Vancouver General Hospital). In all studies, patients were treated with manualized brief psychodynamic group psychotherapy (12 sessions, either interpretive or supportive). Piper et al. (2009) studied four different kinds of outcomes based on evaluation of clinically significant change and found that 50% had changed significantly after therapy and at 6-month follow-up (maintenance); 25% had changed only at follow-up (delayed recovery); a few changed during therapy, but were not changed at follow-up (relapse); while almost 25% did not change at all (nonrecovery). Joyce et al. (2010) wanted to replicate results from an earlier study (Ogrodniczuk et al., 2002), which had reported that three distinct indices of interpersonal relatedness, quality of object relations, current social functioning, and attachment insecurity, each had significant relationships with measures of treatment outcome. Only the key finding (attachment insecurity) was verified in this study. Hernandez et al. (2016) investigated whether referential language predicted decrease in post-treatment general and grief symptoms, and found that higher use of self-referential statements predicted higher levels of general symptoms at post-treatment. Contrary to this, higher use of references to the group members independently predicted lower post-treatment levels of grief symptoms. Kealy et al. (2017a) studied the relationship between the patients' capacity for Psychological Mindedness (PM) and aspects of the group process, and concluded that PM was positively associated with several group process variables (therapeutic work, alliance, expression of emotion), as rated by the therapist and other group members. Kealy et al. (2017b) investigated the relationship between patients' psychodynamic work versus supportive work and outcomes in two types of short-term group psychotherapy, at termination and at 6-month follow-up. They conclude that psychodynamic work, that is, a focus on the development of insight and self-reflection can contribute to further benefits after the group therapy for complicated grief, suggesting that it may reflect a general curative mechanism of group treatments.

An RCT Protocol, but No Implementation

Suszek et al. (2015) produced an RCT study protocol on how to investigate potential differences in outcome between intensive, psychodynamic, and cognitive-behavioral therapy. The project has not been implemented, but is still included here for didactic purposes. Their *objectives* are to: (1) investigate the effectiveness of each treatment in a day-care setting, (2) demonstrate the respective short- and long-term effectiveness of the treatments, (3) investigate the predictors and moderators of treatment response, and (4) carry out a preliminary examination of the mediators of therapeutic change. *Methods/design*: 199 patients will be randomly assigned to one of three conditions: (1) psychodynamic group therapy; (2) cognitive-behavioral group therapy; or (3) wait-list control group. The manualized therapies will last 12 weeks. Primary outcome measures will include self-reported symptoms of anxiety, observer-rated symptoms of anxiety, global improvement, and recovery rate.

Five Observational Studies (One Based on Group Analytic Theory)

Østergård et al. (2022) investigated the effectiveness of focused time-limited group analytic psychotherapy (Lorentzen, 2014), and they also examined whether outcomes were predicted by the client's psychological mindedness and personality structure as measured by Operationalized Psychodynamic Diagnosis (OPD). Sixty-six student counseling clients were treated in nine groups for about 6 months (mean 15.5 sessions). Results: pre-post effect sizes were large for symptoms (GSI) and interpersonal problems (IIP-64), and moderate for the Social Adjustment Scale. Psychological mindedness significantly predicted lower GSI and IIP, and higher personality structure was associated with fewer symptoms (GSI).

Zajenkowska et al. (2019) wanted to compare the effectiveness of intensive CBGT (Cognitive Behavioral Group Therapy) and PDGT (Psychodynamic Group Psychotherapy) conducted in the day clinic of a public hospital in Warsaw, Poland. The outcome variables were *depressive symptoms* as measured by The Patient Health Questionnaire (PHQ-9; Kroenke & Spitzer, 2002) and *hostile attributions*, as evaluated by The Ambiguous Intentions and Hostility Questionnaire (AIHQ; Combs et al., 2007). The PHQ-9 is a self-report based on the Diagnostic and Statistical Manual of Mental Disorders (DSM-IV) criteria for depressive disorders, while in AIHQ, patients are asked to read five different situations with ambiguous causes, to place themselves in the various situations, and score on a dimensional scale (from 1–5): whether the other person in the scenario acted intentionally; how angry the patient felt; and finally, how much the other person is blamed. Thirty-seven patients were evaluated at the start and after the end of 12 weeks of intensive group therapy (five times a week). Results: the general conclusion was that hostile attribution decreased in both types of groups, but depressive symptoms decreased more in the CBT group. One limitation of the study is the low number of participants, due to a dropout rate of 26%.

In a day ward, 139 patients with anxiety and personality disorders were assessed with the Eysenck Personality Questionnaire before and after 12 weeks of treatment in short-term group psychodynamic psychotherapy (Sieradzki et al., 2017). Results: levels of neuroticism, extraversion, psychoticism, and lie (a control factor) did not change significantly in the group of more neurotic patients. In the group of personality disorders, the level of neuroticism decreased significantly, whereas the level of extraversion increased. The levels of psychoticism and lie (control) did not change in any of the groups.

Leirvåg et al. (2010) compared the effectiveness of psychodynamic group therapy (PGT) and body awareness group therapy (BAGT) as a follow-up treatment after 18 weeks of day treatment for personality disorders. Twenty-one female patients given PGT were compared with 29 female patients receiving BAGT, one session a week for about two years, and were assessed as to personality disorders, symptoms, and interpersonal problems (SCID-II, GSI, and CIP, respectively), at admission and discharge from day treatment, and after outpatient group therapy. Results: BAGT patients improved significantly more on GAF, GSI, and CIP, but because of the limitations of this study, the results warrant a larger randomized study.

In a pre-post observational design based on 236 outpatients with diagnoses of mood (9.7%), neurotic (50.8%), and personality disorders (39.4%), Jensen et al. (2010) assessed the effectiveness of short-term psychodynamic group therapy (39 sessions in 3 months) in a public outpatient clinic. Even though many patients reliably improved, a substantial part of the patients were still within the pathological range of Danish norms after therapy, indicating that many of these patients might need an alternative or longer treatment.

Three Treatment Models of Interest (One Group Analytic)

Focused Brief Group Therapy (Whittingham, 2018)

This is an integrative interpersonal approach to brief group therapy (8 sessions) that uses formal assessment to guide and inform treatment. By utilizing assessment as a key part of real-time clinical feedback throughout treatment, multiple therapeutic goals are enhanced. This article addresses two specific uses of assessment within focused brief group therapy: to focus treatment on *interpersonal subtype distress* and to inoculate clients against *self-sabotage.*

Qualitative Study: Retrospective Reflections on Group Experience

Pingitore et al. (2017) selected a qualitative descriptive design for this study of eight adolescents who attended a process-oriented psychotherapy group for three months (12 sessions). Afterwards, they went through semi-structured, open-ended interviews, and the data were analyzed using manifest content analysis. All participants reflected on group events and the meaning of their experiences. Several therapeutic factors that were consistent with Yalom's theoretical framework emerged from the data, and several recommendations for group therapists were identified.

Focused Group Analytic Psychotherapy (FGAP)

Based on some of the results and clinical experiences made during our research, I decided to construct a new, time-limited therapy, Focused Group Analytic Psychotherapy (FGAP; Lorentzen, 2022). One important rationale for this was that patients without PD (less personality pathology) were found to change faster in STG than similar patients did in LTG and had the same *sustained* improvement as LTG patients. While constructing the new therapy, the old manual (Lorentzen, 2014) was taken as a point of departure. Rereading the manuals, I was struck by the lack of instructions on how to evaluate personality and personality pathology, and decided to change it. Members' level of personality organization is strongly related to how well the individual member manages in a group and for the therapeutic quality of the group as a whole, so I updated this issue accordingly. In addition, I wanted to underline the importance of developing a *case formulation*, including a specific *psychodynamic hypothesis.* Elements of the hypothesis can, in concert with aspects of interpersonal problems and symptoms, be formulated (or loosely woven together) as a *therapy focus.* The *pre-therapy preparation* has also been given a more prominent place; i.e., more time is being spent on negotiating different dynamically charged issues (therapy focus) with the patients. Other topics underlined in the new book are *higher therapist activity*, work in the *here-and-now*, and the need to take the group through four more or less clearly defined *phases* (opening, differentiation, interpersonal work, and termination).

FGAP is based on group analytic and psychoanalytic theory, and I have included some of Otto Kernberg's psychoanalytic theories (1980) to vitalize FGAP. He has, over the decades, systematically developed his theories on personality integration, including aspects from several areas of psychoanalysis like ego-psychology, object relations theory, and self-psychology. Combining group analytic theory with central aspects of his rich theoretical framework (see, e.g., Caligor et al., 2018) makes it possible to continue Foulkes' tradition of running heterogeneous (transdiagnostic) groups, at least within certain limits. Kernberg operates with five levels of personality organization: (1) Normal, (2) Neurotic, (3) High-level, (4) Moderate- level, and (5) Low-level borderline. Only patients from the first three levels are suitable for FGAP. Patients with a lower level of personality organization will need longer time in treatment, probably also input of more supportive and psychoeducational elements in the treatment.

The evaluation should be thorough and based on information that is obtained in a combined clinical/psychodynamic interview by a relatively experienced clinician. This evaluation should focus on the quality/impairment in the following personality domains: sense of identity, quality of object relations, maturity of defenses, affect tolerance/control (aggression), moral values, and degree of pathological narcissism (Caligor et al., 2018, p. 552). Each domain is rated on a scale from 1–5, and the mean decides the level. Patient suitability for this therapy can be decided through a thorough evaluation/preparation (3–5 sessions). A structured interview (STIPO-R; Clarkin et al., 2016) also exists but is mostly used in research. This interview is informative, however, as to how questions can be formulated to expose different aspects of the diversity of personality domains, and can thus be useful for training less experienced clinicians. A profile of interpersonal problems, using the Inventory of Interpersonal Problems Circumplex (Alden et al., 1990), should also be teased out for each patient, and so should a clinical diagnosis. More detailed instructions can be found in Lorentzen (2022), a book that also includes basic theory, describes the stages in the group process, therapist interventions, plus offers a multitude of relevant clinical vignettes.

Summing Up

This narrative may appear as a random wandering through the field of group analytic research, more than a tidy overview of what has been done and what remains to be done. I have, however, attempted to systematically incorporate elements from central sources of group research, including history, handbooks, research literature, and clinical experience. Even though the Sheffield report contains few high-quality outcome studies, the conclusion was that several studies supported the use of psychodynamic group and group analytic psychotherapy as effective approaches across diverse conditions, participants, groups, and settings. That group analytic (and other psychodynamic) therapies, both short- and long-term, are efficacious for patients treated in trans-diagnostic groups has also been verified by external evaluators (Burlingame & Strauss, 2021, p. 614). The data gave, however, no information as to the types of patients for whom GA and A/D group therapies were most effective. The same verdicts were confirmed through the literature search described above, which ended up with 24 papers. Almost one-half of these were built on group analytic theory (one RCT, represented by nine papers, one observational study, and one new therapy model, Focused Group Analytic Psychotherapy). The rest of the studies represented A/D theory (six RCTs, four observational studies, one qualitative study, and one ultra-brief interpersonal therapy model). Given that our data search gives a true picture of existing group analytic research, the growth in the field has been scarce since the Sheffield report was published. There are, however, two novelties: (1) The appearance of a new RCT studying, amongst other questions, the efficacy of *long-term GA* (Lorentzen et al., 2013), and (2) A newly constructed model for *time-limited group analytic therapy*, suitable for patients with a higher level of personality organization (Lorentzen et al., 2022). Such a therapy could easily be reworked or modified into a manual (guidelines) for use in specific group analytic research to ensure that investigators use replicable approaches. In order to adapt the therapy (and research) to subjects with more serious personality pathology, specific elements can also be added or subtracted (types of interventions, psychoeducational elements, individual sessions), and the duration of therapy or frequency of sessions can be manipulated.

What Kind of Studies Does GA Need?

Generally speaking, all sorts of quantitative outcome studies are needed: RCTs, otherwise controlled studies, observational studies, and case studies. The same goes for qualitative research that may be on all levels of sophistication, from unstructured interviews of patients about their experiences of a session, to systematically mapping and grading of interpersonal behaviors over time, to be used in search of associations between these and positive outcomes of therapy. On the other hand, needs may be very different between countries because of diversity in culture, politics, tradition, standard of living, etc., which speaks to the value of a book like this.

Research may take place on several levels, for example, as quality assurance in private practice or public outpatient units, clinicians using structured questionnaires that give them feedback from their own therapies/patients. Larger projects that require more money, administration, or know-how may have to be organized by universities, eventually by inviting clinicians into cooperative networks.

Conclusion

I would like to end this chapter with two wishes for our profession: firstly, I think more explicit standards for evaluation and clinical research should become a part of all formal training programs in group analysis. Next, I would suggest that we more systematically use our knowledge of unconscious motivations to explore *why* there is such a scarcity of research in group analysis. Maybe a report from four seasoned group analysts of experiences with integrating a randomized clinical trial with everyday clinical work can give hints about where to start (Horneland et al., 2012)?

References

Alden, L.E., Wiggin, J. S., & Pincus, A.L. (1990). Construction of circumplex scales for the inventory of interpersonal problems. *Journal of Personality Assessment*, 55, 521–536.

Alldredge, C.T., Burlingame, G.M., Yang, C., & Rosendahl, J. (2021). Alliance in group therapy: A meta-analysis. *Group Dynamics: Theory, Research, and Practice*, 25(1): 13–28.

Bakali, J.V., Baldwin, S.A., & Lorentzen, S. (2009). Modeling group process constructs at three stages in group psychotherapy. *Psychotherapy Research*, 19(3), 332–343.

Bakali, J.V. (2013). Group processes in short- and long-term psychodynamic group psychotherapy. PhD thesis University of Oslo, Norway.

Bakali, J.V., Wilberg, T., Klungsøyr, O., & Lorentzen, S. (2013). Development of group climate in short- and long-term psychodynamic group psychotherapy. *International Journal of Group Psychotherapy*, 63(3), 366–393.

Bednar, R.L., & Kaul, T.J. (1978). Experimental group research: Current perspectives. In S.L. Garfield & A.E. Bergin (Eds.), *Handbook of Psychotherapy and Behavior Change: An Empirical Analysis* (pp. 769–815.). New York: Wiley.

Blackmore, C., Beecroft, C., Parry, G., Booth, A., Tantam, D., Chambers, E., Simpson, E., Roberts, E., & Saxon, D. (2009). *The Sheffield Report*. Sheffield: Centre for Psychological Services Research, School of Health and Related Research. University of Sheffield, UK.

Blackmore, C., Tantam, D., Parry, G., & Chambers, E. (2012). Report on a systematic review of the efficacy and clinical effectiveness of group analysis and analytic/dynamic group psychotherapy. *Group Analysis*, 45, 46–69.

Bormann, B., & Strauss, B. (2007). Group climate, cohesion, alliance, and empathy as components of the therapeutic relationship within group psychotherapy: Test of a multilevel model. *Gruppenpsychotherapie und Gruppendynamik*, 43(1), 1–20.

Burchard, E., Michaels, J., & Kotkov, B. (1948). Criteria for the evaluation of group therapy. *Psychosomatic Medicine*,10, 257–277.

Burlingame, G.M., MacKenzie, R.K., & Strauss, B. (2004). Small-group treatment: evidence for effectiveness and mechanisms of change. In M.J. Lambert (Ed.), *Handbook of Psychotherapy and Behavior Change* (pp. 647–696). New York: Wiley.

Burlingame, G.M., Seebeck, J.D., Janis, R.A., Whitcomb, K.E., Barkowski, S., Rosendahl, J., & Strauss, B. (2016). Outcome differences between individual and group formats when identical and nonidentical treatments, patients, and doses are compared: A 25-year meta-analytic perspective. *Psychotherapy*, 53(4), 446–461.

Burlingame, G.M., McClendon, D.T., & Yang, C. (2018a). Cohesion in group therapy: A meta-analysis. *Psychotherapy*, 55(4), 384–398.

Burlingame, G.M., Whitcomb, K.E., Woodland, S.C., Olsen, J.A., Beecher, M., & Gleave, R. (2018b). The effects of relationship and progress feedback in group psychotherapy using the group questionnaire and outcome questionnaire-45: A randomized clinical trial. *Psychotherapy*, 55(2), 116–131.

Burlingame, G.M., & Strauss, B. (2021). Efficacy of small group treatments: Foundation for evidence-based practice. In M. Barkham, W. Lutz, & L.G. Castonguay (Eds.), *Handbook of Psychotherapy and Behavior Change* (pp. 583–624). New York: Wiley.

Caligor, E., Kernberg, O.F., Clarkin, J.F., & Yeomans, F.E. (2018). *Psychodynamic Therapy for Personality Pathology: Treating Self and Interpersonal Functioning*. Washington, DC: American Psychiatric Association Publishing.

Clarkin, J.F., Caligor, E., Stern, B.L., & Kernberg, O.F. (2016). The Structured Interview of Personality Organization: STIPO-R. The Personality Studies Institute. www.borderlinedisorders.com.

Combs, D.R., Penn, D.L., Wicher, M., & Waldheter, E. (2007). The Ambiguous Intentions Hostility Questionnaire (AIHQ): A new measure for evaluating hostile social-cognitive biases in paranoia. *Cognitive Neuropsychiatry*, 12(2), 128–143.

Emrick, C. (1975). A review of psychologically oriented treatment of alcoholism. *Journal for the Study of Alcoholism*, 36, 88–108.

Fjeldstad, A., Høglend, P.A., & Lorentzen, S. (2016). Presence of personality disorder moderates the long-term effects of short-term and long-term psychodynamic group therapy: A 7-year follow-up of a randomized clinical trial. *Group Dynamics: Theory, Research, and Practice*, 20(4), 294–309.

Fjeldstad, A., Høglend, P., & Lorentzen, S. (2017). Patterns of change in interpersonal problems during and after short-term and long-term psychodynamic group therapy: A randomized clinical trial. *Psychotherapy Research*, 27(3), 350–361.

Fjeldstad, A. (2019). The role of treatment duration in psychodynamic group psychotherapy. PhD thesis. University of Oslo, Norway.

Flückiger, C., Del Re, A.C., Wampold, B.E., & Horvath, A.D. (2018). The alliance in adult psychotherapy: A meta-analytic synthesis. *Psychotherapy*, 55(4), 316–340.

Foulkes, S.H. (1977). *Therapeutic Group Analysis.* New York: International University Press. First published, 1964.

Foulkes, S.H. (1986). *Group Analytic Psychotherapy: Method and Principles.* London: Maresfield Library. First published 1975.

Foulkes, S.H., & Anthony, E.J. (1984). *Group Psychotherapy: The Psychoanalytical Approach.* 2nd edition. London: Maresfield Reprints. First published 1957.

Fuhriman, A., & Burlingame, G.M. (1998). *Handbook of Group Psychotherapy: An Empirical and Clinical Synthesis.* New York: Wiley.

Gleave, R.L., Burlingame, G.M., Beecher, M.E., Griner, D., Hansen, K., & Jenkins, S. A. (2017). Feedback-informed group treatment: Application of the OQ–45 and group questionnaire. In D.S. Prescott, C.L. Maeschalck, & S.D. Miller (Eds.), *Feedback-informed Treatment in Clinical Practice: Reaching for Excellence* (pp. 141–166. Washington, DC: American Psychological Association.

Hernandez, C.A., Piper, W.E., Ogrodniczuk, J.S., Joyce, A.S., & Weideman, R. (2016). Use of referential language in short-term group psychotherapy for complicated grief. *Group Dynamics: Theory, Research, and Practice*, 20(1), 1–15.

Horneland, M., Sande Børnes, D., Høbye, K., Knutsen, H., & Lorentzen, S. (2012). Can the clinician-researcher gap be bridged? Experiences from a randomized clinical trial in analytic/dynamic group psychotherapy? *Group Analysis*, 45(1), 84–98.

Jensen, H.H., Mortensen, E.L., & Lotz, M. (2010). Effectiveness of short-term psychodynamic group therapy in a public outpatient psychotherapy unit. *Nordic Journal of Psychiatry*, 64(2), 106–114.

Johnson, J.E., Burlingame, G.M., Olsen, J.A., Davies, D.R., & Gleave, R.L. (2005). Group climate, cohesion, alliance, and empathy in group psychotherapy: Multilevel structural equation models. *Journal of Counseling Psychology*, 52, 310–321.

Joyce, A.S., Ogrodniczuk, J.S, Piper, W.E., & Sheptycki, A.R. (2010). Interpersonal predictors of outcome following short-term group therapy for complicated grief: a replication. *Clinical Psychology & Psychotherapy*, 17(2), 122–135.

Kernberg, O.F. (1980). *Internal World and External Reality: Object Relations Theory Applied*. New York and London: Jason Aronson.

Kealy, D., Sierra-Hernandez, C.A., Piper, W.E., Joyce, A.S., Weideman, R., & Ogrodniczuk, J. S. (2017a). Psychological mindedness and psychotherapy process in short-term group therapy. *Psychodynamic Psychiatry*, 45(3), 343–361.

Kealy, D., Sierra-Hernandez, C.A., Piper, W.E., Joyce, A.S., Weideman, R., & Ogrodniczuk, J.S. (2017b). Short-term group therapy for complicated grief: The relationship between patients' in-session reflection and outcome. *Psychiatry*, 80(2), 125–138.

Kealy, D., Hewitt, P.L., Söchting, I., Mikail, S.F., Smith, M.M., Flett, G.L., et al. (2025). A comparison of the effect of two types of brief psychodynamic group therapy on perfectionism-related attitudes, self-relatedness, and self-esteem. *Psychotherapy Research*, 35(2), 319–336.

Kroenke, K., & Spitzer, R.L. (2002). The PHQ-9: A new depression diagnostic and severity measure. *Psychiatric Annals*, 32(9), 509–515.

Krogel, J., Burlingame, G.M., Chapman, C., Renshaw, T., Gleave, R., Beecher, M., & Macnair-Semands, R. (2013). The Group Questionnaire: A clinical and empirically derived measure of group relationship. *Psychotherapy Research*, 23(3), 344–354.

Kösters, M., Burlingame, G.M., Nachtigall, C., & Strauss, B. (2006). A meta-analytic review of the effectiveness of inpatient group psychotherapy. *Group Dynamics: Theory, Research, and Practice*, 10(2), 146–163.

Lau, M., & Kristensen, E. (2007). Outcome of systemic and analytic group psychotherapy for adult women with a history of intrafamilial childhood sexual abuse: A randomized controlled study. *Acta Psychiatrica Scandinavica*, 116(2), 96–104.

Leirvåg, H., Pedersen, G., & Karterud, S. (2010) Long-term continuation treatment after short-term day treatment of female patients with severe personality disorders: Body awareness group therapy versus psychodynamic group therapy. *Nordic Journal of Psychiatry*, 64(2), 115–122.

Lieberman, M. (1976). Change induction in small groups. *Annual Review of Psychology*, 27, 217–250.

Lorentzen, S., Bøgwald, K.P., & Høglend, P. (2002). Change during and after long-term analytic group psychotherapy. *International Journal of Group Psychotherapy*, 52(3), 419–429.

Lorentzen, S. (2003). Long-term analytic group psychotherapy with outpatients: Evaluation of process and change. Doctoral thesis, University of Oslo, Norway.

Lorentzen, S. (2006). Contemporary challenges for research in group analysis. *Group Analysis*, 39(3), 321–340.

Lorentzen, S., & Høglend, P.A. (2008). Moderators of the effects of treatment length in long-term psychodynamic group psychotherapy. *Psychotherapy and Psychodynamics*, 77, 321–322.

Lorentzen, S., Bakali, J.V., Hersoug, A.G., Hagtvet, K.A., Ruud, T., & Høglend, P. (2012). Psychodynamic group psychotherapy: Impact of group length and therapist professional characteristics on development of therapeutic alliance. *Clinical Psychology & Psychotherapy*, 19(5), 420–433.

Lorentzen, S., Ruud, T., & Fjeldstad, A. (2013). Comparison of short-and long-term dynamic group psychotherapy: Randomised clinical trial. *The British Journal of Psychiatry*, 203(4), 280–287.

Lorentzen, S. (2014). *Group Analytic Psychotherapy: Working with Affective, Anxiety and Personality Disorders.* LondonandNew York: Routledge.

Lorentzen, S., Fjeldstad, A., Ruud, T., & Høglend, P.A. (2015a). Comparing short- and long-term group therapy: Seven-year follow-up of a randomized clinical trial. *Psychotherapy and psychosomatics*, 84(5), 320–321.

Lorentzen, S., Ruud, T., Fjeldstad, A., & Høglend, P.A. (2015b). Personality disorder moderates outcome in short- and long-term group analytic psychotherapy: A randomized clinical trial. *British Journal of Clinical Psychology*, 54(2), 129–146.

Lorentzen, S., Fjeldstad, A., Ruud, T., Marble, A., Klungsøyr, O., Ulberg, R., & Høglend, P. (2015c). The effectiveness of short- and long-term psychodynamic group psychotherapy on self-concept: Three years follow-up of a randomized clinical trial. *International Journal of Group Psychotherapy*, 65(3), 362–385.

Lorentzen, S., Strauss, B., & Altmann, U. (2018). Process-outcome relationships in short-and long-term psychodynamic group psychotherapy: Results from a randomized clinical trial. *Group Dynamics: Theory, Research, and Practice*, 22(2), 93–107.

Lorentzen, S. (2022). *Focused Group Analytic Psychotherapy. An Integration of Clinical Experience and Research*. London and New York: Routledge.

Lorentzen, S. (2025). Research in group analysis. What works for whom? *Group Analysis*, 58(3), 299–316.

Luborsky, L., Singer, B., & Luborsky, L. (1975). Comparative studies of psychotherapy. *Archives of General Psychiatry*, 32, 995–1008.

Marmarosh, C.L., Markin, R.D., & Spiegel, E.B. (2013). *Attachment in Group Psychotherapy.* Washington, DC: American Psychological Association.

Marmarosh, C.L. (2017). Attachment in group psychotherapy: Bridging theories, research, and clinical techniques. *International Journal of Group Psychotherapy*, 67 (2), 157–160.

Meltzoff, J., & Kornreich, M. (1970). *Research in Psychotherapy.* New York: Atherton Press.

Ogrodniczuk, J.S., Piper, W.E., McCallum, M., Joyce, A.S., & Rosie, J.S. (2002). Interpersonal predictors of group therapy outcome for complicated grief. *International Journal of Group Psychotherapy*, 52(4), 511–535.

Østergård, O.K., Frandsen, C.R., & Valbak, K. (2022). Psychological mindedness, personality structure, and outcomes in short-term group analytic psychotherapy. *International Journal of Group Psychotherapy*, 72(2), 113–142.

Pines, M. (1983). *The Evolution of Group Analysis.* London: Routledge and Kegan Paul.

Pingitore, F., & Ferszt, G.G. (2017). The "voice" and perspectives of adolescents participating in a short-term group. *International Journal of Group Psychotherapy*, 67 (3): 360–382.

Piper, W.E., Ogrodniczuk, J.S., Joyce, A.S., & Weideman, R. (2009). Follow-up outcome in short-term group therapy for complicated grief. *Group Dynamics: Theory, Research, and Practice*, 13(1), 46.

Rosendahl, J., Alldredge, C.T., Burlingame, G.M., & Strauss, B. (2021). Recent developments in group psychotherapy research. *American Journal of Psychotherapy*, 74(2), 52–59.

Sieradzki, A., Szechiński, M., & Małyszczak, K. (2017). The effects of short-term group psychodynamic psychotherapy on the personality traits of patients treated in a day ward. *Psychiatria Polska*, 51(4), 633–646.

Smith, M.L., & Glass, G.V. (1977). Meta-analysis of psychotherapy outcome studies. *American Psychologist*, 32, 752–760.

Suszek, H., Holas, P., Wyrzykowski, T., Lorentzen, S., & Kokoszka, A. (2015). Short-term intensive psychodynamic group therapy versus cognitive-behavioral group therapy in day treatment of anxiety disorders and comorbid depressive or personality disorders: study protocol for a randomized controlled trial. *Trials*, 16(1), 319.

Thomas, G.W. (1943). Group psychotherapy: A review of the recent literature. *Psychosomatic Medicine*, 17, 166–180.

Whittingham, M. (2018). Innovations in group assessment: How focused brief group therapy integrates formal measures to enhance treatment preparation, process, and outcomes. *Psychotherapy*, 55(2), 186–190.

Zajenkowska, A., Rajchert, J., Macianowicz, O., Holas, P., & Murawic, S. (2019). Cognitive-behavioral (CBT) and psychodynamic (PDT) group psychotherapy and their impact on depressive symptoms and hostile attributions. *International Journal of Group Psychotherapy*, 69(4), 383–407.

Index

For Product Safety Concerns and Information please contact our EU representative GPSR@taylorandfrancis.com
Taylor & Francis Verlag GmbH, Kaufingerstraße 24, 80331 München, Germany

www.ingramcontent.com/pod-product-compliance
Ingram Content Group UK Ltd.
Pitfield, Milton Keynes, MK11 3LW, UK
UKHW021724240926
475702UK00030BA/2660

9781032982205